OXFORD ASSESS AND PROGRESS

Series Editors

Katharine Boursicot
Director, Health Professional Assessment Consultancy (HPAC)
Honorary Reader in Medical Education St George's,
University of London

David Sales
Consultant in Medical Assessment

T0202126

OXFORD ASSESS AND PROGRESS

Also available and forthcoming titles in the Oxford Assess and Progress series

OXFORD ASSESS AND PROGRESS

Clinical Dentistry

Nicholas Longridge BSc (Hons), BDS (Hons), MFDS RCSEd

Academic Clinical Fellow/Specialty Registrar in Endodontics
Liverpool University Dental Hospital, United Kingdom

Peter Clarke BDS (Hons), MFDS RCSP (Glasg)

Specialty Registrar in Restorative Dentistry
University Dental Hospital of Manchester, United Kingdom

Raheel Aftab BDS, MJDF RCSEng, PgCert Primary Dental

General Dental Practitioner, Educational Supervisor
Kent, United Kingdom

Tariq Ali MB ChB, MRCS, DOHNS RCSEng, MRCEM, BDS, MJDF RCSEng

Associate Lecturer, Faculty of Medicine, University of Queensland
Registrar Oral and Maxillofacial Surgery
Queensland, Australia

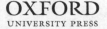
OXFORD
UNIVERSITY PRESS

OXFORD
UNIVERSITY PRESS

Great Clarendon Street, Oxford, OX2 6DP,
United Kingdom

Oxford University Press is a department of the University of Oxford.
It furthers the University's objective of excellence in research, scholarship,
and education by publishing worldwide. Oxford is a registered trade mark of
Oxford University Press in the UK and in certain other countries

© Oxford University Press 2019

The moral rights of the authors have been asserted

First Edition published in 2019

Published in the United States of America by Oxford University Press
198 Madison Avenue, New York, NY 10016, United States of America

British Library Cataloguing in Publication Data
Data available

Library of Congress Control Number: 2019931586

ISBN 978–0–19–882517–3

Printed and bound in Great Britain by Ashford Colour Press Ltd.

Series editor preface

The *Oxford Assess and Progress* series is a groundbreaking development in the extensive area of self-assessment texts available for dental and medical students. The questions were specifically commissioned for the series, written by practising clinicians, extensively peer-reviewed by students and their teachers, and quality-assured to ensure that the material is up-to-date, accurate, and in line with modern testing formats.

The series has a number of unique features and is designed to be as much a formative learning resource as a self-assessment one. The questions are constructed to test the same clinical problem-solving skills that we use as practising clinicians, rather than only to test theoretical knowledge. These skills include:

* gathering and using data required for clinical judgement
* choosing the appropriate examination and investigations
* applying knowledge and interpreting findings
* demonstrating diagnostic skills
* ability to evaluate undifferentiated material
* ability to prioritize
* making decisions and demonstrating a structured approach to decision-making.

Each question is bedded in reality and is typically presented as a clinical scenario, the content of which has been chosen to reflect the common and important conditions that most dentists and doctors are likely to encounter both during their training and in exams! The aim of the series is to build the reader's confidence in recognizing important symptoms and signs and suggesting the most appropriate investigations and management, and, in so doing, to aid the development of a clear approach to patient management which can be transferred to the clinical environment.

The content of the series has deliberately been pinned to the relevant *Oxford Handbook* but, in addition, has been guided by a blueprint which reflects the themes identified in the General Dental Council's *Preparing for practice—Dental teams learning outcomes for registration*, including an evidence-based approach to learning, along with clinical, managerial, and professionalism scenarios.

Particular attention has been paid to giving learning points and constructive feedback on each question, using clear fact- or evidence-based explanations as to why the correct response is right and why the incorrect responses are less appropriate. The question editorials are clearly referenced to the relevant sections of the accompanying *Oxford Handbook* and/or more widely to medical literature or guidelines. They are designed to guide and motivate the reader, being multi-purpose in nature and covering, e.g. exam technique, approaches to difficult subjects, and links between subjects.

Another unique aspect of the series is the element of competency progression from being a relatively inexperienced student to being a more experienced junior dentist. We have suggested the following four degrees of difficulty to reflect the level of training, so that the reader can monitor their own progress over time:

- graduate should know ★
- graduate nice to know ★★
- foundation dentist should know ★★★
- foundation dentist nice to know ★★★★

We advise the reader to attempt the questions in blocks as a way of testing their knowledge in a clinical context. The series can be treated as a dress rehearsal for life as a clinician by using the material to hone clinical acumen and build confidence by encouraging a clear, consistent, and rational approach, proficiency in recognizing and evaluating symptoms and signs, making a rational differential diagnosis, and suggesting appropriate investigations and management.

Adopting such an approach can aid not only success in examinations, which really are designed to confirm learning, but also—more importantly—being a good dentist and doctor. In this way, we can deliver high-quality and safe patient care by recognizing, understanding, and treating common problems, but at the same time remaining alert to the possibility of less likely, but potentially catastrophic, conditions.

David Sales and Kathy Boursicot
Series Editors

A note on single best answer questions

Single best answer questions are currently the format of choice being widely used by most undergraduate and postgraduate knowledge tests, and therefore, the questions in this book follow this format.

Single best answer questions have many advantages over other machine-markable formats, such as extended matching questions (EMQs), notably the breadth of sampling or content coverage that they afford.

Briefly, the single best answer or 'best of five' question presents a problem, usually a clinical scenario, before presenting the question itself and a list of five options. These consist of one correct answer and four incorrect options, or 'distractors', from which the reader has to choose a response.

All of the questions in this book, which are typically based on an evaluation of symptoms, signs, results of investigations, or material interactions, either as single entities or in combination, are designed to test *reasoning* skills, rather than straightforward recall of facts, and utilize cognitive processes similar to those used in clinical practice.

The peer-reviewed questions are written and edited in accordance with contemporary best assessment practice, and their content has been guided by a blueprint pinned to all areas of the General Dental Council's document *Preparing for practice—Dental teams learning outcomes for registration*, which ensures comprehensive coverage.

The answers and their rationales are evidence-based and have been reviewed to ensure that they are absolutely correct. Incorrect options are selected as being plausible, and indeed they may appear correct to the less knowledgeable reader. When answering questions, the reader may wish to use the 'cover' test, in which they read the scenario and the question but cover the options.

Kathy Boursicot and David Sales
Series Editors

Author preface

Dental school can be a challenging and emotional time. The breadth of experiences gained both professionally and socially cannot be rivalled, and in hindsight, most come to look upon their time at university as a thoroughly enjoyable experience. Needless to say, preparing for the multitude of examinations and assessments throughout the programme is never a favourite pastime, but a necessary evil nonetheless. Whether it is the prospect of finals or postgraduate examinations on the horizon, we remember the constant pressure to read and revise only too well. Our own experiences frequently involved discussing a range of possible questions which lacked informative answers. This led us to the Oxford Assess and Progress Series and to the production of this book.

The *Oxford Handbook of Clinical Dentistry* (*OHCD*) was never far from reach during dental school, and within this book, we have attempted to provide a series of single best answer questions that link the *OHCD* with real-life practical scenarios to test reasoning and application of knowledge. Where possible, recommended reading and references to seminal papers have been provided to encourage further reading and to support evidence-based practice. Within the book, we have selected *Keywords*, where relevant, to help highlight specific clues or words that can assist with recall in those high-pressure situations. All questions have been written and peer-reviewed by clinicians working within each specialty, and we have endeavoured to provide in-depth justification for correct and incorrect answers. Undoubtedly, some topics will remain contentious, but, where necessary, we have explained our reasoning and hope that this highlights the 'grey' areas in many dental scenarios. Chapters are formatted by specialty, and we have attempted to maintain a clear focus on clinically oriented scenarios that will be beneficial for finals and beyond. A selection of questions on 'Law and ethics' have been written and combined into the clinical specialty for which they are relevant.

As previously mentioned, we started this book with the hope of providing an informative and supportive revision tool that encourages further reading and evidence-based practice. Looking back, we all remember dental school with fond memories, and we hope that you find this book useful and wish you the very best for your finals and future careers beyond.

**Nicholas Longridge, Peter Clarke,
Raheel Aftab, and Tariq Ali**

Acknowledgements

The authors would like to thank all of the contributors for their hard work in producing the content for this book. Special thanks must go to the authors of the *Oxford Handbook of Clinical Dentistry* David and Laura Mitchell, for allowing us to use their excellent book as a guiding framework and revision source. We would like to thank all reviewers—students and specialists—for their detailed feedback and discussion points, which we hope to have reflected in the final book. We are also indebted to Geraldine Jeffers and Rachel Goldsworthy at Oxford University Press for their support, guidance, and patience throughout the entire project. Nick would like to thank his wife, Sarah, and his parents for their endless support. Peter would like to thank his wife, Tess, for her patience and understanding throughout the process. Tariq would like to thank his family, friends, and colleagues for their constant support throughout his career. Raheel would also like to thank his family.

All four authors would like to dedicate the book to their good friend Andy Jones, who was taken from this world too soon and sadly passed away in 2017.

Publisher's acknowledgement

Thank you to the 27 dental lecturers and clinicians who participated in our anonymous peer-review process and kindly gave their time to this project.

Thank you to Dr Karolin Hijazi, Clinical Lecturer in Oral Medicine, University of Aberdeen Dental School, who reviewed the oral medicine chapter.

Thank you to Professor Balvinder Khambay, School of Dentistry, University of Birmingham, and Mr P J Turner, Consultant Orthodontist, Birmingham School of Dentistry, who reviewed the orthodontic chapter.

Thank you to David and Laura Mitchell who gave their kind permission for the reuse of a table and figure from the *Oxford Handbook of Clinical Dentistry*.

Publisher's acknowledgement

Contents

Contents

About the authors

Nicholas Longridge is an Academic Clinical Fellow/Specialty Trainee in Endodontics at Liverpool University Dental Hospital. Alongside his specialist training, Nicholas is completing a 3-year Doctorate in Dental Sciences (DDSc) in Endodontics. His current research interests are in regenerative endodontics and pulp biology. Prior to commencing his specialist training, Nicholas worked as a dental core trainee in a variety of hospital settings across different specialties. He is a member of the Royal College of Surgeons of Edinburgh and has a Bachelor of Science degree in Anatomy and Human Biology.

Peter Clarke is a Specialty Registrar in Restorative Dentistry at the University Dental Hospital of Manchester. Having completed his undergraduate training, he proceeded to undertake a number of core training jobs, covering a variety of disciplines. Having been involved at various levels in undergraduate teaching and examining throughout his career, he now plays an active role in coordinating the regional teaching programme for dental core trainees.

Raheel Aftab is a general dental practitioner working within a multi-disciplinary dental team in Kent. Following his undergraduate training, Raheel passed the Membership of Joint Dental Faculties from the Royal Colleague of Surgeons England examinations and soon after completed a Postgraduate Certificate in Primary Dental Care from the University of Kent. He is currently undergoing further training at King's College London in fixed and removable prosthodontics. Alongside his clinical duties, Raheel is an Educational Supervisor for Health Education London and Kent, Surrey, and Sussex. Raheel takes a particular interest in digital dentistry, incorporating digital workflow and CAD/CAM as part of routine dental care for his patients.

Tariq Ali is a dual-qualified Oral and Maxillofacial Surgery Registrar currently working in Queensland, Australia. He undertook both his undergraduate degrees in the United Kingdom, having first completed Medicine at the University of Birmingham and later completing Dentistry at the University of Liverpool. He has worked in a broad range of surgical specialties and emergency medicine, having completed his memberships in Dentistry, Surgery, and Emergency Medicine. Tariq has also completed his Diploma in Head and Neck Surgery at the Royal College of Surgeons England, a prerequisite to otorhinolaryngology training. He now plays an active role in clinical teaching for medical and dental students at the University of Queenland.

Series editors

Katharine Boursicot BSc MBBS MRCOG MAHPE NTF SFHEA FRSM is a consultant in health professions education, with special expertise in assessment. Previously, she was Head of Assessment at St George's, University of London, Barts and the London School of Medicine and Dentistry, and Associate Dean for Assessment at Cambridge University School of Clinical Medicine. She is consultant on assessment to several UK medical schools, medical Royal Colleges, and international institutions, as well as an assessment advisor to the General Medical Council.

David Sales trained as a general practitioner and has been involved in medical assessment for 30 years. Previously he was the convenor of the MRCGP knowledge test, chair of the Professional and Linguistics Assessment Board (PLAB) Part 1 panel, and consultant to the General Medical Council Fitness to Practise knowledge tests across all medical and surgical specialties. He has run item writing workshops for a number of undergraduate medical schools, medical royal colleges including the Diploma of Membership of the Faculty of Dental Surgery (MFDS) and internationally in Europe, South East Asia, South Asia, and South Africa.

Contributors

Nadia M Ahmed
Specialist Orthodontist
Kettering General Hospital
Northamptonshire, UK

Gurpreet Singh Jutley
Rheumatologist
University Hospital Birmingham
West Midlands, UK

Thomas Albert Park
Clinical Dental Officer
Pennine Care NHS
Foundation Trust
Greater Manchester, UK

Normal and average values

Haematology: reference intervals

Measurement	Reference interval
White cell count (WCC)	$4.0–11.0 \times 10^9/L$
Red cell count	M: $4.5–6.5 \times 10^{12}/L$; F: $3.9–5.6 \times 10^{12}/L$
Haemoglobin	M: 13.5–18.0 g/dL; F: 11.5–16.0 g/dL
Packed red cell volume (PCV) or haematocrit	M: 0.4–0.54 l/L; F: 0.37–0.47 l/L
Mean cell volume (MCV)	76–96 fL
Mean cell haemoglobin (MCH)	27–32 pg
Mean cell haemoglobin concentration (MCHC)	30–36 g/dL
Neutrophil count	$2.0–7.5 \times 10^9/L$; 40–75% WCC
Lymphocyte count	$1.3–3.5 \times 10^9/L$; 20–45% WCC
Eosinophil count	$0.04–0.44 \times 10^9/L$; 1–6% WCC
Basophil count	$0.0–0.1 \times 10^9/L$; 0–1% WCC
Monocyte count	$0.2–0.8 \times 10^9/L$; 2–10% WCC
Platelet count	$150–400 \times 10^9/L$
Reticulocyte count	$25–100 \times 10^9/L$; 0.8–2.0%
Erythrocyte sedimentation rate	<20 mm/hour (but depends on age; see OHCM 10th edn, p. 372)
Activated partial thromboplastin time (VIII, IX, XI, XII)	35–45 seconds
Prothrombin time	10–14 seconds

International normalized ratio (INR)	Clinical state (see OHCM 10th edn, p. 351)
2.0–3.0	Treatment of deep vein thrombosis (DVT), pulmonary emboli (treat for 3–6 months)
2.5–3.5	Embolism prophylaxis in atrial fibrillation (see OHCM, p. 335)
3.0–4.5	Recurrent DVT and pulmonary embolism; arterial disease, including myocardial infarction; arterial grafts; cardiac prosthetic valves (if caged ball, aim for 4–4.9) and grafts

Biochemistry	
Alanine aminotransferase (ALT)	5–35 IU/L
Albumin	35–50 g/L
Alkaline phosphatase (ALP)	30–150 IU/L
Amylase	0–180 U/dL
Aspartate aminotransferase (AST)	5–35 IU/L
Bilirubin	3–17 µmol/L
Calcium (total)	2.12–2.65 mmol/L
Chloride	95–105 mmol/L
Cortisol	450–750 nmol/L (a.m.) 80–280 nmol/L (midnight)
C-reactive protein (CRP)	<10 mg/L
Creatine kinase	M: 25–195 IU/L F: 25–170 IU/L
Creatinine	70–<150 µmol/L
	Normal value
Ferritin	12–200 µg/L
Folate	2.1 µg/L
Gamma glutamyl transpeptidase (GGT)	M: 11–51 IU/L F: 7–33 IU/L
Lactate dehydrogenase (LDH)	70–250 IU/L
Magnesium	0.75–1.05 mmol/L
Osmolality	278–305 mOsmol/kg
Potassium	3.5–5 mmol/L

Biochemistry	
Protein (total)	60–80 g/L
Sodium	135–145 mmol/L
Thyroid-stimulating hormone (TSH)	0.5–5.7 mU/L
Thyroxine (T4)	70–140 nmol/L
Thyroxine (free)	9–22 pmol/L
Urate	M: 210–480 mmol/L F: 150–39 mmol/L
Urea	2.5–6.7 mmol/L
Vitamin B12	0.13–0.68 mmol/L
Arterial blood gases	
pH	7.35–7.45
Arterial oxygen partial pressure (PaO_2)	>10.6 kPa
Arterial carbon dioxide partial pressure ($PaCO_2$)	4.7–6.0 kPa
Base excess	± 2 mmol/L
Urine	
Cortisol (free)	<280 nmol/24 hours
Osmolality	350–1000 mOsmol/kg
Potassium	14–120 mmol/24 hours
Protein	<150 mg/24 hours
Sodium	100–250 mmol/24 hours

The index of orthodontic treatment need*

Grade 1 (none)

1 Extremely minor malocclusions, including displacements of <1 mm.

Grade 2 (little)

2a Increased overjet 3.6–6 mm with competent lips.
2b Reverse overjet 0.1–1 mm.
2c Anterior or posterior crossbite with up to 1 mm discrepancy between retruded contact position and intercuspal position.
2d Displacement of teeth 1.1–2 mm.
2e Anterior or posterior openbite 1.1–2 mm.
2f Increased overbite 3.5 mm or more, without gingival contact.
2g Pre-normal or post-normal occlusions with no other anomalies. Includes up to half a unit discrepancy.

Grade 3 (moderate)

3a Increased overjet 3.6–6 mm with incompetent lips.
3b Reverse overjet 1.1–3.5 mm.
3c Anterior or posterior crossbites with 1.1–2 mm discrepancy.
3d Displacement of teeth 2.1–4 mm.
3e Lateral or anterior openbite 2.1–4 mm.
3f Increased and complete overbite without gingival trauma.

Grade 4 (great)

4a Increased overjet 6.1–9 mm.
4b Reversed overjet >3.5 mm with no masticatory or speech difficulties.
4c Anterior or posterior crossbites with >2 mm discrepancy between retruded contact position and intercuspal position.
4d Severe displacement of teeth, >4 mm.

*Reproduced from Peter H. Brook, William C. Shaw; The development of an index of orthodontic treatment priority, *European Journal of Orthodontics*, Volume 11, Issue 3, 1 August 1989, Pages 309–320. Copyright © 1989, by permission of Oxford University Press.

4e Extreme lateral or anterior openbites, >4 mm.
4f Increased and complete overbite with gingival or palatal trauma.
4h Less extensive hypodontia requiring pre-restorative orthodontic space closure to obviate the need for a prosthesis.
4l Posterior lingual crossbite with no functional occlusal contact in one or both buccal segments.
4m Reverse overjet 1.1–3.5 mm with recorded masticatory and speech difficulties.
4t Partially erupted teeth, tipped and impacted against adjacent teeth.
4× Supplemental teeth.

Grade 5 (very great)

5a Increased overjet >9 mm.
5h Extensive hypodontia with restorative implications (more than one tooth missing in any quadrant) requiring pre-restorative orthodontics.
5i Impeded eruption of teeth (with the exception of third molars) due to crowding, displacement, the presence of supernumerary teeth, retained deciduous teeth, and any pathological cause.
5m Reverse overjet >3.5 mm with reported masticatory and speech difficulties.
5p Defects of cleft lip and palate.
5s Submerged deciduous teeth.

Cephalometric values

Table 1 Cephalometric values: analysis of lateral skull tracings*

SNA	$= 81° (\pm 3)$
SNB	$= 79° (\pm 3)$
ANB	$= 3° (\pm 2)$
1-Max	$= 109° (\pm 6)$
1-Mand	$= 93° (\pm 6)$ or 120 minus MMPA
MMPA	$= 27° (\pm 4)$
Facial proportion	$= 55\% (\pm 2)$
Inter-incisal angle	$= 133° (\pm 10)$

* Reproduced from Mitchell D, Mitchell L, *Oxford Handbook Clinical Dentistry*, 6th Edition, Table 4.1, page 130, (2014). By permission of Oxford University Press.

NORMAL AND AVERAGE VALUES

Adult Dental Health Survey 2009 (some facts)*

- The proportion of adults in England who were edentate (no natural teeth) has fallen by 22% from 28% in 1978 to 6% in 2009.
- Only 17% of dentate adults had very healthy periodontal (gum) tissues and no periodontal disease (i.e. no bleeding, no calculus, no periodontal pocketing of 4 mm or more, and in the case of adults aged 55 or above, no loss of periodontal attachment of 4 mm or more anywhere in their mouth).
- Overall 45% of adults had periodontal (gum) pocketing exceeding 4 mm, although for the majority (37%), disease was moderate, with pocketing not exceeding 6 mm.
- Just under one-third of dentate adults (31%) had obvious tooth decay in either the crown or root of their teeth.
- There are social variations in dental decay, with adults from routine and manual occupation households being more likely to have decay than those from managerial and professional occupational households (37% compared with 26%)
- The prevalence of decay (using the natural tooth crowns as the measure) in England has fallen from 46% to 28% since 1998, and this reduction is reflected in all age groups.
- Moderate tooth wear has increased from 11% in 1998 to 15% in 2009, although severe wear remains rare.
- 75% of adults said that they cleaned their teeth at least twice a day and a further 23% of adults said that they cleaned their teeth once a day.
- 8% of dentate adults had one or more untreated teeth with unrestorable decay, and those who did had an average of 2.2 teeth in this condition.
- The majority of dentate adults (85%) had a tooth affected by restoration. Among people with at least one restoration, 9% had some secondary decay.
- Almost two-thirds (61%) of dentate adults said that the usual reason they attended the dentist is for a regular check-up; 12% of adults who had ever been to a dentist had an MDAS (Modified Dental Anxiety Scale) score of 19 or more, which suggests extreme dental anxiety.

*Contains public sector information licensed under the Open Government Licence v3.0.
[http://www.nationalarchives.gov.uk/doc/open-government-licence/version/3/]

Abbreviations

3D	Three-dimensional
Aa	*Aggregatibacter actinomycetemcomitans*
ACE	Angiotensin-converting enzyme
ADJ/EDJ	Amelodentinal junction/enamodentine junction
ADP	Adenosine diphosphate
AED	Automated external defibrillator
AFP	Atypical facial pain
AI	Amelogenesis imperfecta
AIDS	Acquired immune deficiency syndrome
ALL	Acute lymphoblastic leukaemia
ALP	Alkaline phosphatase
ALT	Alanine aminotransferase
AML	Acute myeloblastic leukaemia
ANB	A point, nasion, and B point
ANOVA	Analysis of variance
ANS	Autonomic nervous system; anterior nasal spine
ANUG	Acute necrotizing ulcerative gingivitis
AO	Atypical odontalgia
AST	Aspartate aminotransferase
BD	Twice daily
BEC	Bioactive endodontic cement
BLS	Basic life support
BNF	*British National Formulary*
BOP	Bleeding on probing
BP	Bullous pemphigoid
BPE	Basic periodontal examination
BPPV	Benign paroxysmal positional vertigo
CAD/CAM	Computer-aided design/computer-aided manufacture
CBCT	Cone beam computed tomography
CCD	Charge-coupled device
CEA	Cost-effectiveness analysis
CEJ	Cemento-enamel junction
CH	Calcium hydroxide
CHC	Chronic hyperplastic candidiasis

CKD	Chronic kidney disease
Cl⁻	Chloride ion
CLL	Chronic lymphocytic leukaemia
CML	Chronic myeloblastic leukaemia
CN	Cranial nerve
CoCr	Cobalt-chromium
COPD	Chronic obstructive pulmonary disease
CPA	Cerebellopontine angle
CPD	Continuing professional development
CPP-ACP	Casein phosphopeptides–amorphous calcium phosphates
CRP	C-reactive protein
CUA	Cost utility analysis
CVA	Cerebrovascular accident
DCP	Dental Care Professional
DI	Diabetes insipidus
DIGO	Drug-induced gingival overgrowth
dL	Decilitre
DLE	Discoid lupus erythematosus
DMFT	Diseased, Missing, Filled Teeth
DPH	Dental public health
DPT	Dental panoramic tomogram/dentopantomogram
DVT	Deep vein thrombosis
EAL	Electronic apex locator
ECG	Electrocardiogram
ED	Emergency department
EDTA	Ethylenediaminetetraacetic acid
ENA	Extractable nuclear antibody
ENT	Ear, nose, and throat
ESR	Erythrocyte sedimentation rate
ESRF	End-stage renal failure
EWL	Estimated working length
FBC	Full blood count
FG	Free gingival
fL	Femtolitre
FPM	First permanent molar
FWS	Freeway space
g	Gram
GA	General anaesthesia
GCS	Glasgow coma scale

GDC	General Dental Council
GDPR	General Data Protection Regulation
GGT	Gamma glutamyl transpeptidase
GHIH	Growth hormone inhibitory hormone
GIC	Glass-ionomer cement
GMP	General medical practitioner
GORD	Gastro-oesophageal reflux disease
GP	Gutta percha
GTN	Glyceryl trinitrate
Gy	Gray
HEBP	1-hydroxyethylidene-1,1-bisphosphonate
HHV	Human herpesvirus
HIV	Human immunodeficiency virus
HSW	Health and Safety at Work etc. Act
IAN	Inferior alveolar nerve
ICDAS	International caries detection and assessment system
ICP	Intercuspal position
IgA	Immunoglobulin A
IgE	Immunoglobulin E
IgG	Immunoglobulin G
IHD	Ischaemic heart disease
IHS	Inhalation sedation
IL-1	Interleukin-1
IM	Intramuscularly
IMCA	Independent Mental Capacity Advocate
INR	International normalized ratio
IOTN	Index of orthodontic treatment need
IRCP	International Commission on Radiological Protection
IR(ME)R	Ionising Radiation Medical Exposure) Regulations
IRR	Ionising Radiation Regulations
IU	International unit
IV	Intravenous
JE	Junctional epithelium
JSNA	Joint strategic needs assessment
kPa	Kilopascal
kV	Kilovolt
L	Litre
LDH	Lactate dehydrogenase
LL4	Lower left first premolar

LL6	Lower left first molar
LL7	Lower left second molar
LL8	Lower left third molar
LLD	Lower left first deciduous molar
LLE	Lower left second primary molar
LMN	Lower motor neurone
LMWH	Low-molecular-weight heparin
LPS	Lipopolysaccharide
LR4	Lower right first premolar
LR6	Lower right first molar
LR7	Lower right second molar
LR8	Lower right third molar
mA	Milliampere
MAC	Membrane attack complex (immunology)
MAF	Master apical file
MCH	Mean cell haemoglobin
MCHC	Mean cell haemoglobin concentration
MCV	Mean cell volume
MDAS	Modified Dental Anxiety Scale
MDMA	3,4-Methylenedioxymethamphetamine
MHRA	Medicines and Healthcare Products Regulatory Agency
MI	Myocardial infarction
mm	Millimetre
mmol	Millimole
MMP	Mucous membrane pemphigoid
MOCDO	Missing teeth, overjets, crossbites, displacement of contact points, overbites
mOsmol	Milliosmole
MPa	Megapascal
MPTS	Methacryloxypropyl-trimethoxysilane
MRONJ	Medication-related osteonecrosis of the jaw
MTA	Mineral trioxide aggregate
MTAD	Mixture of tetracycline, citric acid, and a detergent
mU	Milliunit
NADH	Nicotinamide adenine dinucleotide
NAI	Non-accidental injury
NaOCl	Sodium hypochlorite
NHS	National Health Service
NIDDM	Non-insulin-dependent diabetes mellitus

NiTi	Nickel titanium
nmol	Nanomole
NOAC	New oral anticoagulant
NSAID	Non-steroidal anti-inflammatory drug
NSTEMI	non-ST segment elevation myocardial infarction
OD	Once daily
OHCM	*Oxford Handbook of Clinical Medicine*
OHNA	Oral health needs assessment
OJ	Overjet
OM	Occipitomental
OM10O	Occipitomental 10
OM30O	Occipitomental 30
OMFS	Oral and maxillofacial surgery
OPG	Oral pantomogram
OPT	Orthopantomogram
OVD	Occlusal vertical dimension
PA	Periapical; posteroanterior
PaCO$_2$	Arterial partial pressure of carbon dioxide
PaO$_2$	Arterial partial pressure of oxygen
PCV	Packed cell volume
PD	Peritoneal dialysis
PDL	Periodontal ligament
PE	Pulmonary embolism
PEFR	Peak expiratory flow rate
pg	Picogram
PHG	Primary herpetic gingivostomatitis
PJP	*Pneumocystis jirovecii* pneumonia
PMC	Preformed metal crown
pmol	Picomole
PMR	Polymyalgia rheumatica
PP	Pancreatic polypeptide
ppm	Parts per million
PRR	Pathogen recognition receptor
PSP	Photostimulable phosphor
PVS	Polyvinylsiloxane
QDS	Four times daily
RANK	Receptor activator of nuclear factor kappa-B
RAP	Retruded axis position
RAS	Recurrent aphthous stomatitis

RBB	Resin-bonded bridge
RCA	Root cause analysis
RCP	Retruded contact point/position
RCRG	Royal College of Radiologists Guidelines
RCT	Randomized controlled trial
ReRCT	Revision root canal treatment
RFH	Resting face height
RHP	Radiation and Health Protection
RIDDOR	Reporting of Injuries, Diseases and Dangerous Occurrences Regulations 1995
RMGIC	Resin-modified glass-ionomer cement
RPA	Radiation Protection Advisor
RPD	Removable partial denture
RSD	Root surface debridement
SAH	Subarachnoid haemorrhage
SCC	Squamous cell carcinoma
SIRS	Systemic inflammatory response syndrome
SJS	Stevens–Johnson syndrome
SLE	Systemic lupus erythematosus
SLM	Selective laser melting
SNA	Sella turcica, nasion, and A point
SNB	Sella turcica, nasion and A point
spp.	Species
SSC	Stainless steel crown
STEMI	ST segment elevation myocardial infarction
StR	Specialty registrar
T4	Thyroxine
TB	Tuberculosis
TBSA	Total body surface area
TEGMA	Tri-ethylene glycol dimethacrylate
TEN	Toxic epidermal necrolysis
THA	Terminal hinge axis
TIA	Transient ischaemic attack
TMD	Temporomandibular dysfunction
TMJ	Temporomandibular joint
TON	Traumatic optic neuropathy
TPHA	*Treponema pallidum* haemagglutination assay
TSH	Thyroid-stimulating hormone
U	Unit

UK	United Kingdom
UL1	Upper left permanent central incisor
UL2	Upper left lateral incisor
UL5	Upper left second premolar
UL6	Upper left first permanent molar
ULA	Upper left primary central incisor
UMN	Upper motor neurone
UR1	Upper right central incisor
UR3	Upper right permanent canine
UR5	Upper right second premolar
UR6	Upper right first permanent molar
USO	Upper standard occlusal
WBC	White blood cell
WCC	White cell count
WHO	World Health Organisation
WSN	White sponge naevus
ZOE	Zinc oxide eugenol

How to use this book

Oxford Assess and Progress, Clinical Dentistry has been carefully designed to ensure you get the most out of your revision and are prepared for your exams. Here is a brief guide to some of the features and learning tools.

Organization of content

Chapter editorials will help you unpick tricky subjects, and when it is late at night and you need something to remind you why you are doing this, you will find words of encouragement!

Answers can be found at the end of each chapter, in order.

How to read an answer

Unlike other revision guides on the market, this one is crammed full of feedback, so you should understand exactly why each answer is correct, and gain an insight into the common pitfalls. With every answer, there is an explanation of why that particular choice is the most appropriate. For some questions, there is additional explanation of why the distractors are less suitable. Where relevant, you will also be directed to sources of further information such as the *Oxford Handbook of Clinical Dentistry*, websites, and journal articles.

Progression points

The questions in every chapter are ordered by level of difficulty and competence, indicated by the following symbols:

★   *Graduate 'should know'*—you should be aiming to get most of these correct.

★★   *Graduate 'nice to know'*—these are a bit tougher, but not above your capabilities.

★★★   *Foundation dentist 'should know'*—these will really test your understanding.

★★★★   *Foundation dentist 'nice to know'*—give these a go when you are ready to challenge yourself.

Oxford Handbook of Clinical Dentistry

The OHCD page references are given with the answers to some questions (e.g. OHCD 6th edn → p. 340). Please note that this reference is the **sixth edition** of the OHCD, and that subsequent or previous editions are unlikely to have the same material in exactly the same place.

Chapter 1

Anatomy of the head and neck

Nicholas Longridge

'Which nerves do you need to anaesthetize?'
'Which vessel are you trying to avoid?'

Both are routine questions encountered by students during their time in dental school, and both require sound knowledge of the anatomy of the head and neck. From wrestling with basic anatomical concepts and planes to tracing the branches of the external carotid artery, anatomy will underpin the rest of your practising career and is a fundamental building block on which all other knowledge can be laid down. Basic anatomical knowledge begins with the osseous structures of the head and neck, blood vessels, lymphatics, and nerves. Interpretation of this knowledge is required for functional and clinical applications, which is a daily occurrence for practising dentists and dental care professionals. Such a large subject is difficult to assess in a small number of questions, but this chapter touches on aspects of developmental embryology and tooth formation, along with functional anatomical questions designed to test the theory behind some common dental procedures and clinical presentations. Undoubtedly, excellent knowledge of the innervation and blood supply to the teeth and surrounding structures will be most beneficial for dentists and dental care professionals during their practising careers.

Key topics include:

- Anatomical planes and terminology
- Craniofacial development
- The musculoskeletal system, including ossification and bony remodelling
- Innervation and vascular supply to the head and oral cavity, including the cranial nerves
- Structure of the eye, ear, nasal cavity, and oral cavity
- Odontogenesis
- Histology of the oral cavity.

QUESTIONS

1. A 25-year-old man attends for review. He has clinical signs of Treacher–Collins syndrome, and the consultant is discussing the first and second pharyngeal arch syndromes. A junior dental student asks which cranial nerve develops with, and goes on to innervate, the second pharyngeal arch. Which is the single most appropriate response? ★

A Abducens—VI

B Facial—VII

C Glossopharyngeal—IX

D Mandibular branch of the trigeminal—V₃

E Vagus—X

2. A 22-year-old man undergoes a bimaxillary osteotomy to correct a severe reverse overjet (Class III skeletal relationship). During the procedure, the consultant asks the specialty registrar what single type of ossification is involved in the formation of the mandible during embryological development. ★

A Ectopic

B Endochondral

C Endosteal

D Intramembranous

E Periosteal

3. A 23-year-old woman returns to the surgery 5 days after surgical extraction of her lower right third molar. She reports loss of sensation from the floor of the mouth on the right-hand side. Which single nerve is most likely to have been damaged during her extraction? ★

A Chorda tympani

B Hypoglossal

C Inferior alveolar

D Lingual

E Nerve to the mylohyoid

4. A 45-year-old man is receiving an inferior alveolar nerve block for the restoration of a lower right first molar from a dental student, who is administering the injection for the first time. They are using the direct technique (over the contralateral premolar teeth), and their supervisor asks them which single muscle will the needle pass through. ★

A Buccinator

B Masseter

C Medial pterygoid

D Palatoglossus

E Superior constrictor

5. A 25-year-old man attends with a buccal swelling next to the lower right first molar. Incision and drainage of the abscess is planned. Which single branch of the external carotid artery should be avoided, whilst conducting this treatment? ★

A Ascending pharyngeal

B Facial

C Lingual

D Maxillary

E Parotid

6. An 18-year-old man is having a cranial nerve assessment performed after a traumatic incident. Upon protrusion of his tongue, the tongue deviates to the left-hand side. Which single nerve has been affected? ★

A Glossopharyngeal

B Hypoglossal

C Lingual

D Mandibular branch of the trigeminal

E Pharyngeal plexus

7. A 33-year-old woman attends for extraction of the upper left second premolar. The clinical tutor asks the student to anaesthetize the patient using infiltrations prior to the procedure. Which nerves require anaesthetizing? (Select one from the options listed below.) ★

A Anterior superior alveolar nerve + middle superior alveolar nerve

B Middle superior alveolar nerve + greater palatine nerve

C Middle superior alveolar nerve + nasopalatine nerve

D Posterior superior alveolar nerve + greater palatine nerve

E Posterior superior alveolar nerve + lesser palatine nerve

8. A 73-year-old man has Paget's disease and develops trigeminal neuralgia in the lower jaw region. Compression of which single cranial foramen is most likely to be causing his neuralgia? ★★

A Foramen lacernum

B Foramen ovale

C Foramen rotundum

D Foramen spinosum

E Stylomastoid foramen

9. A 45-year-old woman attends with localized right-sided facial pain of an aching nature and trismus. The pain has been present for 4 weeks and is localized to the pre-auricular region. It was preceded by recurrent clicking, with no restriction on opening. The patient is now unable to open her mouth beyond 20 mm. Which single component of condylar head movement is inhibited? ★★

A Abduction

B Circumduction

C Protrusion

D Rotation

E Translation

10. The presence of the anatomical attachment of which single muscle visible in Figure 1.1 may obscure radiographic assessment of the root apices? ★★

A Buccinator

B Lateral pterygoid

C Medial pterygoid

D Mylohyoid

E Posterior belly of the digastric

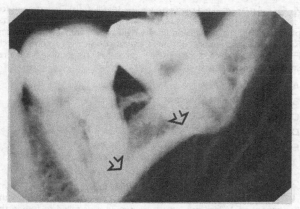

Figure 1.1
Reproduced from Whaites, E, *Essentials of Dental Radiography and Radiology* 5th Ed.
Copyright 2013, Fig 21.7a, Page 274, with permission from Elsevier.

11. A 24-year-old man who has undergone a low-volume cone beam computed tomography (CBCT) scan of a tooth with a complex dens invaginatus is being assessed (Oehler's classification 3b). The CBCT sofware is used to scroll through the full series of images in a corono-apical direction, to enable visualization of the complex anatomy of the root in cross-section. Using the method described above, which single anatomical plane is being utilized to assess the image? ★ ★

A Coronal

B Frontal

C Longitudinal

D Sagittal

E Transverse

12. A 25-year-old woman has an intraoral swelling that has been present for 2 days. The differential diagnosis for this swelling would differ, based on its location. Other than the gingiva, which location in the oral cavity would you be able to exclude salivary gland pathology from the differential diagnosis? ★ ★ ★

A Anterior hard palate

B Buccal sulcus

C Floor of the mouth

D Soft palate

E Tongue

13. An 18-year-old man attends the Maxillofacial Department, following an alleged assault to the right side of his head. He has pain, bruising, and depression of the right cheek, with limited opening. Radiographic assessment confirms a fracture of the right zygomatic arch. Entrapment of which single muscle is most likely responsible for the restricted opening? ★★★

A Buccinator

B Lateral pterygoid

C Medial pterygoid

D Masseter

E Temporalis

14. A 1-day-old boy has been born at full term in hospital with a unilateral cleft lip. The parents are concerned and ask how this has happened. Which two structures would have failed to fuse in this scenario? (Select one answer from the options listed below.) ★★★

A Frontonasal prominence and the intermaxillary segment

B Frontonasal prominence and the maxillary prominence

C Lateral nasal prominence and the maxillary prominence

D Medial nasal prominence and the intermaxillary segment

E Medial nasal prominence and the maxillary prominence

15. A 7-year-old boy presents with signs of amelogenesis imperfecta (AI). Clinically, the enamel is of normal thickness but is comparatively soft. Radiographically, the enamel is of similar radiodensity to the dentine. Which single stage of tooth development is the disorder most likely to have affected? ★★★★

A Bell

B Bud

C Cap

D Crown maturation

E Root development

16. An 82-year-old woman fails to attend her review appointment at the dry mouth clinic. The consultant takes this opportunity to discuss the autonomic nerve supply to the parotid gland with junior staff. Parasympathetic nerve supply to the parotid gland is via the otic ganglion. Which single cranial nerve supplies pre-ganglionic parasympathetic nerve fibres to the otic ganglion? ★★★★

A Accessory nerve

B Facial nerve

C Glossopharyngeal nerve

D Vagus nerve

E Vestibulocochlear nerve

17. A 68-year-old woman with unilateral facial paralysis is assessed by a maxillofacial doctor in the Emergency Department (ED). Her mouth and cheek are drooping on the right-hand side, and she cannot bare her teeth or purse her lips on that side when asked. However, she can still wrinkle the skin of her forehead to command. What is the single most likely cause for the signs that have been described? ★★★★

A Acoustic neuroma

B Bell's palsy

C Otitis media

D Parotid tumour

E Stroke

18. A 34-year-old woman requires root canal treatment on an asymptomatic lower left first permanent incisor (LL1), which has two canals. Having been given two buccal infiltrations for anaesthesia, she can still feel pain. Which single nerve is most likely to be providing accessory innervation to the tooth? (Select one answer from the options listed below.) ★★★★

A Hypoglossal

B Lingual

C Long buccal

D Nerve to the mylohyoid

E Right inferior alveolar

6. B ★

CN assessments are an important part of a junior dentist's clinical knowledge. If asked to assess the CNs, the twelfth nerve (hypoglossal—XII) deviates to the affected side, i.e. if the patient had a large malignant lesion at the base of the left side of their tongue, the tongue would deviate to the left side. The glossopharyngeal nerve supplies sensory function to the posterior part of the tongue. The lingual nerve is a branch of the mandibular nerve of the trigeminal nerve (CN V), which does not provide motor function to the tongue. The pharyngeal plexus supplies the palatoglossus muscle of the tongue, which is a small extrinsic muscle of the tongue that passes from the soft palate into the tongue. Motor fibres of the pharyngeal plexus supply the majority of the muscles of the soft palate and the constrictor muscles. The motor fibres travel to the muscles via the vagus nerve but are derived from the cranial root of the accessory nerve (CN XI).

Keywords: tongue, deviation.

7. B ★

Nerve supply to the maxillary teeth is via the maxillary branch of the trigeminal nerve (CN V_2). The nerve enters the pterygopalatine fossa via the foramen rotundum. At this point, the posterior superior alveolar nerve bifurcates and passes inferiorly along the infratemporal surface of the maxilla to innervate the maxillary molars. The majority of the maxillary nerve continues as the infraorbital nerve, which continues through the pterygopalatine fossa and inferior orbital fissure to enter the infraorbital canal. The middle superior alveolar nerve branches along this course and runs to supply to upper premolars and, on occasions, the mesiobuccal root of upper first molars. The anterior superior alveolar nerve branches further along this course to supply the canine and upper incisors. Collectively, these branches form a plexus which can be referred to as the superior dental plexus. The upper anterior teeth can also be anaesthetized using an infraorbital block.

For extractions, it is also necessary to anaesthetize the gingival tissues. The palatine gingivae are supplied by the greater palatine nerves, and the buccal and labial gingivae are supplied by the same superior alveolar branch that supplies the tooth. Buccal or labial infiltration will therefore anaesthetize the tooth and its labial or buccal gingivae, so only the palatal gingivae require additional infiltration. Knowledge of these nerve pathways is essential for all dental practitioners and can assist in the diagnosis of poorly localized, irreversible pulpitis when other special investigations have failed. See Figure 1.4 which shows the arterial supply and innervation of the palate.

Keywords: upper, premolar, infiltrations, nerves.

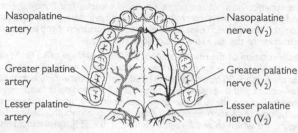

Figure 1.4

Reproduced from Scully C, *Oxford Handbook Applied Dental Sciences*, figure 4.1, page 54, Copyright (2003) by permission of Oxford University Press.

8. B ★★

Paget's disease of bone is a rare chronic disease that involves disorganized bone remodelling. The disease can result in pain, fractures, and arthritis. It most commonly affects bones of the axial skeleton and is often localized to a small number of bones, including the pelvis. It can occasionally affect the cranial bones, with potential compression of neural tissue at the cranial foramina. Good knowledge of nerve pathways is therefore important during diagnosis and assessment of symptoms. In this particular scenario, trigeminal neuralgia is affecting the mandibular distribution of the trigeminal nerve. See Figure 1.5 (see Colour Plate section) which shows a superior view of the cranial base.

Foramen and associated CNs include:

- Optic canal—*optic nerve (CN II)*
- Superior orbital fissure—*oculomotor (CN III), trochlear (CN IV), abducens (CN VI), ophthalmic branches of the trigeminal nerve*
- Foramen rotundum—*maxillary branches of the trigeminal nerve*
- Foramen ovale—*mandibular branch of the trigeminal nerve*
- Stylomastoid foramen—*facial nerve (CN VII)*
- Jugular foramen—*glossopharyngeal (CN IX), vagus (CN X), branches of the accessory nerve (CN XI)*
- Hypoglossal canal—*hypoglossal nerve*

Keywords: cranial foramina.

9. E ★★

The temporomandibular joint (TMJ) comprises the mandibular fossa and articular eminence of the temporal bone and the head of the mandibular condyle. An articular disc separates the two bones, and the joint is surrounded by a joint capsule which contains synovial fluid. The articulating surfaces are lined with fibrocartilage, and the articular disc is attached to the capsule and to bone by anterior and posterior fibroelastic bands. The anterior aspect of the articular disc and joint capsule is attached to the superior head of the lateral pterygoid muscle. The condylar head undergoes two major components of movement during opening: rotation and translation. These allow elevation, depression, protrusion, and retraction of the mandible to take place.

Initial rotation of the mandible about the terminal hinge axis (THA) occurs within the inferior compartment of the joint capsule and accounts for the first 15–20 mm of opening (total 45 mm). Following this, translation occurs in the upper compartment, and the mandibular head moves anteriorly onto the articular eminence. Therefore, in the absence of pathology, translation accounts for the majority of mouth opening. See Figure 1.6 which shows a sagittal section of the TMJ, (a) the mandible elevated, and (b) the mandible depressed.

Keywords: pain, pre-auricular, preceded, recurrent click, 20 mm, condylar head.

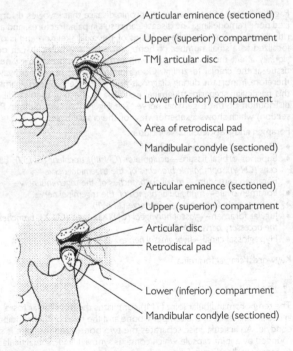

Articular eminence (sectioned)
Upper (superior) compartment
TMJ articular disc
Lower (inferior) compartment
Area of retrodiscal pad
Mandibular condyle (sectioned)

Articular eminence (sectioned)
Upper (superior) compartment
Articular disc
Retrodiscal pad
Lower (inferior) compartment
Mandibular condyle (sectioned)

Figure 1.6
Reproduced from Scully C, *Oxford Handbook Applied Dental Sciences*, Figure 4.2 b & c, pg 63, Copyright (2003) by permission of Oxford University Press.

10. D ★★

The bony attachment of the mylohyoid (mylohyoid ridge) is often seen on lower posterior periapicals adjacent to, or overlapping, the root apices of the posterior teeth. It is often visualized as a radio-opaque line within the premolar–molar region. Knowledge of the anatomical attachment of this muscle is important when diagnosing pathology and assessing the proximity of the inferior dental nerve. Furthermore, the location of the mylohyoid ridge can have significant ramifications with regard to the spread of periapical infections. As the mylohyoid represents the inferior boundary of the mouth, roots that lie above the mylohyoid ridge are more likely to produce a sublingual swelling, as infection is likely to remain above the mylohyoid. By comparison, roots that pass below the mylohyoid attachment are more likely to enable spread of infection below the floor of the mouth into the sub-mandibular region, i.e. a submandibular space swelling. The origins and insertions of the other muscles can be found in the recommended reading.

Keywords: anatomical muscle attachment, lower posterior periapical.

→ Atkinson M. *Anatomy for Dental Students* (4th ed.). Oxford University Press, Oxford; 2013.

11. E ★★

The anatomical planes are key references used to describe and document clinical findings (see Figure 1.7 for anatomical position and planes). More recently, in dentistry, the use of advanced radiography techniques, such as CBCT, has gained popularity due to their ability to provide high-quality, three-dimensional (3D) images of complex anatomical structures. The technology is now frequently encountered in everyday scenarios, e.g. when assessing impacted teeth, root canal anatomy, and residual bone for implant placement. Whilst CBCT images can be reformatted to provide a 3D reconstruction, they are frequently viewed individually in each of the three anatomical planes:

1. Coronal (frontal)—a vertical plane that divides the body into anterior and posterior segments
2. Sagittal (longitudinal)—a vertical plane that divides the body into left and right segments
3. Transverse (axial)—a horizontal plane that divides the body into superior and inferior segments.

Keywords: CBCT, corono-apical, cross-section, anatomical plane.

→ Devlin H, Craven R. *Oxford Handbook of Integrated Dental Biosciences.* Oxford University Press, Oxford; 2018.

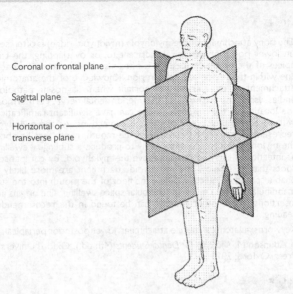

Coronal or frontal plane

Sagittal plane

Horizontal or
transverse plane

Figure 1.7
Reproduced from Scully C, *Oxford Handbook Applied Dental Sciences*, Figure 2.1, pg 12,
Copyright (2003) by permission of Oxford University Press.

12. **A** ★★★

There are three pairs of major salivary glands: the parotid, submandibular, and sublingual glands. As well as this, several hundreds of minor
salivary glands are located within the submucosa of the mouth. These
glands can become blocked or traumatized to form mucoceles or can
undergo neoplastic change to become benign or malignant neoplasms.
However, minor salivary glands are absent from the anterior hard palate
and the gingivae. As a result, swellings identified in these regions are
unlikely to have developed from salivary tissue, and this can be excluded
from the differential diagnosis. Understanding the histology of the oral
mucosa and soft tissues is important during assessment and diagnosis
of disease.

Keywords: salivary gland pathology, location.

13. **E** ★★★

General signs and symptoms of facial bone fractures include pain,
swelling, bruising, haematomas, and bony steps. Specific signs related to

the local anatomy may include unilateral epistaxis (e.g. if an antral wall is fractured), visual disturbances (if the orbit is fractured), paraesthesiae (if nerves are damaged), or limited opening (if muscles are involved). Limited opening may be as a result of muscle entrapment or muscular spasm or purely due to localized swelling and discomfort. Fracture of the zygomatic arch may occur in isolation or, more commonly, in combination with a zygomatic complex fracture. The origin of the temporalis muscle is the temporal line at the superior aspect of the parietal bone of the skull. From here, it passes medial to the zygomatic arch and inserts onto the coronoid process of the mandible. If the zygomatic arch is depressed, the inferior fibres or the tendon of the temporalis will be impinged at the insertion to the coronoid process, therefore limiting the normal range of opening of the mandible on that side. Of the remaining options, only the masseter muscle attaches directly to the zygoma. However, its origin is the external surface of the zygomatic arch and, as such, depression would not lead to entrapment. The remaining options do not attach or pass under the zygomatic arch and therefore would not be affected.

Keywords: limited opening, zygomatic arch, depression.

14. E ★★★

Children can be born with various kinds of cleft, which are reported to occur in approximately 1 in 700. There is a 2:1 male-to-female ratio when it comes to clefts involving the lip alone, and the ratio is inverted for cleft palates alone. This may be due to the fact that the palatine shelves elevate a week earlier in boys than girls.

The face derives from five facial prominences that form during facial development:

- Two mandibular processes
- Two maxillary processes
- Frontonasal process.

The frontonasal process gives rise to the lateral and medial nasal processes, which fuse with the bilateral maxillary prominences to form the upper lip, nose, and philtrum. The two medial nasal prominences fuse together at the midline to form the intermaxillary segment. As the maxillary prominence grows inwards, it fuses with the lateral nasal prominence to form the nasolacrimal groove. Failure of the maxillary prominence to fuse with the medial nasal process (or intermaxillary segment) results in a cleft lip, which can be uni- or bilateral.

Inadequate fusion of the two nasal processes can result in a very rare median cleft lip. See Figure 1.8 which illustrates facial development.

Keywords: unilateral cleft lip, failed to fuse, embryological development.

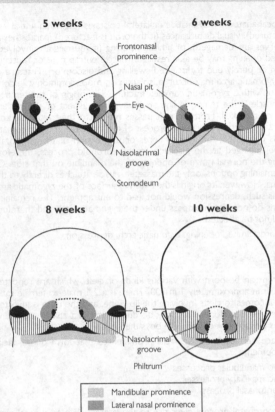

5 weeks

6 weeks

Frontonasal
prominence

Nasal pit

Eye

Nasolacrimal
groove

Stomodeum

8 weeks

10 weeks

Eye

Nasolacrimal
groove

Philtrum

	Mandibular prominence
	Lateral nasal prominence
	Medial nasal prominence
	Maxillary prominence

Figure 1.8

15. D ★★★★

Oral epithelial and mesenchymal cells, along with migrating neural crest cells, are responsible for tooth formation. The interaction between these cell layers is essential for tooth development. These cell layers form the dental lamina, and within this lamina, the various stages of tooth development occur. These stages are named the bud, cap, and bell. During the bud and cap stages, the epithelial and mesenchymal cells proliferate to form the enamel organ and the dental papilla, respectively. The bell stage is defined by cell morphodifferentiation and histodifferentiation when enamel- and dentine-producing cells develop. Enamel-forming ameloblasts develop from the cells of the inner enamel epithelial cells, whilst odontoblasts (dentine-producing cells) differentiate from ectomesenchymal cells (neural crest cells) that lie adjacent to the inner enamel epithelium. The resultant crown shape is determined by the inner enamel epithelium. Ameloblasts begin depositing enamel after dentine has begun to form, and this site of initial dentinogenesis and amelogenesis is referred to as the amelodentinal junction (ADJ). Ameloblasts subsequently pass through several stages, including a secretory and maturation phase. AI is a group of hereditary conditions that can present with multiple phenotypic variations.

The crown maturation (primary epithelial band) stage involves growth of the enamel crystals that have been deposited, and this phase accounts for the majority of the mineral found in enamel. Defects in the crown maturation stage are likely to present with hypomaturation AI, which would typically present in the manner described in the scenario. See Figure 1.9 which shows the initiation stage of human tooth development.

Keywords: tooth development, amelogenesis.

→ Gadhia K , McDonald S, Arkutu N, Malik K. Amelogenesis imperfecta: an introduction. *British Dental Journal*. 2012;**212**:377–9.

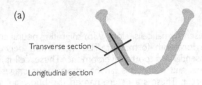

(a)

Transverse section

Longitudinal section

Longitudinal section   **Tranverse section**

Preodontogenesis

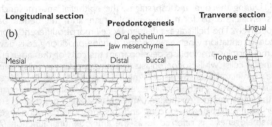

(b)

Oral epithelium
Jaw mesenchyme

Mesial   Distal   Buccal

Lingual

Tongue

Tongue

Initiation

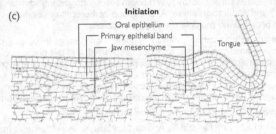

(c)

Oral epithelium
Primary epithelial band
Jaw mesenchyme

Tongue

Dental lamina

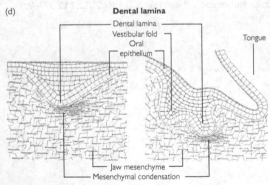

(d)

Dental lamina
Vestibular fold
Oral
epithelium

Tongue

Jaw mesenchyme
Mesenchymal condensation

Figure 1.9

16. C ★★★★

The glossopharyngeal nerve provides parasympathetic fibres to the otic ganglion via the lesser petrosal nerve. Post-synaptic parasympathetic fibres then pass to the parotid gland via the auriculotemporal nerve. The otic ganglion is one of four parasympathetic ganglia of the head, along with the submandibular, ciliary, and pterygopalatine ganglia. These ganglia are the site of synapse for parasympathetic fibres of the autonomic nervous system (ANS). The ANS can be subdivided into the sympathetic, parasympathetic, and enteric nervous system. Of these subdivisions, the sympathetic (fight or flight) and parasympathetic (rest and digest) divisions are heavily involved in everyday functions such as heart rate, breathing, salivation, and swallowing. In the head, these ganglia are primarily secretomotor in function, i.e. they induce secretions from various glands (with the exception of the ciliary ganglion). Functions of the parasympathetic ganglia of the head include:

- Pterygopalatine ganglion—secretomotor to the lacrimal gland and mucous glands of the mouth, palate, and nose. Known colloquially as the 'hay fever' ganglion. Supplied by CN VII—facial
- Otic ganglion—secretomotor to the parotid gland
- Submandibular ganglion—secretomotor to the sublingual and submandibular glands. Supplied by CN VII—facial
- Ciliary ganglion—motor to the constrictor muscle of the eye and the ciliary body (responsible for adjusting the shape of the lens in the eye to enable focusing on objects at various distances). Supplied by CN III—oculomotor.

All the other answers listed are CNs that carry out important functions throughout the body, particularly the head and neck.

Keywords: autonomic, cranial nerve, otic ganglion, parasympathetic.

17. E ★★★★

The first action in this case would be to fast-bleep the stroke registrar! The signs and symptoms described indicate an upper motor neuron (UMN) lesion because the forehead has been spared, which is most likely to have been caused by an intracranial tumour or stroke. Knowledge of neuroanatomy is fundamental for this question, specifically the facial motor nucleus. The concept of UMN and lower motor neuron (LMN) lesions can be complicated to grasp. A UMN is any neuron carrying information within the central nervous system between the motor areas and CN nuclei. An LMN is any neuron carrying motor information from the CN nucleus to the target muscles and is the same as the peripheral nerve. When put simply, the area of the facial motor nucleus controlling the upper face receives its nerve supply from both sides of the cerebral hemispheres, whilst the part controlling the lower face receives its supply only from the contralateral hemisphere. Therefore, when a right UMN lesion occurs, the patient retains some control over the left forehead (from the left side of the brain), but loses motor control of the left lower face. However, when an LMN injury occurs, all neurons leaving

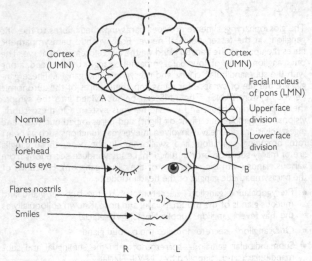

Cortex
(UMN)

Cortex
(UMN)

Facial nucleus
of pons (LMN)

A

Upper face
division

Normal

Lower face
division

Wrinkles
forehead

Shuts eye

B

Flares nostrils

Smiles

R   L

Figure 1.10

the facial motor nucleus in the brainstem are affected, and as a result, all five peripheral branches of the facial nerve on the same side are affected. This results in complete paralysis of all the muscles on the same side. Therefore, a left LMN lesion would affect the muscles on the left-hand side, rendering the left side of the face completely paralysed, e.g. Bell's palsy, which is a diagnosis of exclusion when all other causes have been eliminated. See Figure 1.10 which shows: label A—UMNs from the right side are affected, but innervation from the left UMN remains; label B—both LMNs are affected, and therefore, there is no innervation to the muscles.

Keywords: unilateral facial paralysis, retained use of forehead ('forehead sparing').

18. D ★★★★

The normal innervation of the mandibular teeth is from the incisive branch of the inferior alveolar nerve (IAN). The teeth on the left side are supplied by the left IAN, and the teeth on the right side by the right IAN. In reality, there is often crossover of innervation at the midline of anatomical structures, and the mandible is no exception. It has been reported that in 42% of patients, there is crossover of innervation of the lower mandibular incisors from the contralateral IAN. However, given that, in this scenario, a buccal infiltration has been given, crossover supply from the contralateral IAN is unlikely, as the local anaesthetic has been deposited locally and this should anaesthetize both teeth. Although the nerve to the mylohyoid is classified as a motor nerve, a number of studies have identified that mandibular teeth can receive sensory innervation from sensory fibres travelling within this branch. They are thought to enter the mandible through the retromental foramina located on the lingual aspect of the mandible, superior to the genial tubercles. A lingual infiltration will help to anaesthetize accessory sensory neurons. The lingual and long buccal nerves may supply accessory nerves to the third mandibular molar teeth.

The hypoglossal nerve is a purely motor nerve and not known to carry accessory sensory neurons.

Keywords: LL1, buccal infiltration, accessory innervation.

→ Rosella LF, Buffoli B, Labanca M, Rezzani R. A review of the mandibular and maxillary nerve supplies and their clinical relevance. *Archives of Oral Biology*. 2012;**57**:323–34.

Preventative and paediatric dentistry

Nicholas Longridge

'Prevention is better than the cure.'

The child patient can be a challenging and daunting proposition for the junior dentist and dental student. Whilst children can be anxious, unco-operative, and unpredictable, they also present an extremely rewarding opportunity, which, if managed correctly, may go on to influence their healthcare experiences for the rest of their lives. Excellent behavioural management of the child patient (and their parents!) is fundamental to a successful clinical and patient-reported outcome.

Aside from possible behavioural issues, paediatric patients may present with a series of unique clinical presentations that require additional skills and knowledge above and beyond those required for adult patients. Differences in the micro- and macro-structures of primary and permanent teeth, coupled with variations in eruption dates, lead to an evolving mixed dentition that can lead to some difficult diagnostic and treatment planning scenarios. Furthermore, dental anxiety and the pre-ponderance for dento-alveolar trauma in children and young adults may exacerbate the patient management of an already complex situation.

Prevention is central to paediatric dentistry. However, whilst significant progression has occurred in some areas, poor dietary habits and suboptimal oral hygiene regimes remain significant concerns for the profession, with large numbers of dental extractions still performed under general anaesthesia each year.

Key topics include:

- Tooth anatomy and eruption patterns
- Abnormalities of structure and form
- Prevention and management of dental caries, including pulp therapy
- Dental trauma
- Dental extractions and space management
- Behavioural management
- Safeguarding
- Pharmacological management.

QUESTIONS

1. A 15-year-old boy attends your surgery for a routine examination. His upper right permanent canine is yet to erupt. His upper left permanent canine erupted at the appropriate age. At approximately what age would you expect this tooth to have erupted? (Select one answer from the options listed below.) ★

A 6–7.4 years

B 7.5–8.9 years

C 9–10.4 years

D 10.5–11.9 years

E 12–13.4 years

2. A 14-month-old girl is brought to the surgery by her mother. She is concerned that a gap is present between some of her child's developing upper teeth. Which teeth would you expect to have erupted in the maxillary arch of this child? (Select one answer from the options listed below.) ★

A As and Bs

B As, Bs, and Ds

C As, Bs, Cs, and Ds

D As, Bs, Ds, and Es

E As, Bs, Cs, Ds, and Es

3. The babysitter of a 4-year-old boy telephones the practice, as the child fell down a staircase and has knocked out his upper right deciduous central incisor. The boy was momentarily unconscious but appears normal now. Which is the single most appropriate advice to give to the babysitter over the phone? ★

A Bring the child to the practice to have it re-implanted by a dentist

B Do not re-implant, and reassure the babysitter not to worry

C Do not re-implant, and take the child to the local Emergency Department

D Re-implant the tooth at home, and bring the child to the practice

E Re-implant the tooth, and take the child to the local Emergency Department

4. A 3-year-old girl attends, following a recent fall. The crown of the upper left primary central incisor (ULA) is significantly displaced labially (protruded). The tooth is non-mobile. A radiograph confirms the clinical diagnosis of lateral luxation. Which is the single most appropriate treatment? ★

A Extract the ULA

B Orthodontic repositioning

C Refer for specialist care

D Reposition the ULA

E Review after 2–3 weeks

5. A 9-year-old girl attends for a single routine restoration with her father. When asked, the father says that he was not married to the child's mother at birth, but that they subsequently married and that he is named on the birth certificate. Which is the single most appropriate option for obtaining consent for this procedure? ★

A Father and mother

B Father only

C Mother only

D No consent required

E The patient can consent for themselves

6. A 13-year-old girl attends for a routine dental examination, and multiple white spot lesions are noted around the cervical region of the upper and lower incisors. She reports frequent intake of sugary carbonated beverages (2 L per day). In this scenario, what is the single most appropriate management to reduce her caries risk? ★

A Brushing the lesion

B Chewing sugar-free gum

C Prescribing fluoride supplements

D Reducing the frequency of sugar attacks

E Topical fluoride

7. A 10-year-old girl has marked plaque-induced gingivitis. A 'simplified basic periodontal examination (BPE)' is performed. This procedure involves assessment of selective teeth termed 'index teeth'. These teeth include all permanent first molars. Which other teeth are included in the simplified BPE? (Select one answer from the options listed below.) ★

A Upper left and lower right permanent central incisors

B Upper permanent central incisors and lower permanent central incisors

C Upper primary incisors and lower primary incisors

D Upper right and lower left lateral incisors

E Upper right and lower left permanent central incisors

8. A subdued 5-year-old boy is seen in the practice. He has multiple injuries on his hands, knees, chin, and back of the neck. The parents report that the patient recently fell in the park. Injury to which single region would raise the most suspicion of a non-accidental injury (NAI)? ★★

A Behind the ears

B Chin

C Forehead

D Hands

E Knees

9. A 7-year-old girl has had a pulpotomy performed on her lower right second primary molar. Which single coronal restoration is considered the most appropriate? ★★

A Amalgam

B Compomer

C Composite

D Glass ionomer cement (GIC)

E Preformed metal crown (PMC)

10. A grossly carious lower right permanent first molar (LR6) is extracted from a 9-year-old boy. The child's parents are keen to know how likely the lower permanent second molar (LR7) is to fill the gap created. Which is the single best predictor that the LR7 will erupt into a good clinical position? ★★

A Age of the patient

B Atraumatic extraction technique

C Early calcification at the LR7 root bifurcation

D Lack of periapical pathology around the LR6

E Presence of a space maintainer following LR6 extraction

11. A 7-year-old girl has been referred for extraction of all of her carious primary molars under general anaesthesia (GA). Extensive oral hygiene instructions and preventive advice were given to the child and her parents prior to their GA appointment. Which is the single most appropriate future management for this child? ★★

A Refer for specialist care due to high caries rate

B Three-month recall for 4-yearly topical fluoride application

C Three-month recall for twice-yearly topical fluoride application

D Three-month recall with fluoride application and fissure sealing of permanent molars

E Three-month recall with high fluoride toothpaste prescription (2800 ppm)

12. A 15-year-old girl has a mid-third root fracture of her upper left permanent central incisor (UL1). It is decided to splint the tooth to reduce the risk of future tooth loss. Which is the single most appropriate length of time for the tooth to be splinted with a flexible splint? ★★

A 2 weeks

B 4 weeks

C 8 weeks

D 4 months

E Indefinitely

13. A 13-year-old adolescent boy is complaining about crooked teeth. Incidentally, a unilateral, severely infraoccluded and ankylosed lower left second primary molar (LLE) is identified. The permanent successor is not present, and the adjacent teeth are tipping. Which is the single most appropriate initial management of the LLE? ★★

A Direct composite restoration

B Extraction followed by restoration of the space

C Indirect onlay

D Orthodontic assessment

E Reassure and monitor

14. An 8-year-old boy has occlusal caries in his lower right first permanent molar. He is an irregular attender. Clinically, the caries is minimal and confined to the distal section of the fissure system. A bitewing radiograph shows the caries extends into the outer third of the dentine. Which is the single most appropriate restorative management strategy for this tooth? (Select one answer from the options listed below.) ★★

A Amalgam restoration

B Composite restoration

C Fissure sealant

D Preformed metal crown (PMC)

E Preventive resin restoration

15. An 8-year-old boy attends, following a recent fall in the playground. His upper right permanent central incisor (UR1) has been intruded by 5 mm. A radiograph confirms the UR1 is present with incomplete root development. Which is the single most appropriate course of action regarding the UR1? ★★★

A Commence immediate root canal treatment

B Extraction

C Orthodontic repositioning

D Review after 2–3 weeks

E Surgical repositioning

16. An 8-year-old cooperative boy has a routine examination, and the patient's mother has brought a 3-year-old sibling with no dental experience to observe their first examination. Which is the single most appropriate definition of this non-pharmacological behaviour management strategy? ★★★

A Behaviour shaping

B Enhanced control

C Live modelling

D Positive reinforcement

E Systematic desensitization

17. An 8-year-old boy has a complicated crown fracture of his upper right permanent central incisor (UR1), which happened the previous morning (>24 hours). The tooth is positive to sensibility testing. Which is the single most appropriate management? ★★★

A Apexification

B Direct pulp cap

C Extraction

D Pulpotomy

E Root canal treatment

18. A 9-year-old boy has deep pitting of the palatal aspect of both permanent maxillary lateral incisors. A diagnosis of dens invaginatus is made. The boy reports no symptoms from the teeth, which respond positively to sensibility testing. Which is the single most appropriate management? ★★★

A Composite restorations of the upper lateral incisors

B Extract the upper lateral incisors

C Fissure-seal the upper lateral incisors

D Oral hygiene instruction and monitor

E Root canal treatment on the upper lateral incisors

19. A 9-year-old boy has an unrestorable, grossly carious lower right first permanent molar (LR6) and a heavily restored upper right first permanent molar (UR6). The remainder of the permanent dentition is present radiographically, caries-free and minimally restored. They have a Class I incisal and molar relationship with well-aligned arches. Due to compliance issues, general anaesthesia is required. For which single treatment should the patient be consented? ★★★★

A Extract the LR6 and all of the remaining first permanent molars (FPMs)

B Extract the LR6 and the contralateral LL6

C Extract the LR6 and the opposing UR6

D Extract the LR6 tooth only

E Extract the UR6 and extirpate the LR6

20. A 9-year-old boy attends for an examination. The enamel on all his primary and secondary teeth appears dull, frosty and pitted. There is considerable post eruptive breakdown of a number of teeth and marked sensitivity. Bitewings show numerous carious lesions and enamel that is less radiopaque than the underlying dentine. Which is the single most likely diagnosis? ★★★★

A Amelogenesis imperfecta (AI)

B Dentinogenesis imperfecta (DI)

C Fluorosis

D Molar incisor hypoplasia (MIH)

E Taurodontism

21. A 5-year-old boy with uncontrolled diabetes has gross caries in all of his primary molars. He is very anxious and considered uncooperative. The teeth are unrestorable and asymptomatic. Which is the single most appropriate treatment strategy to manage his carious molars? ★★★★

A Await natural exfoliation

B Extraction using general anaesthesia (GA) as a day case

C Extraction using GA as an inpatient

D Extraction using inhalation sedation

E Extraction using local anaesthesia

22. A 7-year-old boy attends with his mother for a routine examination where he is assessed by a foundation dentist (first year post-qualification). The child had multiple primary teeth extracted under general anaesthesia (GA) 18 months ago. Occlusal caries is diagnosed in his lower right first permanent molar, which is partially erupted. The boy was not brought to two subsequent appointments for the restoration. What is the single most appropriate management strategy the dentist should take in this scenario? ★ ★ ★ ★

A Contact the child's general medical practitioner (GMP)

B Contact the local safeguarding nurse

C Discharge from the practice

D Discuss with their foundation trainer

E Refer to social services

ANSWERS

1. D ★   OHCD 6th ed. → p. 64

The average age for eruption of the upper permanent canines is between 11 and 12 years. However, a range of 10–12 years has been identified in epidemiological studies. Variation occurs across the population, and each case must be assessed based on the general stage of development and eruption of all permanent teeth. As a very basic mnemonic for assisting in the assessment of canine development, the phrase 'Big Canines for Big School' can be of some help. Knowledge of when the contralateral canine erupted or its degree of eruption would provide crucial information regarding whether the missing canine is likely to erupt spontaneously. Six months is considered a reasonable time period to monitor for contralateral tooth eruption prior to investigation. However, further information should be sought regarding:

• Previous extractions
• Previous trauma, particularly to the primary teeth
• Spacing or crowding in the relevant labial and buccal segments
• Whether the canine can be palpated buccally—this should be documented from the age of 9 years.

Radiographs are likely to provide the greatest information regarding canine location. Parallax periapicals or an orthopantomogram (OPT) with an upper occlusal would enable positioning of the canine to be determined, whilst CBCT can be indicated where tooth resorption or cyst formation is suspected. Table 2.1 shows the chronology of development of primary dentition.

Keywords: upper permanent canine, appropriate age.

Table 2.1 Chronology of eruption of permanent dentition

Tooth	Maxillary	Mandibular
1	6.7–8.1	6.0–6.9
2	7.0–8.8	6.8–8.1
3	10.0–12.2	9.2–11.4
4	9.6–10.9	9.6–11.5
5	10.2–11.4	10.1–12.1
6	6.1–6.7	5.9–6.9
7	11.9–12.8	11.2–12.2
8	17.0–19.0	17.0–19.0

Reproduced from Welbury R, et al, *Paediatric Dentistry* fourth edition, table 2.1, page 12, Copyright (2012) with permission from Oxford University Press.

→ Welbury R, Duggal M, Hosey M. *Paediatric Dentistry* (4th ed.). Oxford University Press: Oxford; 2012.

2. B ★   OHCD 6th ed. → p. 64

It helps to know the eruption dates of all teeth. Knowing which teeth should be present at any given age will help you to identify the teeth when charting and will alert you to abnormal eruption patterns which may have an underlying cause.

In this particular scenario, the mother is likely to be concerned that a gap exists between the Bs and Ds, and only reassurance is required at this stage.

Average normal eruption dates of primary teeth are listed in Table 2.2. The dates in the table are approximate and should be used as a guide-line. The pattern of eruption may be more significant when assessing the developing dentition.

Keywords: developing dentition, 14-month old.

→ Welbury R, Duggal M, Hosey M. *Paediatric Dentistry* (4th ed.). Oxford University Press: Oxford; 2012.

Table 2.2 Chronology of eruption of primary dentition (months)

Tooth	Maxillary	Mandibular
A	8–12	6–10
B	9–13	10–16
C	16–22	17–23
D	13–19	14–18
E	25–33	23–31

Reproduced from Welbury R, et al, *Paediatric Dentistry* fourth edition, table 2.2, pg 13, Copyright (2012) with permission from Oxford University Press.

3. C ★

The child is only 4 years old and will be in the primary dentition. Primary teeth must never be re-implanted, as the apex of the primary tooth may be pushed into the developing permanent tooth germ, causing damage.

Losing consciousness after trauma may be an indicator of an underlying brain injury, so it is important to have the patient examined immediately by a medical professional. Other indicators of neurological damage include vomiting, memory loss, confusion, and headaches.

Checking for neurological damage would take priority over the patient's oral health in most situations.

Reassurance only is incorrect in this scenario. Trauma must always be followed up with a dentist to examine for oral injuries and to allow clinical and radiographic assessment, as symptoms or pathology may have a delayed presentation.

Keywords: 4-year old, unconscious.

→ Malmgren B, Andreasen JO, Flores MT, *et al*. International Association of Dental Traumatology guidelines for the management of traumatic dental injuries: 3. Injuries in the primary dentition. *Dental Traumatology*. 2012;**28**:174–82.

4. A ★   OHCD 6th ed. → p. 98

The history and examination describe a lateral luxation injury. These teeth are often non-mobile due to impaction of the root into the alveolar bone and can be associated with vertical displacement. Dental trauma injuries are common between 1 and 4 years of age. Preservation of the integrity of the permanent successor is a fundamental concept when managing primary dental trauma. Luxation with labial crown displacement carries a high risk of damage to the permanent tooth, as the root is displaced towards the developing tooth germ of the permanent successor, and consequently, they are best managed with extraction. Severity of damage to the permanent tooth has been linked with the age of the child at injury. Radiographs are likely to show the tooth is elongated and would reaffirm the need for extraction. Mild luxation injuries may be monitored when damage to the permanent successor is not suspected. Orthodontic re-positioning is not appropriate for this scenario, but referral to a specialist may be indicated where compliance is challenging and general anaesthesia is necessary, which may frequently be the case within this age bracket.

Keywords: lateral luxation, labially, significantly.

5. B ★   OHCD 6th ed. → p. 674

The Children Act 2004 sets out who has parental responsibility for a child. The information provided in this scenario means that no date of birth is actually required to interpret parental responsibility. Biological fathers who are named on the birth certificate for births registered after 1 December 2003 (in England) or who have subsequently married the mother would be able to give legal consent. Therefore, in this scenario, the father can provide consent for treatment. In addition to this, fathers holding a court order granting them parental responsibility overrides any issues relating to birth certificates and marital status. If a mother were to choose to give her child up for adoption, she would also surrender parental responsibility to the adopting parents. In situations where a patient under the age of 16 presents for treatment, a clinician can use his or her professional judgement to establish whether the patient understands the nature of treatment, along with its benefits and limitations, and whether they can compare alternative treatments to come to a decision. This is called Gillick competence. It is unlikely that a child of this age can truly understand and weigh up the information regarding their dental treatment. Clinicians are advised to exercise caution when determining if a patient is Gillick-competent and, if possible, to delay treatment until an adult with parental responsibility is available.

Keywords: subsequently married, named on birth certificate, consent.

→ Wheeler R. Gillick or Fraser? A plea for consistency over competence in children: Gillick and Fraser are not interchangeable. *BMJ*. 2006;**332**:807.

6. D ★   OHCD 6th ed. → p. 28

Dental caries is a dynamic process. For demineralization to occur, the following four factors must be present.

- Substrate (fermentable carbohydrate)
- Bacteria
- Time
- Host (tooth).

All of the options above may be involved in caries prevention. Clearly, in this scenario, no amount of intervention or preventative advice will reduce the caries risk, unless the frequency of sugar intake is reduced. Each time food or drink (with sugars in) is consumed, substrate will be available to bacteria in dental plaque. The result is a drop in acidity of the local environment at the tooth surface, leading to demineralization. Eventually, saliva buffers the acid formed by fermented carbohydrates and tips the equilibrium in favour of remineralization. The more frequent the intake of sugar, the greater the length of time that demineralization will occur throughout the day. Therefore, in this scenario, it is important to reduce the intake of sugar. Fluoride contained within oral saliva is especially effective at remineralizing enamel when it comes in contact with the enamel–plaque interface. Constant supply of low-level fluoride in liquid form (i.e. topical fluoride) is most effective at preventing caries. Brushing removes plaque and thus helps prevent further demineralization, thus tipping the dynamic process in favour of remineralization. Systemic fluoride is less effective in caries prevention than topical fluoride, and it does not remineralize softened enamel. Systemic fluoride used during tooth formation can help with caries prevention by strengthening the tooth structure and forming shallower fissures, which are less susceptible to caries. Chewing gum will stimulate saliva after consumption of food or drink.

Keywords: white spot lesions, frequent, sugary.

→ Welbury R, Duggal M, Hosey M. *Paediatric Dentistry* (4th ed.). Oxford University Press: Oxford; 2012.

7. E ★

The simplified BPE uses a WHO 621 probe to examine the index teeth of children aged 7–17. The index teeth are all permanent first molars and the upper right and lower left permanent central incisors. It has been recommended that between the ages of 7 and 11, BPE scores—0, 1, and 2—are used to assess gingivae for bleeding, calculus, and plaque retentive factors. Prior to 12 years of age, periodontal false pocketing can be evident, particularly around partially erupted teeth. From 12 to 17 years of age, the full range of BPE scores—0, 1, 2, 3, 4, and *—should be used on index teeth. Assessment of all teeth is considered excessive, as true periodontal disease would be unlikely to present without involving the index teeth described above. Just as in adult patients, further investigations would be required if pocketing is identified, which would include radiographs and more detailed periodontal charting. Specialist referral may be required in these cases.

Keywords: simplified BPE, index teeth.

→ Clerehugh V, Kindelan S. *Executive summary—guidelines for periodontal screening and management of children and adolescents under 18 years of age.* British Society of Periodontology and British Society of Paediatric Dentistry. 2012. Available at: http://www.bsperio.org.uk

8. A ★★   OHCD 6th ed. → p. 96

It is unusual for anybody to hurt themselves behind the ears or the neck. Accidental injuries usually occur on areas of the body that are exposed (hands) or areas which protrude (chin, nose). Therefore, trips and falls can easily traumatize a child's chin, hands, or knees.

Other suspicious injuries include torn frena in non-ambulatory children, bruises of different ages (i.e. various shades and colours), and bruises around the thighs and buttocks.

Assessment of the child's general appearance, including cleanliness, and their social interactions with family and the dental team will provide further information regarding the likelihood of neglect or an NAI. Discussing the injuries with the child's parents or the child themselves may elicit important information regarding the mechanism of injury, which may corroborate the clinical findings.

Escalation and discussion with a more senior clinician, a practice safeguarding lead, or a local safeguarding officer/nurse would be appropriate as a first-line measure. It is not advisable to manage these situations on your own or without additional support. You should always be aware of your local child protection guidelines.

Keywords: subdued, back of the neck, fell in the park.

→ Department for Education, Home Office, Department of Health and Social Care, *et al. Safeguarding children.* Available at: https://www.gov.uk/topic/schools-colleges-childrens-services/safeguarding-children

9. E ★★   OHCD 6th ed. → p. 86

PMCs or stainless steel crowns (SSCs) are the restoration of choice in teeth that have been pulp-treated, either with pulpotomy or pulpectomy. Asymptomatic carious primary molars with marginal wall breakdown or caries involving two surfaces are also recommended for restoration with a PMC. A systematic review of five randomized controlled trials concluded that teeth restored with PMCs were less likely to develop problems such as pain and abscess formation, as well as being less uncomfortable to the patients during treatment. Plastic restorations with amalgam, composite, compomer, and GIC generally record a poorer performance by comparison to PMCs, which show lower failure rates in many studies.

Keywords: pulpotomy, primary molar, coronal restoration.

→ Innes NP, Ricketts D, Chong LY, et al. Preformed crowns for decayed primary molar teeth. *Cochrane Database of Systematic Reviews.* 2015;**12**:CD005512.

10. C ★★

Unplanned early or late loss of a lower first molar can create numerous occlusal problems and exacerbate malocclusions. The timing of the extraction is therefore very important. The best predictor for this is when there is radiographic evidence showing calcification of dentine at the root bifurcation of the lower second molar. This is thought to occur between 8 and 10 years. Analysis of the developing dentition and orthodontic consultation should be sought, if possible. However, removal of pain and infection should take priority, if present. Early loss of a lower first permanent molar is associated with:

- Distal drifting, tipping, and rotation of the second premolar
- Potential for premolar spacing.

Late loss of a lower first permanent molar is associated with:

- Mesial tipping and mesio-lingual rotation of the lower second molar. This results in poor occlusal contacts and buccal segment spacing
- The second premolar can drift distally.

Orthodontic consultation is required, as skeletal classification and crowding can impact upon the designated treatment plan. See Figure 2.1 which shows severe tipping of the lower secondary and over-eruption of

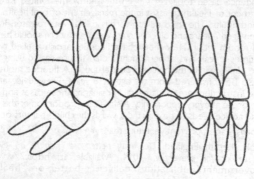

Figure 2.1

Reproduced from Welbury R, et al, *Paediatric Dentistry* fourth edition, Figure 14.13b, page 286, Copyright (2012) by permission of Oxford University Press.

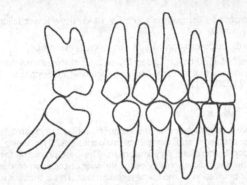

Figure 2.2

Reproduced from Welbury R, et al, *Paediatric Dentistry* fourth edition, Figure 14.14b, page 286, Copyright (2012) by permission of Oxford University Press.

the upper first molar. Figure 2.2 prevents over-eruption of the opposing first molar and reduces mesial tilting of the lower second molar.

Keywords: lower permanent second molar, erupt, predictor.

→ Cobourne M, Williams A, Harrison M. *A guideline for the extraction of first permanent molars in children.* Royal College of Surgeons of England. 2014. Available at: https://www.rcseng.ac.uk/dental-faculties/fds/publications-guidelines/clinical-guidelines

11. D ★★

This child has a high caries rate and should be managed accordingly. An evidence-based toolkit has been devised by the United Kingdom's Department of Health to assist in the management of oral health in children and adults. The third edition of this toolkit was released in 2014. Children aged 7 years and older who are causing concern should be placed on a 3-month recall. They should have fluoride varnish applied twice or more times a year, and all permanent molars fissure-sealed using a resin sealant, ideally within the first year post-eruption. A fluoride mouth rinse may also be considered from the age of 8 years. Diet advice and oral hygiene instructions are fundamental in managing these cases and should be reinforced at every opportunity. A significant proportion of this education and advice needs to be directed towards the child's parents or carers.

Keywords: caries, preventive, future management.

→ Public Health England. *Delivering better oral health: an evidence-based toolkit for prevention.* 2014. Available at: https://www.gov.uk/government/publications/delivering-better-oral-health-an-evidence-based-toolkit-for-prevention

12. B ★★

When trauma causes a tooth to become mobile, splinting can provide stability to allow periodontal healing and comfort for the patient. Splinting for too long can result in the tooth becoming ankylosed, and not splinting for long enough may result in less favourable healing outcomes. Generally, the type of healing is classified as: calcific healing (dentine and cementum), fibrous healing (connective tissue), osseous healing (bone and connective tissue), and non-healing. The chances of calcific healing are likely improved with good apposition of the fractured segments—potentially more so than the length of time for which the tooth is splinted. Patient advice should include a soft diet for a week, good oral hygiene, and short-term use of chlorhexidine mouthwash for optimal prognosis. Follow-ups are recommended at 4 weeks, 8 weeks, 4 months, 6 months, 1 year, and 5 years.

Keywords: mid-third root fracture, splint.

→ DiAngelis AJ, Andreasen JO, Ebeleseder KA, et al. International Association of Dental Traumatology guidelines for the management of traumatic dental injuries: 1. Fractures and luxations of permanent teeth. *Dental Traumatology.* 2012;**28**:2–12.

13. D ★★

Treatment depends upon multiple factors, including the severity and rate of infraocclusion and the patient's age. However, an orthodontic assessment is nearly always indicated to enable the correct long-term treatment plan to be decided, particularly when there is concomitant malocclusion. Early diagnosis of infraoccluded teeth can help to reduce potential complications. Delayed treatment can result in: tipping of adjacent teeth, loss of arch space, over-eruption of opposing teeth, insufficient development of alveolar width or height, increased risk of developing caries, and localized periodontal attachment loss. As a permanent successor is not present, orthodontics could help to close the space, without the need for restorative treatment, or to maintain the space to facilitate restorative treatment in the future. Reassurance and monitoring of an infraoccluded tooth are only advised in the short term if the tooth is not ankylosed, the successor is present, the tooth is not having a detrimental effect on the patient's oral health, and the degree of infraocclusion is slight. This is usually more relevant in late-presenting adult patients. Composite build-ups and indirect onlays can be used in the medium term to maintain occlusal stability in cases of slight or moderate infraocclusion. In this scenario, extraction will be likely due to the severity and the patient's age, but an orthodontic opinion is needed first. Definitive restoration of the resulting space would typically be delayed until dento-alveolar development is complete, or it may not be necessary.

Keywords: 13-year old, successor not present, crooked teeth, severely infraoccluded.

→ Arhakis A, Boutiou E. Etiology, diagnosis, consequences and treatment of infraoccluded primary molars. *Open Dentistry Journal*. 2016;**10**:714–19.

14. E ★★

Minimal occlusal caries with evidence of dentine involvement requires exploration and removal. Preventive resin restoration enables caries to be identified and removed, whilst remaining minimally invasive. Furthermore, fissure sealing of the remaining fissure pattern will protect the tooth from further occlusal caries in the pits and fissures. Amalgam is a suitable restorative material, but it is more destructive due to cavity design requirements for retention and the need for a minimum thickness of approximately 2 mm. Implementation of the Minamata Convention recommendations is also decreasing amalgam usage. From 1 July 2018, in England, regulations state that amalgam should not be used in children under 15 years of age and pregnant or breastfeeding women (unless deemed strictly necessary by the clinician). A conventional composite restoration may be required if the caries extends over a significant proportion of the occlusal surface or through the marginal ridge. Dentists using truly minimally invasive procedures have presented evidence for sealing caries with resin fissure sealants alone. Theoretically, sealing the carious lesion blocks substrate from reaching the bacteria. However, caution is required during placement of the sealant, with careful long-term maintenance. Fissure sealants alone in irregular attendees would not be advised.

Keywords: minimal caries, outer third of dentine.

→ Welbury R, Duggal M, Hosey M. *Paediatric Dentistry* (4th ed.). Oxford University Press, Oxford; 2012.

15. D ★★★   OHCD 6th ed. → p. 104.

In this case, the UR1 is considered to be moderately intruded and importantly, root development is incomplete.

Severity of intrusion:

- Mild <3 mm
- Moderate 3–6 mm
- Severe >6 mm.

Initial management for permanent incisors that have incomplete root development is to allow for passive repositioning for 2–3 weeks. However, each clinical situation differs and some severe intrusions can be managed surgically.

Active repositioning, including surgical and orthodontic repositioning, should be considered if no movement is evident within the first 2–3 weeks or if passive eruption ceases and the tooth remains infraoccluded. Teeth with complete root development that are mildly intruded can be monitored for passive repositioning for 2–3 weeks prior to active repositioning. Moderate and severe intrusions are best managed with either orthodontic or surgical repositioning and may be best referred for specialist care. Appropriate special investigations and trauma charts should be carried out to monitor the vitality of the intruded tooth and its adjacent teeth. It is likely that root canal treatment will be required, especially in teeth with complete root development, and regular radiographic analysis should occur to confirm no inflammatory resorptive changes.

Keywords: permanent tooth, incomplete root development, 5 mm.

→ Albadri S, Zaitoun H, Kinirons MJ; British Society of Paediatric Dentistry. UK National Clinical Guidelines in Paediatric Dentistry: treatment of traumatically intruded permanent incisor teeth in children. *International Journal of Paediatric Dentistry.* 2010; **20**(Suppl 1):1–2.

16. C ★★★   OHCD 6th ed. → p. 60

Modelling is a branch of observational psychology that involves a behaviour being learnt through imitation. Specifically to dentistry, the young or inexperienced child observes a non-fearful child, or 'model', having a positive experience at the dentist. This approach is thought to work best if the patient can observe a 'live' model with whom they can closely relate, i.e. they are a relative or friend of similar age. In reality, the model is often an older sibling, parent, or family member. Behaviour shaping utilizes selective reinforcement, in which positive reinforcement is provided for behaviours that are closer to the desired behaviour, e.g. praising a child for sitting nicely in the chair, even though they will not open their mouth. Enhanced control is designed to empower the child, so they feel in control of the situation. A stop signal or a countdown are useful examples of this. Systematic desensitization is one approach to achieving a desired goal in phobic patients. A hierarchy of steps are outlined, with each step getting progressively closer to the ultimate desired goal. Positive reinforcement is a branch of operant conditioning whereby a behaviour is strengthened, based on its association with a positive stimulus.

Keywords: sibling, observe, behaviour management.

17. D ★★★

At the age of 8 years, the UR1 would be expected to have incomplete root development, as completion occurs typically 2–3 years after eruption. Although the coronal pulp has been contaminated, inflammation is usually fairly localized due to the cellular structure of the pulp. If the inflamed/infected pulp tissue is removed, there is potential for healing to occur and pulp vitality to be retained. The resulting benefits include continued root development and maintenance of normal repair, defence, and sensory functions. The clinical technique for this is called a pulpotomy (complete or partial). The tooth should be kept under review, as in the long term, there is a risk of losing vitality. Where the apex is immature, the potential for healing is considered to be better. A direct pulp cap could be attempted if pulp exposure is not so severe (<1 mm and <24 hours). Extraction would not be an ideal first-line treatment in this case as the tooth is still restorable, and root canal treatment is inappropriate as the tooth is still vital. Apexification is useful when a tooth with incomplete root formation has lost vitality. Non-setting calcium hydroxide can be used to induce a calcific barrier at the apex before root canal treatment can be performed, but more commonly a bioceramic barrier technique is now employed.

Keywords: 8-year old, complicated crown fracture, >24 hours, positive sensibility testing.

→ Cvek M. A clinical report on partial pulpotomy and capping with calcium hydroxide in permanent incisors with complicated crown fracture. *Journal of Endodontics*. 1978;**4**:232–7.

18. C ★ ★ ★   OHCD 6th ed. → p. 72

This developmental defect is caused by invagination of the enamel epithelium into the dental papilla during tooth formation. It is most commonly associated with the upper lateral incisors and sometimes the premolars. In this instance, the patient is young and has no symptoms, so a more conservative approach would be suitable. Good-quality fissure sealants would reduce the chances of developing caries without sacrificing tooth tissue. Flowable composite may be considered a suitable alternative. However, fissure sealants are considered a more suitable first-line management strategy (many of which are resin-based anyway). Depending on severity, teeth with dens invaginatus are highly susceptible to caries, so simple oral hygiene instructions are unlikely to prevent decay. As the patient is asymptomatic, with positive sensibility tests and no evidence of active caries, more complex restorative treatment is not necessary at this stage. Teeth with dens invaginatus can be challenging to perform root canal treatment on, with CBCT frequently used to diagnose and help plan treatment.

Keywords: palatal aspect of upper lateral incisors, no symptoms.

→ Bishop K, Alani A. Dens invaginatus. Part 2: Clinical, radiographic features and management options. *International Endodontic Journal*. 2008;**41**:1137–54.

19. C ★ ★ ★ ★

An unrestorable molar tooth will require extraction. Therefore, root canal treatment is not appropriate. When extracting FPMs, there is a risk of undesirable tooth movement of adjacent teeth, which may provide unfavourable over-eruption or changes to tooth alignment. This should be taken into account when planning treatment for the patient. Due to the risks involved with a general anaesthetic, treatment plans are frequently more radical in order to try and prevent repeat operations. It is suggested that, with FPMs, when a lower molar is removed, removal of the opposing upper FPM should be given close consideration to prevent over-eruption (i.e. a compensating extraction). Where a local anaesthetic can be used, these extractions are hard to justify and removal is indicated only if there is unfavourable movement at review. Balancing extractions (removal of the contralateral tooth) is unwarranted, as there is no evidence to suggest removal of FPMs affects the midline. In the case of severe crowding or complex malocclusions, orthodontic input is suggested. The evidence supporting this is fairly weak, and each case should be assessed individually.

Keywords: 9-year old, unrestorable lower first permanent molar, general anaesthetic.

→ Cobourne M, Williams A, Harrison M. *A guideline for the extraction of first permanent molars in children.* Royal College of Surgeons of England. 2014. Available at: https://www.rcseng.ac.uk/dental-faculties/fds/publications-guidelines/clinical-guidelines

20. A ★★★★ OHCD 6th ed. → p. 68

AI describes a number of genetically controlled conditions that affect the structure of enamel. The conditions are hereditary but can occur following spontaneous genetic mutations and can present in numerous different forms. Enamel derived from epithelial tissue in the developing tooth germ is produced by ameloblasts. The timing of the defect with regard to enamel development is fundamental to the type of enamel formed, and ultimately the defect observed. The process is intimately linked with genetics and can be classified based on the mode of inheritance. However, the type of defect is often used to classify the condition.

• Hypoplastic—enamel is often thin or translucent. Radiographically, normal enamel–dentine contrast is observed.
• Hypocalcified—this results from inappropriate calcification and, as such, the enamel is of normal thickness but is weak or chalky. This structural change results in enamel that appears more radiolucent than the underlying dentine.
• Hypomaturation—this results from inappropriate resorption of the enamel matrix. The enamel is stronger, by comparison to hypocalcified AI, but is generally softer than normal and is prone to wear. Mottling can occur, and similar enamel–dentine radiodensity can be observed.

Keywords: enamel, all, teeth, frosty, pitted, less radio-opaque.

→ Gadhia K, McDonald S, Arkutu N, Malik K. Amelogenesis imperfecta: an introduction. *British Dental Journal.* 2012;**212**:377–9.

21. C ★★★★

GA should be reserved as a last resort; however, in this case, the main concerns are the patient's medical status and level of anxiety; for this reason, a GA referral would be appropriate. Poorly controlled diabetes would warrant extra precaution during the GA procedure; for this reason, it is often best to keep the patient in overnight. However, this decision is made at the discretion of the treating anaesthetist, and in some cases, this may be managed as day-case GA, providing inpatient facilities are available, should they be required.

Good cooperation is needed from patients during inhalation sedation, as the patient is conscious during the procedure. This may be difficult for a patient of such young age.

Performing extractions using local anaesthesia in multiple quadrants in anxious patients may be difficult, as they may not wish to return after the first appointment.

Keywords: uncontrolled diabetes, very anxious, unrestorable.

→ Adewale L, Morton N, Blayney M. *Guidelines for the management of children referred for dental extractions under general anaesthesia.* Association of Paediatric Anaesthetists of Great Britain and Ireland. 2011. Available at: https://www.rcoa.ac.uk/document-store/guidelines-the-management-of-children-referred-dental-extractions-under-general

22. **D** ★★★★   OHCD 6th ed. → p. 96

The scenario describes a potential case of dental neglect. At 7 years of age, the child will rely on parents to attend appointments and, as such, the term 'was not brought' is preferred over 'did not attend'. As a junior clinician, the foundation trainer should be the first port of call to discuss the case. It is more than likely that the foundation trainer will have experience in handling such cases, with pragmatic advice to assist in handling the issue.

It is important to adhere to your local safeguarding policy and any guidance provided by your local safeguarding children board. However, repeated failure to comply with reasonable appointment requests would be a cause for concern, and your practice or local safeguarding nurse would be an appropriate second step. This may require follow-up with the patient's GMP or local Social Services Department, as the family may be known to social services and may already have a designated support worker assisting the family.

Keywords: foundation dentist, multiple extractions, GA, caries, not brought, two, appointments.

→ Harris J, Sidebotham P, Welbury R. *Child protection and the dental team: an introduction to safeguarding children in dental practice.* Committee of Postgraduate Dental Deans and Directors (COPDEND), Sheffield; 2006.

Orthodontics

Nadia Ahmed

'Straightening things out.'

Orthodontics is 'the specialty of dentistry concerned with growth of the face, the development of dentition, and the prevention and correction of occlusal anomalies. A malocclusion can be defined as 'a deviation from the ideal that may be aesthetically or functionally unsatisfactory, with a wide range of occlusal traits'.

Orthodontics is a constantly evolving specialty, with ever changing principles and techniques continuing to be developed. There has been huge progress in orthodontics in recent times, with changes in the types of brackets, archwire materials, and appliance systems (such as temporary anchorage devices and aligner technology).

The key principles of orthodontics date back to 1899 when Edward Angle described 'the key to a normal occlusion as the anteroposterior relationship between the upper and lower first molars'. In 1972, Lawrence Andrews described 'six keys to an ideal static occlusion'. This was the basis of early orthodontic treatment planning.

Knowledge of craniofacial development and growth is required as a foundation for understanding the aetiology of a patient's malocclusion, to reach a diagnosis, and to plan orthodontic treatment. A basic understanding of the types of orthodontic appliances is beneficial (mainly fixed appliances, functional appliances, some use of removable appliances, and retainers).

In addition to the management of a malocclusion, orthodontic treatment is often required in conjunction with other specialties, including oral and maxillofacial surgery, paediatric and restorative dentistry

Key topics discussed in this chapter include:

- Fixed appliances
- Functional appliances
- Removable appliances
- Retention
- Index of treatment need
- Orthodontic assessment and diagnosis
- Cephalometric analysis
- Malocclusion
- Ectopic canines
- Dental anomalies.

QUESTIONS

1. A 12-year-old boy attends for a check-up. He has the following features in his malocclusion:

Class II division 1 incisors

Overjet of 6 mm

Incompetent lips

Contact point displacement of 4.5 mm between LR3 and LR4

Contact point displacement of 3 mm between UL1 and UL2

Overbite of 70% complete to tooth.

What is his index of orthodontic treatment need (IOTN)? (Select one answer from the options listed below.) ★

A 3a

B 3d

C 3f

D 4a

E 4d

2. A 9-year-old girl attends for a review appointment. Six months ago, her upper left permanent central incisor had not erupted, and it is still not present today. A radiograph reveals the presence of a supernumerary overlying the unerupted tooth. She presents with the following clinical features:

- Class II division 1 incisor relationship
- Overjet of 5 mm
- Increased overbite
- Lingual displacement of the partially erupted lower right lateral incisor (LR2)
- Upper left first permanent molar (UL6) is in crossbite

Which single feature of the child's dentition would lead you to score a grade 5 in her IOTN? ★

A A midline supernumerary tooth

B An increased overbite

C An overjet of 5 mm

D Severe crowding of 4 mm associated with the LR2

E UL6 is in crossbite

3. A 21-year-old female, who is undergoing fixed orthodontic treatment, attends for a routine examination. Her plaque control is particularly poor. Which single most important risk would encourage you to contact the orthodontist to discuss discontinuing treatment? ★

A Decalcification

B Loss of vitality

C Pericoronitis

D Root resorption

E Tooth mobility

4. A 12-year-old girl attends for assessment. Her upper right central incisor overlaps the coronal one-third of the lower incisor crown height, and there is contact between the lower incisal edges and the palatal surface of the upper incisors. Which single option best describes the patient's overbite in this scenario? ★

A Increased and complete

B Increased and incomplete

C Normal and complete

D Reduced and complete

E Reduced and incomplete

5. An 11-year-old girl with a posterior crossbite is undergoing orthodontic treatment with a removable appliance. Which single tooth movement would a removable appliance not be able to achieve? ★ ★

A Bodily movement

B Canine retraction

C Reduction of an increased overbite

D Space maintenance

E Tipping of teeth

6. A 10-year-old boy is undergoing the initial stages of his orthodontic treatment. He has a crossbite and has been provided with a removable appliance in order to expand the maxillary arch. Which single component should be adjusted to achieve the desired movement? ★ ★

A Acrylic base plate

B Adam's clasps

C Midline expansion screw

D Offset southend clasp

E Posterior bite plane

7. A 17-year-old woman attends for a routine check-up with her general dental practitioner, having been discharged from her orthodontist following comprehensive orthodontic treatment. She reports that she has lost the instructions for wearing her vacuum-formed retainers. What is the single most appropriate piece of advice to give in this scenario? ★★

A Wear the retainers full-time

B Wear the retainers only during the day and remove for eating/drinking

C Wear the retainers for 2–3 hours per day

D Wear the retainers only at night

E Wear the retainers only during the day and keep them in if eating/drinking

8. A 9-year-old boy has a Class II skeletal discrepancy and would benefit from a functional appliance. What would be the most ideal age range at which to begin his treatment in order to utilize his pubertal growth spurt? (Select one answer from the options listed below.) ★★

A 10–11 years

B 12–13 years

C 14–15 years

D 16–17 years

E Over 17 years

9. A 15-year-old boy with a palatally impacted canine is having a closed exposure to enable alignment of the tooth, using a gold chain and fixed appliances. The tooth requires significant three-dimensional tooth movement. Which single type of tooth movement requires the highest force? ★★

A Bodily movement

B Extrusion

C Intrusion

D Rotation

E Tipping

10. A 12-year-old boy has an orthodontic assessment and his incisor relationship is to be classified. His lower incisor edges are posterior to the cingulum plateau of his upper incisors. The overjet is 2 mm, and the upper incisors are retroclined. Which is the single most appropriate British Standards Institute Incisor classification? ★★

A Class I

B Class II

C Class II division 1

D Class II division 2

E Class III

11. A 13-year-old boy attends the Orthodontic Department. His upper right permanent canine erupted six months ago. However, the upper left permanent canine is still unerupted and not palpable buccally. What would be the most appropriate radiographic investigation to assess the developing dentition and locate the upper left permanent canine? (Select one answer from the options listed below.) ★★★

A A cone beam computed tomogram (CBCT)

B A lateral cephalogram and an orthopantomogram (OPT)

C A periapical (PA) and an upper standard occlusal (USO)

D An OPT and a PA

E An OPT and a USO

12. A 14-year-old girl has had a cephalometric tracing performed as part of her orthodontic assessment. Using this tracing, how would her skeletal relationship be identified? (Select one answer from the options listed below.) ★★★

A Measure the angle formed by the A point, glabella, and B point

B Measure the angle formed by the A point, nasion, and B point

C Measure the angle formed by the A point, porion, and B point

D Measure the angle formed by the A point, sella turcica, and nasion

E Measure the angle formed by the anterior nasal spine, nasion, and sella turcica

13. An 9-year-old girl has been referred due to rotation and displacement of her upper left central incisor. A periapical radiograph of the central incisors reveals an unusual radio-opacity in the midline. What is the single most likely cause of the presenting complaint in this scenario? ★★★

A Complex odontome

B Compound odontome

C Conical supernumerary

D Supplemental supernumerary

E Tuberculate supernumerary

14. A 12-year-old boy attends your practice. The clinical features of his malocclusion include:

- A 10-mm overjet
- Class II division 1 incisor relationship
- A moderate Class II skeletal base
- Class II buccal segments
- Proclination of the upper incisors
- Well-aligned upper and lower arches.

You decide to refer him to an orthodontist. What is the most likely management for his malocclusion? (Select one answer from the options listed below.) ★★★★

A Delay treatment until facial growth has completed, then provide orthognathic surgery

B Extraction of one unit in all four quadrants and fixed appliances

C Extraction of two units in the maxilla and non-extraction in the mandible prior to fixed appliances

D Headgear retraction of upper buccal segments

E Provision of a twin block functional appliance

15. A 13-year-old girl has an increased, complete overbite that is traumatizing the palatal mucosa. The intraoral orthodontic assessment shows the patient is in the permanent dentition and has an overjet of 8 mm, upper incisors of average inclination, mild upper and lower arch crowding, and an increased curve of Spee in the lower arch. Which single type of appliance is most appropriate in managing the first stage of orthodontic treatment? ★ ★ ★ ★

A Lower removable appliance with a posterior bite plane

B Upper removable appliance with a flat anterior bite plane

C Upper removable appliance with a labial bow

D Upper removable appliance with a Robert's retractor

E Upper removable appliance with Z springs on the upper incisors

16. A local dental practice is reviewing its storage requirements and looking to dispose of old study models. The practice manager has identified study models taken 4 years ago for a patient who received orthodontic treatment at the age of 11 years, who is no longer seen at the practice. What single piece of advice should be given to manage these models? ★ ★ ★ ★

A Dispose of the models as clinical waste

B Dispose of the models as hazardous waste

C Securely send the models to her new dentist

D Store the models for a further 10 years

E Store the models for a further 14 years

ANSWERS

1. E ★   OHCD 6th ed. → p. 126

The index of orthodontic treatment need (IOTN) comprises a dental health component and an aesthetic component. The acronym MOCDO (Missing teeth; Overjet; Crossbite; Displacement of contact points; Overbite) can be used to help prioritize the single worst feature of a malocclusion, in order to score the dental health component. The order of the acronym is hierarchical. A score of 4d indicates severe displacement of teeth of >4 mm.

- 3a—increased overjet 3.6–6mm with incompetent lips
- 3d—displacement of teeth 2.1–4mm
- 3f—increased and complete overbite without gingival trauma
- 4a—increased overjet 6.1–9mm.

Keywords: IOTN, displacement of 4.5 mm.

2. A ★   OHCD 6th ed. → p. 126

The dental health component of the IOTN was developed from an index used by the Dental Health Board in Sweden to reflect these occlusal traits. Grade 5 indicates a very great need for treatment:

- 5a—increased overjet *greater* than 9 mm
- 5h—extensive hypodontia with restorative implications (>1 tooth missing in any quadrant), requiring pre-restorative orthodontics
- 5i—impeded eruption of teeth (except third molars) due to crowding, displacement, the presence of supernumerary teeth, retained deciduous teeth, and any pathological cause
- 5m—reverse overjet *greater* than 3.5 mm, with reported masticatory and speech difficulties
- 5p—defects of cleft lip and palate and other craniofacial anomalies
- 5s—submerged deciduous teeth.

The clinical scenario describes a 9-year-old child with delayed eruption of a permanent central incisor. With the exception of the midline supernumerary tooth impeding eruption, none of the other options would score grade 5. Moreover, this patient is very young and not all of her permanent dentition will have erupted. Therefore, an accurate assessment of her IOTN is difficult, but a midline supernumerary tooth would be picked up at around this time frame.

Delayed eruption of a permanent maxillary incisor tooth can be considered in the following circumstances:

- Eruption of the contralateral incisor occurred >6 months previously
- The maxillary incisors remain unerupted >1 year after the eruption of mandibular incisors
- There is a significant deviation from the normal eruption sequence, i.e. lateral incisors erupting prior to the central incisor.

Keywords: feature, IOTN, dental health component, grade 5.

→ Yaqoob O, O'Neill J, Patel S, *et al. Management of unerupted maxillary incisors*. Royal College of Surgeons (England). 2016. Available at: https://www.rcseng.ac.uk/dental-faculties/fds/publications-guidelines/clinical-guidelines/

3. A ★   OHCD 6th ed. → p. 132

Decalcification occurs when cariogenic plaque is present with a high-sugar diet. A fixed appliance predisposes to plaque accumulation, as cleaning around the fixed appliance can be difficult. Demineralization of the enamel can occur if patients do not follow dietary advice and do not brush their fixed appliances adequately, leaving a white outline around the brackets. Some degree of tooth mobility during treatment is normal. Other common risks discussed include relapse, root resorption and gingival recession. Rarely, pulpal necrosis might occur if rapid and excessive force is applied to the teeth that are already compromised.

Keywords: poor oral hygiene.

4. C ★   OHCD 6th ed. → p. 146

Overbite is described as the vertical overlap of the lower incisors by the upper incisors, along with a description of the contact that the lower incisor edge makes with the upper incisors or palate. The normal vertical overlap is described as the upper incisor teeth covering one-third to one-half of the lower incisor crown height. Less than this is described as reduced, and greater than this is described as increased. An overbite is complete if the edge of the lower incisors make contact with the upper incisors or palatal mucosa, and incomplete if the edge of the lower incisors do not make contact with the tooth surface or palatal mucosa.

An increased overbite is more commonly associated with Class II division 2 cases where the upper central incisors are retroclined.

An increased overbite does not necessarily require treatment, unless it is causing trauma to the palatal mucosa.

Keywords: overlaps the coronal one-third to half.

5. A ★★   OHCD 6th ed. → pp. 158 and 160

Fixed appliances can offer a wider range of tooth movements in comparison to removable appliances. Greater control over tooth movement can be achieved, as brackets not only provide vertical or tilting movements on the tooth surface, but also a force couple can be generated by the interaction between the bracket and the archwire. Rotational and apical movements are also possible. Removable appliances are capable of the following tooth movements:

1. Tipping
2. Movement of a block of teeth
3. Influencing eruption of opposing teeth, i.e. flat anterior bite plane, buccal capping.

Keywords: removable appliance, tooth movements.

6. C ★★   OHCD 6th ed. → pp. 146 and 158

A removable appliance typically comprises four parts: one or more active component, retention, anchorage, and a base plate. The active component exerts the force required for the desired movement and can be a spring, an elastic, or a screw, or a combination of any of these components. For arch expansion, a midline expansion screw is commonly used. There are various types of springs and screws that can be used, depending on the tooth movement required.

- An acrylic base plate provides the framework of the appliance to which all other components attach and provide anchorage.
- Adam clasps are a non-active component which provide retention by engaging undercuts, generally on the posterior teeth.
- An alternative retentive component is a southend clasp on the anterior teeth.
- A posterior bite plane allows some disclusion to aid crossbite correction.

Keywords: expand, maxillary arch, component, movement.

7. D ★★

Orthodontists may differ in the retention regime prescribed; however, in the absence of clear instructions, vacuum-formed retainers should be worn every night (12 hours). There is a high risk of relapse if the patient does not consistently wear them. There is a risk of caries and damage to the enamel if food and drinks are consumed whilst wearing the retainers. Only water can be consumed safely. The patient should return to their orthodontist to seek clarification of their retention regime if they are unsure.

Keywords: instructions, vacuum-formed retainer.

→ Littlewood SJ, Millett DT, Doubleday B, Bearn DR, Worthington HV. Retention procedures for stabilising tooth position after treatment with orthodontic braces. *Cochrane Database of Systematic Reviews*. 2016;**1**:CD002283

8. B ★★   OHCD 6th ed. → p. 162

The ideal ages for the use of functional appliances to achieve the desired jaw growth vectors is 10–12 years for girls, and 12–14 years for boys. Studies have shown that an earlier treatment start with a twin block prolongs treatment time for patients and can result in losing patient compliance with lengthened treatment. Following a twin block (approximately 9 months if worn well), fixed appliances are provided, which is a further 18–24 months of treatment. Cases where a twin block may be fitted early include occasions when a child is being bullied about their malocclusion or when a child is at increased risk of trauma.

Keywords: pubertal growth, age.

9. A ★★

Bodily movement requires 50–120 g force, similar to the force required to torque teeth into position, which is 50–100 g. Rotational movement and extrusion require a force of 35–60 g. Tipping movements require 25–60 g.

Bodily movement requires the highest force, as a greater area of the periodontal ligament is involved, so the force is dissipated over a greater area, and therefore, more force needs to be applied in order for optimal force levels to be obtained.

Keywords: tooth movement, highest force.

10. D ★★

The definitions for Classes 1, II (1), II (2), and III should be known, in order to be able to do an orthodontic assessment in practice and make appropriate referrals.

Class I—the lower incisor edges lie immediately below the cingulum plateau of the upper incisors.

Class II, division 1—the lower incisor edges lie posterior to the cingulum plateau of the upper incisors and the upper central incisors are proclined or of average inclination with an increased overjet.

Class II, division 2—the lower incisor edges lie posterior to the cingulum plateau of the upper incisors and the upper central incisors are retroclined. The overjet is usually minimal or may be increased.

Class III—the lower incisor edges lie anterior to the cingulum plateau of the upper incisors. The overjet is reduced or reversed.

Class II is always classified with a respective subdivision.

In this scenario, the lower incisors occlude posterior to the cingulum plateau, indicating a Class II relationship, and the upper incisors are retroclined.

Keywords: posterior to the cingulum plateau, retroclined.

→ Mitchell L. An Introduction to Orthodontics (4th ed.). Oxford University Press, Oxford; 2013.

11. E ★★★

Parallax is a technique used to identify the position of an unerupted tooth relative to a reference point such as an adjacent tooth. Two radiographs must be taken, with a change in the position of the X-ray tube between the two radiographs. The object farthest away from the X-ray beam will move in the same direction as the tube shift. Two periapical radiographs can be used for horizontal parallax, and an OPT and a USO for vertical parallax. In this scenario, an OPT is also required to assess the developing dentition.

The 'SLOB' rule can be used as a memory aid for this (same lingual, opposite buccal). When using the parallax technique, if a tooth moves in the same direction as the change in direction of the X-ray beam, then that tooth is lingually/palatally positioned.

CBCT is a very useful contemporary tool for assessing impacted teeth. However, due to the higher dose of radiation, it is not a first-line imaging technique and is reserved for cases where resorption of the adjacent teeth is suspected or further information is required for surgical exposure of the canine.

Keywords: canine, unerupted, radiographic investigation.

12. B ★★★   OHCD 6th ed. → p. 130

The angle ANB represents the relationship of the maxilla and the mandible to the anterior cranial base and is obtained by subtracting the angle formed by the sella turcica, nasion, and B point (SNB) from the sella turcica, nasion, and A point (SNA).

ANB = SNA − SNB

The average value is 3° ± 2°, indicating a Class I skeletal relationship. An increased ANB value is indicative of a Class II skeletal relationship, and a decreased ANB is indicative of a Class III skeletal relationship. Broad classification is as follows:

- ANB <2°: Class III
- 2° ≤ ANB ≤ 4°: Class I
- ANB > 4°: Class II.

Keywords: cephalometric, skeletal relationship.

13. C ★★★

Supernumerary teeth occur in 2% of the population in the permanent dentition and are more common in males. Supernumerary teeth can be described according to their morphology or position in the arch. Conical supernumerary teeth are the most common form, and when a conical supernumerary tooth is located in the midline, this is known as a mesiodens.

Conical supernumerary teeth can cause displacement or failure of eruption of a maxillary central incisor, or crowding. In some cases, supernumerary teeth have no effect on adjacent teeth.

Typically, they require removal to facilitate alignment.

Complex and compound odontomes are disorganized masses of mineralized tissue that can impede eruption of teeth.

Keywords: rotated upper central incisor, radio-opacity, midline.

→ Garvey MT, Barry HJ, Blake M. Supernumerary teeth—an overview of classification, diagnosis and management. *Journal of the Canadian Dental Association.* 1999;**65**:612–16.

14. E ★★★★   OHCD 6th ed. → p. 162

A twin block is a type of functional appliance. These guide the forces of muscle function, tooth eruption, and growth to encourage correction of a malocclusion. Commonly, twin blocks are used in growing patients to correct Class II malocclusions with an increased overjet. A twin block will correct a deep overbite by differential eruption of the posterior teeth. As this patient is young, it is possible to utilize his growth in the management of his malocclusion. The timing of twin block appliances is important, and preferably they should be used just before the adolescent growth spurt begins. However, they require adequate retention such as using Adam's clasps, labial bows, and ball hooks. Correction of the malocclusion has been attributed to roughly 30% of skeletal and 70% of dento-alveolar change.

Orthognathic surgery is reserved for when facial growth is complete but the skeletal pattern is too severe to consider orthodontic camouflage alone.

Keywords: 12-year old, 10 mm, Class II skeletal.

→ O'Brien K, Wright J, Conboy F, et al. Effectiveness of early orthodontic treatment with the twin block appliance: a multicenter, randomized, controlled trial. Part 1: dental and skeletal side effects. *American Journal of Orthodontics and Dentofacial Orthopedics*. 2003;**124**:234–43.

15. B ★★★★

In a growing patient, an upper removable appliance with a flat anterior bite plane allows eruption of the posterior teeth and reduction of a deep overbite. The resultant reduction in vertical overlap of the teeth (overbite) will allow a lower fixed appliance to be placed simultaneously, without the lower brackets being in traumatic occlusion.

Keywords: complete traumatic overbite, removable appliance, Class II, division 2.

16. D ★★★★   OHCD 6th ed. → p. 684

Study models are an important part of case planning and assessment in orthodontics. They are part of a patient's clinical records and, as such, should be kept for a minimum of 11 years or until the patient is 25 years old (whichever is longer). In this scenario, as the patient was 11 years old at the time of the impressions, they should be stored until the age of 25 because this is longer than the standard 11 years for adults. As they have already been stored for 4 years, they need to be kept for a further 10 years. This also applies to clinical notes, clinical photographs, and radiographs, which all form part of a patient's medical records.

With the digital revolution in dentistry, scanning and storing models electronically can save vast amounts of space, but it is important to ensure adequate security systems are in place and the data are regularly backed up. The guidelines below illustrate time to keep records.

Keywords: study models.

Dental Protection. *Record keeping in England*. 2017. Available at: https://www.dentalprotection.org/uk/articles/record-keeping-in-the-uk

Periodontics

Peter Clarke

'We can give you a clean slate, but ultimately, it's your job to keep it clean.'

Periodontitis is estimated to be the sixth most prevalent disease in the world, and clinicians are likely to encounter this disease and other gingival conditions on a regular basis. It is therefore important to have a sound understanding of both the pathophysiology and management of periodontitis and related conditions.

Periodontal disease may also be seen as a manifestation of systemic disease, so it may provide a window into the patient's general health. Common conditions, such as diabetes mellitus, have a well-established relationship with the progression of periodontal disease, but rare genetic conditions, such as Ehlers–Danlos syndrome, may produce unusual findings. Therefore, the clinician should have a good breadth of knowledge and be able to examine the patient as a whole, relating oral signs to systemic symptoms in order to diagnose and manage appropriately.

The general dental practitioner's role will focus mainly on diagnosis and non-surgical management of these patients, but awareness of the more advanced treatment will ensure appropriate referral and allow an informed discussion with the patient. A key challenge in the successful management of these patients is often getting them to obtain a suitable level of plaque control to stabilize the disease and maintain health. Ability to communicate this effectively and encourage excellent oral care is an invaluable asset.

The questions in this chapter will test the readers' knowledge of the fundamentals of periodontal diagnosis and practical skills. Moreover, questions are also presented examining the relationship with systemic disease and advanced treatment concepts. It is hoped that the questions in this chapter will test the readers' baseline knowledge and promote further reading around complex or contentious subjects.

Key topics include:

- Diagnosis/disease classification
- Aetiology
- Systemic conditions
- Non-surgical management/cause-related therapy
- Adjunctive therapies
- Surgical management/corrective therapy
- Supportive therapy.

QUESTIONS

1. A 45-year-old man is being reviewed, following a course of non-surgical periodontal therapy. His current full mouth plaque score is 15%, and he has had a good response to the treatment. Following repeat periodontal indices, he still has a number of isolated probing depths of 5 mm, which have reduced from 8 mm. Additional recession is present in these areas, varying from 1 to 2 mm. There is no bleeding present at these sites, and the root surfaces feel smooth. Which single clinical indicator would suggest these sites are stable? ★

A Absence of bleeding on probing
B Plaque scores of <20%
C Presence of plaque-retentive factors
D Recession
E Reduction in probing pocket depth

2. A 44-year-old woman is having non-surgical root surface debridement for chronic periodontitis. The instrument in Figure 4.1 is being used to remove a subgingival calculus from a deep periodontal pocket. These instruments have single cutting edges on the working tip to enable more efficient removal of deposits and to avoid iatrogenic damage. What is the optimal angle between the cutting edge and the tooth surface when in function? ★

A 15°
B 30°
C 45°
D 70°
E 90°

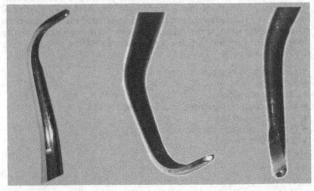

Figure 4.1

3. A 28-year-old man presents for a routine examination. He is a smoker (10 pack years) but is otherwise fit and well. His previous clinical notes report a diagnosis of plaque-induced gingivitis. However, following clinical examination today, his diagnosis has changed to generalized stage I, grade B periodontitis. Which single clinical finding is fundamental in differentiating between these two diagnoses? ★

A Gingival bleeding

B Loss of attachment

C Mobility

D Periodontitis only occurs after gingivitis has been present for 3 weeks

E Recession

4. A 78-year-old man complains of loose teeth. He has not attended the dentist in many years, and a detailed examination reveals:

- Poor plaque control
- Widespread periodontal probing depths of >8 mm
- Furcation involvement of a number of teeth
- Generalized horizontal bone loss of up to 70%.

He is a smoker of 15 pack years (currently smoking five cigarettes a day) but is otherwise fit and well. What is the single most appropriate diagnosis? ★

A Generalized stage III, grade A periodontitis

B Generalized stage III grade C periodontitis

C Generalized stage IV, grade B periodontitis

D Localized stage III, grade A periodontitis

E Localized stage IV, grade B periodontitis

5. A basic periodontal examination is performed on a 42-year-old woman. Her oral hygiene is generally good, but generalized recession of 2–3 mm is noted. In the upper right posterior sextant, a 2* is recorded. What single meaning does the * indicate in this context? ★

A Furcation involvement

B Loss of attachment of >7 mm

C Previous severe periodontal disease

D Probing depths of between 4 and 6 mm

E Probing depths of >6 mm

6. A 27-year-old man attends, complaining of loose teeth. He is medically fit and well and has never smoked. He reports rapid development of mobility, affecting all of his lower anterior teeth and lower right first permanent molar. Periapical radiographs provided by his general dental practitioner show progression of horizontal bone loss from 20% to 50% in the last 12 months. His oral hygiene is good, and he is aware that his father and paternal grandfather suffered from pyorrhoea. Which single bacteria is most commonly associated with the disease above? ★ ★

A *Aggregatibacter actinomycetemcomitans*

B *Fusobacterium nucleatum*

C *Porphyromonas gingivalis*

D *Prevotella intermedia*

E *Tannerella forsythia*

7. A 56-year-old man has swollen gums. Despite suboptimal oral hygiene, the appearance of the gingivae is suggestive of gingival overgrowth. He has controlled type 2 diabetes and hypertension. Which single common medication is most likely to be responsible for this clinical situation? ★ ★

A Amlodipine

B Bendroflumethiazide

C Glipizide

D Metformin

E Simvastatin

8. A 22-year-old woman has bleeding gums and severe pain around her lower front teeth. She has type 1 diabetes mellitus, and she is a heavy smoker (5 pack years). Her gingivae around the lower incisors are acutely tender and inflamed, and there is ulceration, combined with loss of the papilla. No significant probing depths or associated bone loss on the radiographs are noted, but there is an unpleasant odour. Which is the single most likely diagnosis? ★ ★

A Plaque-induced gingivitis

B Molar–incisor, grade C periodontitis

C Necrotizing gingivitis

D Periodontal abscess

E Periodontitis as a manifestation of systemic disease

9. A 52-year-old man has generalized stage II, grade B periodontitis. Oral hygiene instruction was instigated immediately, along with non-surgical periodontal therapy, providing full mouth root surface debridement (RSD). Upon a 3-month review, he has demonstrated no improvement in oral hygiene and his lack of motivation is apparent; heavy plaque deposits are present on all teeth surfaces. What is the single most appropriate next step in his management? ★★

A Commence a second round of RSD

B Prescribe antibiotics to tackle periodontitis

C Provide another round of RSD and prescribe antibiotics to tackle periodontitis

D Re-address oral hygiene instruction

E Refer to a specialist periodontist for periodontal management

10. A 37-year-old woman has received a course of non-surgical periodontal therapy in the undergraduate clinic. At review, loss of attachment charting demonstrates generalized reduction in periodontal probing depths, combined with only minor amounts of associated recession. The clinical tutor asks the presenting student which type of healing is most likely to have occured in this scenario. (Select one answer from the options listed below.) ★★★

A Regeneration: normal bony and junctional architecture is regained

B Regeneration and repair: mainly new bone and periodontal ligament (PDL) are formed, but some healing results from a long junctional epithelium (JE)

C Regeneration and repair: the majority of reduction is from a long JE, but some new bone height and PDL are formed

D Repair: a fibrous connection of scar tissue has formed

E Repair: a long JE attachment has formed

11. A 15-year-old South Asian adolescent boy has severe periodontal destruction and drifting of the upper incisors. His periodontal disease had previously affected his primary dentition, and he has palmar–plantar keratosis. His sibling also suffers from severe periodontal disease. Which single systemic condition is linked with their periodontal disease? ★★★

A Chèdiak–Higashi syndrome

B Hypophosphatasia

C Kabuki syndrome

D Leucocyte adhesion deficiency

E Papillon–Lefèvre syndrome

12. A 25-year-old man presents with generalized probing depths of >7 mm around the upper incisors, all four first permanent molars, and the lower premolars. Although he is an irregular attender, his plaque score is 20% and he is medically fit and well, with no other periodontal risk factors. What single adjunctive management option would routinely be indicated for this patient? ★ ★ ★

A Antibiotics

B Chlorhexidine

C Complement inhibition therapy

D Photodynamic therapy

E Probiotic therapy

13. A 45-year-old man has severe maxillary anterior toothwear. Marked sclerotic dentine is exposed, with 1 mm of supragingival tooth remaining. Dento-alveolar compensation has occurred, and there is no inter-occlusal space for restorations. The surrounding periodontium appears healthy, with no periodontal bone loss and normal root lengths. Which is the single most appropriate procedure to facilitate the direct restoration of these teeth? ★ ★ ★

A Apically repositioned flap

B Crown lengthening

C Gingivectomy

D Reduction of mandibular incisor height

E Overdenture provision

14. A 24-year-old woman has a Class II Millers recession defect, for which a connective tissue graft and a coronally advanced flap are planned. She has excellent oral hygiene, and all four wisdom teeth. Which is the single most appropriate intraoral site for taking her graft? ★ ★ ★

A Attached gingivae

B Buccal mucosa

C Buccal shelf

D Hard palate

E Retromolar pad

15. A 46-year-old woman requires crown lengthening surgery to facilitate the restoration of a fractured upper premolar. Based on the clinical assessment, resection of 2 mm of gingiva is possible. The junction between which two tissues is used to determine whether a resective approach is possible when crown lengthening? ★ ★ ★

A Attached gingiva and alveolar mucosa

B Free gingiva and attached gingivae

C Free gingiva from sulcular epithelium

D Junctional epithelium and periodontal ligament

E Sulcular epithelium and junctional epithelium

16. A consultant delivers a seminar on the pathogenesis of peri-odontal disease. Complement activation is discussed with regard to innate immunity, and a junior dental student asks how bacteria stimulate the complement cascade. Which single cell surface structure stimulates this cascade? ★ ★ ★ ★

A Immunoglobulin G (IgG)

B Interleukin-1 (IL-1)

C Lipopolysaccharide (LPS)

D Membrane attack complex (MAC)

E Pathogen recognition receptors (PRRs)

17. A 34-year-old man is being reviewed, following two courses of non-surgical periodontal therapy. He has stopped smoking 1 year ago and has no other risk factors. His recent plaque score is 23%, and he has three localized areas of isolated probing depth, which radio-graphically demonstrate angular vertical defects, with up to 50% of bone loss. A range of infrabony defects are identified when probing, and he has been treatment-planned for regenerative surgery. Which single type of defect has the most predictable outcome? ★ ★ ★ ★

A One-walled defect

B Two-walled defect

C Three-walled defect

D Circumferential defect

E No walled defect

18. A 46-year-old woman is reviewed 6 weeks after placing a metallo-ceramic crown on her upper right central incisor. The colour match is reasonable, although the crown appears slightly opaque. She also has marked localized marginal gingivitis, with fine subgingival calculus deposits that were not evident prior to crown cementation. The crown margins are 0.5 mm intra-sulcular and are well adapted and smooth on probing. Which single additional aspect of the prosthodontic treatment is most likely to be responsible for the gingivitis? ★ ★ ★ ★

A Bulbous emergence profile

B Excess cement

C Negative crown margins

D Sensitivity to adhesive resin cement

E Supracrestal attached tissue encroachment

19. A 24-year-old woman complains of a localized recession defect around her lower left central incisor, which she is struggling to keep clean. She has a history of orthodontic treatment. Clinically, 4 mm of recession is present labially on the lower incisor, with no loss of papilla height. A 2-mm probing depth associated with the defect and a high frenal attachment are also evident. Although not sensitive, there is localized plaque build-up around the defect, marginal inflammation, and a thin biotype with a 1-mm band of keratinized tissue present. The vestibular depth is also very shallow. Which is the single most appropriate initial treatment if aesthetics are not a major concern? ★ ★ ★ ★

A Advice and reassurance—no intervention

B Connective tissue graft with coronally repositioned flap

C Free gingival graft

D Frenectomy

E Rotational pedicle graft

20. A 53-year-old man is dissatisfied with his recent privately conducted periodontal treatment. He has submitted a formal complaint to the practice. After working to resolve the complaint locally, no solution has been reached. Which single piece of advice is most appropriate to give the patient in this scenario? ★ ★ ★ ★

A Contact a solicitor

B Contact the Dental Complaints Service

C Contact the General Dental Council (GDC)

D Contact the National Health Service (NHS) Ombudsman

E Contact your indemnifier

ANSWERS

1. A ★   OHCD 6th ed. → p. 88

Research by Lang et al. in the 1980s and 1990s highlighted the link between absence of bleeding on probing (BOP) and periodontal stability. Recession and a reduction in probing pocket depths are likely to represent successful treatment outcomes. However, these factors alone do not indicate periodontal stability, as further periodontal destruction could occur concomitantly.

Plaque retentive factors are likely to encourage biofilm formation and aggravation of periodontal tissues. These should be addressed as part of the overall periodontal management.

Plaque accumulation is a fundamental component in periodontitis. Plaque indices, such as the O'Leary plaque index, are useful tools in the assessment and management of caries and periodontitis. Whilst they are useful in assessing patient compliance and prognosis, a low plaque score does not indicate periodontal health, as plaque accumulation will inevitably lead to gingival inflammation, which, depending on host response, may progress to periodontitis.

Keywords: periodontal stability.

→ Lang NP, Adler R, Joss A, Nyman S. Absence of bleeding on probing an indicator of periodontal stability. *Journal of clinical periodontology*. 1990 Nov;**17**(10):714–21.

→ O'Leary T, Drake R, Naylor J. The plaque control record. *Journal of Periodontology*. 1972;**43**:38.

2. D ★

Gracey curettes are site-specific hand scalers used for subgingival debridement. The lower terminal shank should be inserted parallel to the long axis of the tooth. The working tip is designed with a single lower cutting edge to improve adaptation of the curette to the root surface and the base of the pocket. If inserted correctly, this produces an optimal angle of 70° between the tooth surface and the working tip. Absence of a second cutting surface is designed to reduce trauma to the periodontal tissues when scaling.

Keywords: Gracey site-specific (displayed in image), cutting edge.

3. B ★   OHCD 6th ed. → p. 186

Periodontal disease is extremely prevalent in the population. Traditionally, the disease process was classified into four stages: initial, early, established, and advanced—although ultimately, it is a continuous spectrum. In the first three stages, signs of inflammation develop and the immune response establishes. Vasodilatation occurs, bringing with it various cytokines and leucocytes. As the disease becomes more established, there is a shift from the innate immune response to the adaptive immune response, with T and B cells beginning to predominate.

The next stage is the advanced stage of the disease (periodontitis). In this stage, there is a dense inflammatory infiltrate, with large numbers of inflammatory mediators present. The mechanism of tissue destruction is a complex combination of direct bacterial action and indirectly as a result of the host response. Not all cases progress from gingivitis to periodontitis, but it is known that the host response plays a significant part in the overall clinical picture. Around 10–15% of the population will be hypersensitive and suffer from severe disease, and about 10% of the population will be innately resistant to the disease process. Recession and pocket depth measurements are combined to calculate clinical attachment loss.

Keywords: plaque-induced gingivitis, periodontitis.

→ Palmer RM, Ide M, Floyd PD. *A Clinical Guide to Periodontology* (3rd ed.). BDJ Books, London; 2013.

4. C ★

Until recently, classifications of periodontal disease were based upon the work of Armitage and colleagues at the International Workshop for Classification of Periodontal Diseases and Conditions in 1999. A new classification system was released in summer 2018, based upon updated understanding of periodontal biology, which also allows for incorporation of individual patient factors. It is a more pragmatic multidimensional staging system that not only facilitates future adaption to emerging evidence, but also permits personalized diagnosis that is crucial to constructing a comprehensive care plan. One of the big changes is 'aggressive' disease and 'chronic' disease are no longer distinct entities and have been incorporated into an overall umbrella term of 'periodontitis', which is subsequently modified by the clinical findings for that individual patient.

Periodontal disease is now classified by:*

1. The severity and complexity:

   Stage I: initial periodontitis
   Stage II: moderate periodontitis
   Stage III: severe periodontitis with potential for additional tooth loss
   Stage IV: severe periodontitis with potential for loss of dentition

2. The extent and distribution:

   Generalized: >30% of dentition affected
   Localized: <30% of dentition affected
   Molar–incisor distribution: affecting incisor and molar teeth

3. The risk of progression or anticipated treatment response:

*Reproduced from Caton *et al.* A new classification scheme for periodontal and periimplant diseases and conditions – Introduction and key changes from the 1999 classification. *Journal of Periodontology*. 2018;**89**(Suppl 1):S1–S8. Copyright © 2018, John Wiley and Sons.

Grade A: slow rate of progression
Grade B: moderate rate of progression
Grade C: rapid rate of progression.

Severity is classified based on clinical attachment loss (mild, 1–2 mm; moderate, 3–4 mm; or severe, >5 mm) and modified by the complexity of treatment (e.g. local factors such as deep angular bony defects, root grooves, furcation involvement, etc.).

The rate of progression and response to treatment is decided upon by judging the rate of bone loss over time (if sequential radiographs are present) or by estimating the bone loss/age ratio. This is then adjusted by examining the risk factors of the patient such as glycaemic control, smoking habits, and suspected genetic susceptibility.

In this instance, there is no relevant medical history to link the diagnosis to a systemic disease or any clinical evidence of necrotizing disease, and therefore, the diagnosis would come under the classification of 'periodontitis'. Clinically, there is attachment loss of >5 mm affecting the majority of the mouth and up to 70% of horizontal bone loss. Combined with the increased mobility and the numerous furcation lesions, this puts the dentition at risk of being lost and the patient is classified in the stage IV category. Given that he is 78 but has been a lifelong smoker with chronically suboptimal oral hygiene, the rate of bone loss is at an expected rate, and therefore, he would be in grade B category.

Keywords: poor plaque control, widespread pocketing of >8 mm, bone loss of up to 70%.

→Tonetti M, Greenwell H, Kornman K. Staging and grading of periodontitis: Framework and proposal of a new classification and case definition. *Journal of Periodontology.* 2018;**89**(Suppl 1):S159–S172

→ Caton GJ, Armitage G, Berglundh T, *et al.* A new classification scheme for periodontal and peri-implant diseases and conditions: introduction and key changes from the 1999 classification. *Journal of Periodontology.* 2018;**89**(Suppl 1):S1–8.

5. A ★   OHCD 6th ed. → p. 212

The basic periodontal examination is a widely used screening tool to assess for the presence of periodontal disease. It is conducted with a ball-ended probe that has black bands on it (WHO 621 probe) at 3.5–5.5 mm and 8.5–11.5 mm. When conducting the assessment, the mouth is split into sextants and every tooth (apart from the third molars) is examined; the worst score for each sextant is recorded. The score then gives an indication of what treatment is required. Table 4.1 describes the scoring system. The addition of a star to a sextant score indicates there is furcation involvement. Historically, the star was a standalone score for a sextant indicating either furcation involvement or attachment loss of >7 mm; however, this was changed in 2011.

→ British Society of Periodontology. *Basic periodontal examination (BPE).* 2016. Available at: http://www.bsperio.org.uk/publications

Table 4.1 The basic periodontal examination*

BPE code	Indications
0	Pockets <3.5 mm (first black band completely visible) No bleeding on probing or plaque-retentive factors
1	Pockets <3.5 mm (first black band completely visible) Bleeding on probing is present, but there is no plaque-retentive factors
2	Pockets <3.5 mm (first black band completely visible) Plaque-retentive factors are present (e.g. calculus or overhanging restorations)
3	Pockets 3.5–5.5 mm (first black band partially visible)
4	Pockets >5.5 mm (first black band completely into the pocket)
*	Furcation involvement (NB. A star should be recorded, along with a number, if furcation involvement is present in the sextant)

Reproduced from the British Society of Periodontology. *Basic Periodontal Examination*. March 2016. [Available at] http://www.bsperio.org.uk/publications.

6. A ★★

The scenario describes a young male patient with what was traditionally known as localized aggressive periodontitis but would now be classified as localized, grade C periodontitis (the stage would reflect the amount of destruction at the specific time point). Aggressive periodontal disease described a group of diseases in which there is rapidly progressing destruction of the periodontal attachment. It is classified as either localized, generalized, or molar–incisor, depending on its distribution. In the majority of cases, patients tend to be younger in age with good plaque control. There is also a propensity for familial aggregation, and patients display a non-contributory medical history.

Whilst multiple 'red-complex' pathogens have been implicated in periodontitis, *Aggregatibacter actinomycetemcomitans* (Aa), formerly *Actinobacillus actinomycetemcomitans*, has been identified as a key pathogen in localized aggressive periodontal disease (now more correctly approximated to molar–incisor, stage III, grade C periodontitis), with patients demonstrating serum antibodies against the causative agent. This bacterium possesses numerous virulence factors, enzymes, and endotoxins which upregulate the connective tissue inflammatory response, increase connective tissue destruction, and inhibit polymorphonuclear leucocytes function. Furthermore, this bacterium may also invade epithelial cells of the periodontal pocket, increasing its resistance to root surface debridement.

Keywords: progression, bone loss from 20% to 50%, bacteria, commonly associated.

→ Alani A, Seymour R. Aggressive periodontitis: how does an understanding of the pathogenesis affect treatment? *Dental Update*. 2011;**38**:511–21.

7. A ★★

Diagnosing drug-induced gingival overgrowth (DIGO) requires a thorough history and examination. Suboptimal oral hygiene could precipitate gingival swelling in the form of dental biofilm-induced gingivitis. However, the appearance of gingival overgrowth is generally distinct from that of dental biofilm-induced gingival swelling. Careful consideration of the patient's medications is prudent.

Anticonvulsants (phenytoin), immunosuppressants (ciclosporin), and calcium channel blockers (nifedipine) have all been implicated in the development of DIGO. All the drugs listed above could be used in the management of this patient's medical conditions. Of the drugs listed, amlodipine, a calcium channel blocker, is frequently associated with DIGO.

Whilst nifedipine may have been more widely reported in the literature regarding the development of DIGO, amlodipine is an alternative calcium channel blocker more regularly prescribed and also linked with DIGO. Good knowledge of drug classifications and drug names is important in determining the correct answer in this scenario.

Keywords: gingival overgrowth, commonly prescribed medication, hypertension.

→ Seymour RA, Thomason JM, Ellis JS. The pathogenesis of drug induced gingival overgrowth. *Journal of Clinical Periodontology*. 1996;**23**:165–75.

8. C ★★   OHCD 6th ed. → p. 193

Necrotizing periodontal diseases involve bacterial invasion of the periodontium, leading to necrosis and tissue damage. The condition is usually very painful and associated with distinct malodour. Amongst others, bacteria thought to be associated with this disease are *Prevotella intermedia, Fusobacterium* spp., and *Treponema* spp. Patients may also be immunocompromised. Therefore, risk factors, such as smoking, stress, malnutrition, poorly controlled diabetes, steroid use, and other medical conditions which may compromise the immune system, should be noted. Management of this condition is through a combination of antibiotics and localized mechanical debridement of the biofilm (local anaesthesia is often required in order to do this).

Keywords: smoker, diabetes, acutely tender, loss of the papilla, unpleasant odour.

→ Rowland RW. Necrotizing ulcerative gingivitis. *Annals of Periodontology*. 1999;**4**:65–73.

9. D ★★   OHCD 6th ed. → p. 178

Plaque is the primary cause of periodontitis. If the patient is unable or unwilling to maintain low plaque levels, another round of RSD is unlikely to provide any long-term benefit. Patient education and involvement is fundamental to successful management of periodontal disease. This discussion is dynamic and must adapt to each patient's situation. It is important to emphasize that professional treatment is an adjunct to excellent home care.

Further discussion of the aetiology, management, and progression of periodontal disease, along with further oral hygiene instruction, should take precedence over further treatment.

Referral for periodontal surgery is inappropriate, as periodontal surgery is not suitable for generalized periodontitis in patients with poor compliance. Antibiotics are not routinely used to treat periodontitis, unless disease is rapidly progressing and suggestive of grade C (aggressive) periodontitis.

Specialist periodontists are unable to provide any additional treatment until suitable levels of plaque control are attained.

Keywords: grade B periodontitis, oral hygiene, lack of motivation.

10. E ★★★

The three attachment structures of the periodontium to the tooth are as follows (coronal to apical):

1. The junctional epithelium
2. The connective tissue attachment
3. The periodontal ligament.

In health, the JE is, on average, 0.97 mm and the connective tissue attachment is 1.07mm; together, they comprise the *supracrestal attached tissues* (formally the 'biological width'). During active periodontal disease, the JE becomes ulcerated and there is damage to the connective tissue attachment. As the process progresses, the periodontal pocket deepens and the JE and CT attachments migrate apically. Following successful non-surgical therapy, the epithelial cells migrate the quickest and are the first to colonize the root surface, starting at the apical portion of the pocket and migrating coronally. This leads to the formation of a long JE. The connective tissue repair then helps to stabilize this new attachment. In regenerative therapies, the aim is to restore the original periodontal architecture before disease and facilitate the formation of new cementum, PDL, and bone. Healing following successful non-surgical periodontal therapy is therefore reparative whereby a long JE develops.

Keywords: reduction in probing depths, non-surgical therapy, healing.

→ Gargiulo A, Wentz F, Orban B. Dimensions of relations of the dentogingival junction in humans. *Journal of Periodontology*. 1961;**32**: 261–7.

→ Heasman P, Preshaw P, Robertson P. *Successful Periodontal Therapy: A Non-Surgical Approach*. Quintessence, London; 2004.

11. E ★★★

Various systemic conditions are associated with rapid periodontal destruction. Examples include: Chèdiak–Higashi syndrome, Down's syndrome, Ehlers–Danlos syndrome, hypophosphatasia, leucocyte adhesion deficiency, and Papillon–Lefèvre syndrome.

Papillon–Lefèvre Syndrome is a rare autosomal recessive hereditary condition, most common in the South Asian population. A genetic mutation results in the loss of function of a lysosomal enzyme found in neutrophils called cathepsin C; this has an important function in bacteria destruction. Other clinical findings include: palmar–plantar keratosis, arachnodactyly, recurrent skin infections, pes planus (flat feet), onychogryphosis (hypertrophic nails), and acro-osteolysis (resorption of distal phalanges). Management of these patients is difficult, and there is a high risk of tooth loss and edentulism. Furthermore, implants placed in these patients are high risk for peri-implantitis.

Keywords: palmar–plantar keratosis, sibling.

→ Chapple I, Hamburger J. *Periodontal Medicine: A Window on the Body*. Quintessence, London; 2006.

→ Nickles K, Schacher B, Ratka-Krüger P, Krebs M, Eickholz P. Long-term results after treatment of periodontitis in patients with Papillon–Lefèvre syndrome: success and failure. *Journal of Clinical Periodontology*. 2013;**40**:789–98.

12. A ★★★   OHCD 6th ed. → p. 192

The scenario above describes a typical presentation of a patient with generalized aggressive periodontitis (AP)—now classified as generalized stage III, grade C periodontitis. AP is a relatively rare disease, associated with rapid attachment loss. Plaque levels are often inconsistent with the severity of bone loss, and there are strong familial tendencies. Patients are often young (<35 years) and otherwise fit and well.

Antibiotics are important and often lifesaving medications. There are few indications for antibiotic use within dentistry, especially in the management of periodontal disease, but AP is one indication.

Localized AP is associated with particularly virulent pathogens, e.g. *Aggregatibacter actinomycetemcomitans* (Aa), whereas serum antibodies to infective agents in generalized AP are less robust. These pathogens have been shown to invade local gingival tissues, and this makes elimination with RSD alone challenging.

The timing and use of antibiotics in AP remain controversial. However, contemporary evidence shows a greater outcome with antibiotics provided immediately after the first round of RSD. Prior to commencing any antimicrobial therapy, dentists should be confident in their diagnosis, with referral to a specialist advised.

Complement inhibition therapy limits the effect of the complement system and has been shown to reduce the amount of inflammatory markers and minimize attachment loss and bone destruction in monkey models. There is no current evidence on their use in humans.

Photodynamic therapy is an antimicrobial treatment modality where a photosensitizer is administered to bacteria prior to application of a light source. The photosensitizer then breaks down upon activation to produce free radicals which damage the cell membrane. Clinical data do not show consistent long-term benefit over non-surgical management alone.

Probiotic therapy involves taking a tablet containing primary colonizing bacteria that are more conducive to periodontal health, shifting the ecological environment. Again clinical results show minimal clinical significant difference over non-surgical treatment.

Keywords: 25 years, generalized probing depths of >7 mm, plaque score of 20%.

→ Griffiths S, Ayob R, Guerrero A, et al. Amoxicillin and metronidazole as an adjunctive treatment in generalized aggressive periodontitis at initial therapy or re-treatment: a randomized controlled clinical trial. *Journal of Clinical Periodontology*. 2011;**38**:43–9.

13. B ★★★   OHCD 6th ed. → p. 206

Toothwear is an increasing problem within the adult population. Toothwear resulting in only 1 mm of remaining coronal tooth tissue is severe and has significant consequences in terms of treatment predictability. Composite restorations placed at an increased occlusal vertical dimension (OVD) are now a relatively common treatment modality utilized in toothwear management. To facilitate restorations, crown lengthening can be performed to apically reposition the gingivae and recontour the bone (osseous recontouring). An apically repositioned flap without osseous recontouring will likely result in gingival rebound with inadequate crown height gained.

Gingivectomy alone is also likely to encroach upon the supracrestal attached tissues. Reduction of the mandibular incisors may provide space for maxillary restorations, but no increase in bonding surface would be gained. Direct restorations to manage toothwear are commonly placed at an increased OVD, and the Dahl concept is utilized. Overdenture provision should not be overlooked as a potential management strategy; however, overdenture provision would not facilitate the direct restoration of teeth.

Keywords: 1 mm of supra-gingival tooth remaining, dento-alveolar compensation, periodontium healthy.

14. D ★★★   OHCD 6th ed. → p. 211

Free gingival (FG) or connective tissue grafts involve complete detachment of the graft from its donor site to the recipient site. An FG graft involves removal of keratinized tissue, whilst a connective tissue graft is removal of the subepithelial connective tissue only. Adequate preparation of the recipient site is imperative for successful integration, as is careful handling of the graft during harvest and placement. The palate is the most common site for harvest of a soft tissue graft. Subepithelial connective tissue grafts are most commonly sourced from the palate, as the available volume is greater. The tuberosity can be used, but it often

lacks the necessary width of connective tissue required in graft procedures. These flaps do not maintain their original blood supply and, as such,
rely heavily upon the vascularity of the recipient site for survival. A key
component of graft success is to ensure its immobility during the healing
period and allow undisrupted angiogenesis.

Alternatively, pedicle grafts are not detached and, as such, retain their
blood supply. Retention of blood supply is a significant advantage.
However, these flaps can only be repositioned locally (e.g. rotational flap
or coronal advancement flap) and sometimes lack sufficient volumes of
connective or keratinized tissue.

Keywords: recession, connective tissue graft, intraoral site.

→ Miller P. A classification of marginal tissue recession. *International
Journal of Periodontics and Restorative Dentistry*. 1985;**5**:8–13.

15. A ★★★

The mucogingival junction is a soft tissue landmark where the attached
gingiva meets the alveolar mucosa. The attached gingiva is keratinized
tissue, which results in a distinctly lighter colour than the adjacent, highly
vascular alveolar mucosa. The keratinized attached gingiva serves a vital
protective function during mastication and tooth brushing. Removal of
the entire attached gingiva is not advised for crown lengthening, and if an
inadequate attached gingiva is present (i.e. <2–3 mm), then apical repositioning of the flap is advised.

The free gingival groove corresponds to the cemento–enamel junction
of the tooth. At this point, the free gingiva meets the attached gingiva.
The free gingival groove is present in <50% of patients and is often lost
when periodontal tissues become inflamed. See Figure 4.2 which shows
macroscopic periodontal landmarks.

Keywords: crown lengthening, junction, two tissues, resective.

→ Devlin H, Craven R. *Oxford Handbook of Integrated Dental Biosciences*.
Oxford University Press, Oxford; 2018.

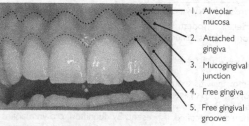

1. Alveolar mucosa
2. Attached gingiva
3. Mucogingival junction
4. Free gingiva
5. Free gingival groove

Figure 4.2

16. C ★★★★

The complement cascade is a general component of innate immunity. Activation of the complement cascade is pro-inflammatory. Activated complement recruits immune cells and assists in bacterial cell destruction. Complement also binds bacteria in a process known as agglutination, which assists in destruction of the pathogens.

The membrane attack complex is formed during complement activation and is heavily involved in the destruction of pathogens. The classical, common, and alternative pathways have been identified. LPS (endotoxin), a component of bacterial cell walls, has been identified as a potent complement activator in periodontal disease.

The classical pathway involves antigen–antibody complex formation, which activates C1 of the complement cascade. The alternative pathway is activated by LPS and bacterial proteases. Both pathways converge at C3 activation where the common pathway begins. IgG is an antibody produced by B cells, whilst IL-1 is a group of immune-regulating cytokines.

Keywords: complement activation, bacteria.

→ Eaton K, Ower P. *Practical Periodontics*. Elsevier, London; 2015.

17. C ★★★★ OHCD 6th ed. → p. 210

Infrabony defects are usually classified by the number of remaining walls surrounding them (i.e. 0 to 3). The predictability of the regenerative outcomes is affected by wound stability and maintaining space for the repopulating cells. Defects that are self-contained are much more likely to maintain both the membrane and regenerative material in position, and therefore provide a stable clot during the healing period. In other words, a three-walled defect will support a membrane or regenerative material better than a one-walled defect. This is most relevant when unreinforced biodegradable membranes or gel formations of growth factor products are utilized, as they will displace more easily. Obviously, titanium-reinforced membranes may negate this problem, as they are self-supporting, but they do require a further surgical procedure to remove them. Furthermore, challenges can arise in producing primary closure with tented membranes, which is another factor that can affect the success of regenerative procedures.

Keywords: infrabony defects, regenerative surgery, predictable.

→ Cortellini P, Tonetti M. Clinical concepts for regenerative therapy in intrabony defects. *Periodontology 2000*. 2015;**68**:282–307.

18. A ★★★★

Localized gingivitis should be carefully examined to consider all possible aetiologies. In this case, recent crown placement is evidently the causative factor. Poor crown margins are extremely common occurrences that should be rectified, if present. By definition, crown margins that are intra-sulcular have not invaded the junctional epithelium and, as such, have not encroached upon the supracrestal attached tissues. Excess cement and poor crown margins were not identified upon clinical examination, and allergy to adhesive resin would be extremely rare.

Poor bulbous emergence profiles can hinder oral hygiene practices and promote plaque and biofilm development. Where insufficient reduction has been provided, the technician has to overbulk the restoration to create sufficient thickness of porcelain for aesthetics and strength. In this scenario, the opaque appearance is potentially suggestive of inadequate reduction. The veneering ceramic is thinner than required for optimal aesthetics, and the more opaque layer becomes visible. Restorations with this design fault could represent a plaque-retentive factor, which would ultimately lead to localized gingivitis.

Keywords: crowns, marginal gingivitis, 0.5 mm intra-sulcular, well adapted.

19. D ★★★★

Gingival recession following orthodontic treatment is relatively common. Camouflage of the malocclusion can occasionally result in a tooth being positioned outside of the bony envelope, leading to dehiscence or fenestration. If there is associated inflammation in the tissue and the biotype is thin, then recession can result. Thicker biotypes with a greater bulk of connective tissue tend to result in less recession, as they are more robust.

When aesthetics is not a major concern and the patient has no complaints of sensitivity, root coverage surgery is not necessary unless the defect is progressing or excessive. If sensitivity is present, then desensitizing agents may be used to remedy this initially. The next consideration relates to the effect of the high frenal attachment. Previous investigations demonstrated little evidence to suggest a frenal pull during muscular activity has any direct effect on gingival recession. However, the high attachment may inhibit effective plaque removal. Some clinicians also suggest there is a plunging effect which drives plaque into the gingival sulcus or an effective gingival seal is prevented, either way perpetuating further local inflammation. Anecdotally, therefore, relieving the frenal attachment can help improve local plaque control and stabilize the situation. Alternatively, if the patient can maintain good plaque control, then surgery may not be warranted. Moreover, where there is little sulcal depth, apical displacement of the frenum during the procedure will help to create greater sulcal depth and facilitate any future root coverage procedures. Some clinicians may do this as a single-stage procedure, combined with root coverage, depending on the situation. It should be appreciated that treatment planning in these situations is contentious and very scenario-specific.

Keywords: recession, high frenal attachment, vestibular depth, shallow.

→ Allen E, Irwin, C, Ziada H, Mullally B, Byrne PJ. Periodontics 6: the management of gingival recession. *Dental Update*. 2007;**34**:534–42.

→ Eaton K, Ower P. *Practical Periodontics*. Elsevier, London; 2015.

20. B ★★★★   OHCD 6th ed. → p. 670

Local resolution should be attempted for all complaints received by the practice—verbal or written. A clear complaints protocol should be in place, which includes the time frame for acknowledgement of receipt of complaint and the time frame for investigation. The GDC's standards for dental professionals state practices require a clear and effective complaints procedure. It is good practice to acknowledge a complaint as soon as possible, and a full response should be given within 10 working days. If the investigation takes longer, then the patient should be updated at least every 10 days.

Where local resolution fails, the NHS ombudsman or the Dental Complaints Service can be utilized for NHS and private treatment, respectively. These services may investigate the complaint and advise actions accordingly. It is unlikely that a well-handled complaint should require escalation to the GDC. However, issues of patient safety, illegal practice, or concerns regarding a registered dentist's or dental care professional (DCP)'s conduct are more serious matters that are more likely to require GDC involvement.

It may be advisable to contact your indemnity provider for advice before responding to complaints, as their guidance can help to resolve matters faster.

Keywords: privately conducted, complaint, no solution.

→ Dental Protection. *Dental Advice Series—Complaints Handling (England)*. 2016. Available at: https://www.dentalprotection.org/docs/librariesprovider4/dental-advice-booklets/dental-advice-booklet-complaints-handling-england.pdf

Endodontics

Nicholas Longridge

'There is a lesion and I need to fix it!'

Endodontics remains a rapidly advancing branch of restorative dentistry. It is highly likely that, by the time this book is published, several new or updated endodontic file systems will have been released. Despite the fairly rapid technological advances that the profession has seen, the key principles of endodontic treatment remain the same:

1. Eliminate microorganisms from the root canal system
2. Prevent reinfection of the root canal system
3. Retain a functional natural tooth.

Whilst these principles are easy to discuss, they are consistently difficult to perform, due, in large part, to the complexity of the root canal system. Multiple theories, principles, and approaches have been discussed to help achieve an optimal technical and clinical outcome. However, evidence to favour one specific stage or system over another is lacking, and as such, a large degree of operator preference and experience will ultimately influence the treatment planning and technical strategy. Much like baking a cake, endodontic treatment relies upon a series of procedural steps to achieve a desirable outcome, which, for the patient, often equates to a functional, pain-free natural tooth.

Good-quality magnification remains a key component of an endodontist's armamentarium, and dental loupes or a dental operating microscope could not be recommended more highly.

Key topics include:

- Endodontic case assessment, including root canal anatomy
- Pain management, including local anaesthesia
- Access and canal identification
- Vital pulp therapy, including caries management
- Canal negotiation and instrumentation
- Root canal irrigation
- Root canal obturation
- Restoration of the endodontically treated tooth.

QUESTIONS

1. A 28-year-old man attends with a continuous aching pain from his upper left first permanent molar (UL6). It occurs spontaneously, disturbs sleep, and is partly relieved by paracetamol. Chewing or biting does not exacerbate the symptoms. The heavily restored UL6 was hyperresponsive to refrigerant (EndoFrost®). All other special investigations were normal. Which is the single most likely diagnosis? ★

A Acute apical abscess

B Atypical facial pain

C Chronic apical periodontitis

D Irreversible pulpitis

E Periodontal abscess

2. A 45-year-old man has sharp pain to cold from his upper right posterior teeth; the pain ceases immediately on removal of the stimulus. He has multiple cervical abrasion cavities. Which single type of sensory nerve fibre is primarily responsible for his pain? ★

A A-β

B A-δ

C C

D Parasympathetic

E Sympathetic

3. A 29-year-old woman is about to have primary root canal treatment on her lower right first permanent premolar (LR4). Figure 5.1 shows burs selected by the clinician during root canal preparation. At which single stage of root canal preparation would it be most appropriate to use these? ★

A Access

B Apical preparation

C Canal identification

D Coronal flaring

E Working length determination

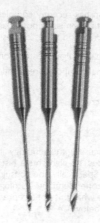

Figure 5.1

4. A 45-year-old man is having root canal treatment on his upper left first premolar. After scouting the canal with a small hand file, a rotary file system is introduced with an ISO 25 tip size and a 10-degree taper (25/.10) until resistance is felt. Subsequently, files with a smaller taper are introduced until the working length is reached (25/.06 → 25/.04). What single concept of endodontic preparation does this technique follow? ★

A Apico-coronal

B Circumferential

C Crown-down

D Modified double flare

E Step back

5. A 52-year-old woman has a sudden onset of severe pain and an altered sensation under her eye, following irrigation during root canal retreatment on a maxillary canine. Which is the single most likely complication? ★

A Extrusion of sodium hypochlorite

B Inadvertent instrumentation of the infraorbital nerve

C Lateral perforation

D Root fracture

E Transportation of apical constriction

6. A 32-year-old man has recently completed root canal treatment on a lower molar that is missing both marginal ridges. Which is the single most appropriate method to restore his tooth? ★★

A A bonded intracoronal amalgam restoration

B A bonded intracoronal composite restoration

C A ceramic inlay

D A full coverage gold crown

E. A gold inlay

7. A consultant is discussing the aetiology and management of dental caries. On his slides, he highlights a histological slice from a progressing carious lesion. Specifically, the consultant discusses the importance of a translucent zone identified histologically within the dentine. A fellow colleague asks what this zone represents. (Select one answer from the options listed below.) ★★

A The caries-infected zone

B The zone of hypermineralized dentine known as tubular sclerosis

C The zone of hypermineralized surface enamel under which the carious process takes place

D The zone of sound dentine immediately adjacent to the pulp complex

E The zone of subsurface caries spread along the amelodentinal junction

8. A foundation dentist is conducting a root canal treatment on the lower right second premolar of a 26-year-old woman. Whilst irrigating with chlorhexidine, she notes that the concentration is only 0.2% and asks her nurse for an alternative irrigant. The nurse goes to see the foundation trainer to see if they can borrow their sodium hypochlorite. The foundation trainer says that it is not advisable to use both solutions concomitantly because it might affect overall bacterial decontamination. What is the single main reason for this advice? ★★

A A precipitate is produced, which can block dentinal tubules from further irrigant effects

B A reaction between the irrigants results in the production of a bacterial growth factor

C Adjunctive sodium hypochlorite has no clinical benefits over chlorhexidine alone

D The combination of solutions causes selective decontamination and overgrowth of the more pathogenic bacteria

E The residual film produced causes degradation of gutta percha, allowing bacterial leakage

9. A 17-year-old adolescent man is referred for root canal treatment of an upper central incisor with an immature apex. The tooth is non-vital and shows comparable root length to the contralateral incisor. Which is the single most appropriate technique to endodontically treat his tooth? ★ ★

A Apexification with repeated dressings of non-setting calcium hydroxide

B Apical plug formation with bioceramic material

C Cvek pulpotomy

D Endodontic surgery

E Regenerative endodontic procedures

10. A 28-year-old man is having an obturation of a permanent upper central incisor. A heated plugger (e.g. System-B®) is being used during the 'downpack'. Which is the single most appropriate description of the obturation technique being used? ★ ★

A Carrier-based thermoplasticized technique

B Cold lateral condensation

C Single cone obturation

D Thermoplasticized injection technique

E Warm vertical compaction

11. A 54-year-old man is having root canal treatment on an upper canine, using stainless steel hand files via the modified double flare technique. An ISO size 25 hand file is the first to bind at the working length. What should be the single most appropriate size of the master apical file (MAF)? ★ ★

A ISO size 20

B ISO size 25

C ISO size 30

D ISO size 35

E ISO size 40

12. A 47-year-old man is having root canal treatment on his upper first molar, which has curved roots. Following coronal preparation of the mesiobuccal canal, an electronic apex locator (EAL) is used and provides a reproducible reading. This is 2 mm shorter than the estimated working length (EWL) from the preoperative radiograph. What is the single most appropriate initial management? ★★

A Obturate to the EWL and review

B Obturate to the EWL, followed by apicectomy

C Prepare using the reading of the EAL

D Take a new radiograph to check for potential perforations

E Take a parallax technique radiograph of the molar to identify the apex

13. A 43-year-old woman has pain from a lower central incisor that has previously received root canal treatment. Radiographically, a small, diffuse periapical lesion is present, but the obturation follows the root anatomy and appears adequate. A parallax radiograph indicates asymmetrical distribution of the obturation. What is the single most likely cause of failure? ★★

A Cyst formation

B Missed canal

C Perforation

D Root fracture

E Transportation of the apex

14. A 58-year-old woman with failed root canal treatment is seen in a new patient consultation clinic. A junior dental student asks about the process of root canal failure. She is aware that certain bacteria have significant dentine adherence capabilities and can survive harsh environments by demineralizing dentine and degrading collagen. Which is the single most likely causative organism in this scenario? ★★

A *Aggregatibacter actinomycetemcomitans* (Aa)

B *Enterococcus faecalis*

C *Neisseria gonorrhoeae*

D *Prevotella intermedia*

E *Streptococcus mutans*

15. A 32-year-old man has pain from his upper right central incisor (UR1), having previously fallen off his bicycle 2 years ago. Radiographically, the UR1 apex appears moth-eaten and is 10% shorter in root length than the adjacent central incisor. Additionally, there is periapical radiolucency. What is the single most likely diagnosis? ★ ★ ★

A External cervical resorption

B External inflammatory resorption

C External replacement resorption

D External surface resorption

E Transient apical breakdown

16. A 58-year-old woman is seen in a new patient clinic, having been referred with a fractured rotary instrument in the upper right first permanent molar. Radiographically, the file has fractured high up, occluding the majority of the canal. The consultant suggests that the use of a reciprocating file system or balanced force technique might have prevented this. For what single primary mechanical reason is this? ★ ★ ★

A Higher rotational speeds, increasing speed of preparation

B Limits heat from friction, increasing the cyclical fatigue limit of nickel titanium (NiTi)

C No longer requires a pecking motion of use, thus reducing flexural fatigue

D Non-continuous rotation prevents file binding and reduces the risk of torsional fracture

E Off-centre rotational pattern, facilitating debris removal

17. An 18-year-old man is having root canal treatment on his lower left first permanent molar. Following access to the pulp chamber, three canals are identified: two mesial canals—mesiobuccal (MB) and mesio-lingual (ML)—and one distal canal. The distal canal is identified as buccally positioned by 2 mm in relation to the mesiodistal midline of the tooth. What is the single most appropriate next step? ★ ★ ★

A Coronal flare all three canals

B Determine the working lengths

C Investigate for a fourth canal orifice

D Place a rubber dam, as access has been achieved

E Take a periapical radiograph to exclude a perforation

18. A 23-year-old man has discomfort from his upper left first pre-molar but is keen to save it, if at all possible. Clinically, the tooth has deficient crown margins but otherwise appears OK. A cone beam computed tomography (CBCT) scan shows a missed palatal canal, a well-obturated buccal canal, and a periapical lesion. What is the single most appropriate management to save the tooth? ★★★

A Antibiotics, a new crown, and monitoring of the apical lesion

B Apicectomy and a new crown

C Extraction

D Obturate the palatal canal and new crown

E Root canal retreatment and new crown

19. A 36-year-old man is having the restoration of a recently endodontically treated permanent molar tooth. Only the pal-atal wall remains in its entirety, but there is 2 mm of supra-gingival den-tine elsewhere. What is the single most appropriate method to retain the core? ★★★

A Multiple dentine pins

B Nayyar core

C Post-preparation in the mesiobuccal canal

D Post-preparation in the palatal canal

E Split post-technique

20. A 34-year-old woman presents having lost an amalgam restor-ation. The tooth was previously painful when biting. The lower right second permanent molar is endodontically treated and has lost a mesio-occluso-distal restoration; an associated deep distal probing pocket is noted. Radiographically, an optimal root filling with furcal radio-lucency is evident. What is the single most likely diagnosis? ★★★★

A Adhesive resin failure

B Corrosion of the amalgam

C Lute dissolution

D Split tooth

E Supra-gingival cusp fracture

21. An undergraduate dental student is conducting re-root canal treatment on a 36-year-old man. During the session, the clinical tutor notices that the student is cycling between sodium hypochlorite (NaOCl) and ethylenediaminetetraacetic acid (EDTA) and advises against doing this. Instead they suggest just to do a penultimate rinse with EDTA prior to obturation. What is the single main reason for changing the irrigation protocol? ★★★★

A Collagen dissolution

B Dentine erosion

C File corrosion

D Root resorption

E NaOCl extrusion

22. A 24-year-old woman has returned to the United Kingdom to get married in 4 weeks. She is interested in whitening her teeth, whilst she prepares for her wedding. She would like to know more about the process of tooth whitening. Which single percentage of hydrogen peroxide is likely to give the quickest results for this patient? ★★★★

A 1%

B 6%

C 10%

D 16%

E 30%

ANSWERS

1. D ★   OHCD 6th ed. → p. 222

An exaggerated response to thermal testing indicates some vitality of the dentino-pulpal complex of the UL6. There is no complaint of tenderness when chewing or biting. These findings should enable you to exclude 'chronic apical periodontitis' and 'acute apical abscess', as these diagnoses would likely result in a negative thermal test and a tooth that is tender to bite. Tenderness when biting, whilst uncommon, has been reported with irreversible pulpitis, more commonly in multi-rooted teeth with an ambiguous pain history, due to the presence of vital and non-vital tissue within different root canals.

The clinical signs clearly indicate a diagnosis of acute pulpitis. Reversible pulpitis would present with sharp pain, which is often difficult to localize. Spontaneous pain which lasts for long periods and can wake a patient would represent irreversible pulpitis—as in this scenario.

Atypical facial pain (or chronic idiopathic facial pain) is a diagnosis of exclusion. It can mimic dental pain, sinusitis, and headaches. However, with careful examination, no pathology is found. These cases must be treated with extreme caution, as extensive unnecessary dental treatment can result.

Keywords: spontaneous, wakes at night, not exacerbated by biting.

2. B ★

A-δ fibres are myelinated nerve fibres responsible for mediating the sharp/shooting pain associated with dentine hypersensitivity and reversible pulpitis. Approximately 90% of A fibres are A-δ. Whilst A-δ fibres are the narrowest A fibres by diameter, they are significantly larger than C fibres, and their size (along with myelination) assists with propagating action potentials through nerves rapidly.

A variety of sensory nerve fibres exist within the human body, with each occupying a specific role in mediating pain, temperature, and proprioception, dependent upon their anatomical composition. The dentino-pulpal complex is innervated by A-β fibres, A-δ fibres, and C fibres, as well as some autonomic sympathetic fibres. Unmyelinated C fibres make up the majority of the innervation of the pulp. They have slow conduction velocities and are responsible for the aching pain associated with irreversible pulpitis. A-β fibres are also believed to be involved in nociception, but to a lesser degree than A-δ fibres.

Parasympathetic nerve fibres within the pulp have been postulated, whilst sympathetic nerve fibres mediate circulation.

Keywords: sharp, ceases immediately.

→ Pashley DH. Dynamics of the pulpo-dentin complex. *Critical Reviews in Oral Biology and Medicine*. 1996;**7**:104–33.

→ Patel S, Barnes J. *Principles of Endodontics* (3rd ed.). Oxford University Press, Oxford; 2019.

3. D ★   OHCD 6th ed. → p. 332

Conducted after access and canal identification, coronal flaring provides a wide range of advantages during root canal preparation, including: improving access to the apical region; removal of infected tissue; improving irrigant placement; and improved accuracy in assessing the working length. It also reduces file separation by decreasing the stress placed upon files when preparing the apical portion of the root canal.

Gates-Glidden burs have non-cutting tips and are available in a range of sizes. Scouting of the canal with some initial hand file flaring can facilitate their introduction. They are not flexible and can lead to endodontic misadventure if used incorrectly, especially in curved canals. Many nickel titanium rotary systems have specific files, or shapers, designed for a similar purpose, which can be more conservative of radicular dentine.

Keywords: root canal preparation, Gates-Glidden bur (pictured).

→ Darcey J, Taylor C, Roudsari RV, Jawad S, Hunter M. Modern endodontic principles Part 3: preparation. *Dental Update*. 2015;**42**:810–22.

4. C ★   OHCD 6th ed. → p. 338

Multiple chemomechanical preparation techniques have been proposed and utilized throughout the years. A large majority of modern rotary systems have adopted a crown-down approach for preparation, which prepares in a stepwise manner from the canal orifice to the apical limit. This is reported to increase access of the irrigant into the apical region of the root canal, eliminate heavily contaminated coronal dentine, assist with straight line access, and reduce instrument separation.

The procedure above describes the technique for a standard taper file system, but others are available which can have variable taper. It is important to understand the file system being used, to avoid iatrogenic damage and to ensure an adequate glide path is created with hand files prior to using automated systems.

Keywords: endodontic preparation, rotary endodontics.

→ Darcey J, Taylor C, Roudsari RV, Jawad S, Hunter M. Modern endodontic principles Part 3: preparation. *Dental Update*. 2015;**42**:810–22.

5. A ★

Sodium hypochlorite's ability to dissolve organic tissue is beneficial in endodontics. However, apical extrusion of irrigant can cause significant soft tissue damage. This is an uncommon occurrence, particularly if care is taken, as irrigant generally only reaches 1–2 mm beyond the needle tip. Safety precautions to prevent extrusion include: using a side-vented needle, gentle irrigation pressure, and not taking the irrigating needle tip closer than 2–3 mm from the working length.

Pain and swelling are the most notable symptoms of a hypochlorite accident. Additional signs such as dysaesthesia or nosebleeds can relate to local anatomy. Management of hypochlorite injuries depends on the severity, but in general, immediate management includes: stopping treatment, removing excess irrigant with paper points or aspirating using an empty syringe, dressing with non-setting calcium hydroxide, and temporizing. Irrigation with saline to try and dilute the hypochlorite is not advised, due to the risk of further extrusion of residual hypochlorite. Pain relief, including a non-steroidal anti-inflammatory drug (if acceptable), should be prescribed, in conjunction with cold compress advice; an early review should then be arranged. For more severe symptoms, liaison with the local maxillofacial unit is advisable, since steroids, antibiotics, and close monitoring of any swelling progression will be required.

Clinicians should be aware of their local policy for managing hypochlorite accidents.

Keywords: severe pain, altered sensation.

→ Baldwin VE, Jarad FD, Balmer C, *et al*. Inadvertent injection of sodium hypochlorite into the periradicular tissues during root canal treatment. *Dental Update*. 2009;**36**:14–19.

→ Farook S, Shah V, Lenouvel D, *et al*. Guidelines for management of sodium hypochlorite extrusion injuries. *British Dental Journal*. 2014;**217**:679–84.

6. D ★★   OHCD 6th ed. → p. 346

Following root canal treatment, teeth that have lost a supporting marginal ridge are at higher risk of fracture. There are multiple proposed reasons for this. Firstly, in non-vital teeth, changes to the physical properties of the dentine can occur by chemical degradation with irrigants and medicaments. Secondly, there is potential for a loss of sensory feedback from root-filled teeth, which can result in higher occlusal forces being transmitted through the tooth. Thirdly, the loss of tooth structure from access cavities or decay (particularly if a marginal ridge is involved), combined with the lost architecture of the pulp chamber roof, can drastically decrease the stiffness of the tooth. This last reason is likely to be the main reason endodontically treated teeth are more prone to fracture.

For these reasons, provision of cuspal coverage restoration has been suggested. A recent study, over a 5-year period, demonstrated lower survival rates for root-filled posterior teeth without cuspal coverage restoration. Modern dentistry has a focus on minimally invasive procedures, and with better bonding systems, many practitioners are now preferring to prescribe onlay restorations, rather than full coverage crowns; either is acceptable, assuming cuspal coverage is provided. Gold remains the most conservative and biocompatible material for posterior teeth. However, the demand for alternative aesthetic restorations has driven an increase in all-ceramic onlay restorations, e.g. monolithic lithium disilicate. Clinically, these restorations require greater preparation.

Keywords: root canal treatment, missing both marginal ridges.

→ MacInnes A, Hall AF. Indications for cuspal coverage. *Dental Update*. 2016;**43**:150–8.

→ Tickle M, Milsom K, Qualtrough A, Blinkhorn F, Aggarwal VR. The failure rate of NHS funded molar endodontic treatment delivered in general dental practice. *British Dental Journal*. 2008;**204**:254–5.

7. B ★★

The carious process, which develops when a bacteria-rich plaque bio-film, fermentable carbohydrates, and a susceptible tooth surface interact over time, is well described in the literature. Histological examination of this process has identified distinct zones which display differing characteristics. In dentine, these are, from outside in: zone of destruction, zone of bacterial invasion, zone of demineralization, and zone of sclerosis (or translucent zone). The translucent zone represents a reparative process, in which odontoblasts deposit dentine in the tubules, as the tooth attempts to reduce insult from the approaching carious process; this is known as tubular sclerosis, which appears translucent under light microscopy because of the reduced light refraction.

Dentine immediately adjacent to the pulp will be the last to undergo the destructive changes of the carious process. It is here that tertiary dentine is produced in response to carious insult. See Figure 5.2 which shows histological changes in enamel and dentine before cavitation of enamel.

Keywords: carious lesion, translucent zone.

→ Kidd E, Fejerskov O. *Essentials of Dental Caries* (4th ed.). Oxford University Press, Oxford; 2016.

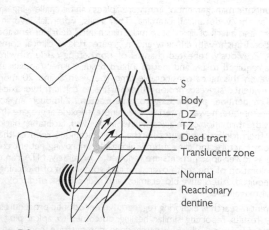

Figure 5.2

Reproduced from Kidd, E. *Essentials of Dental Caries* (3rd Ed). Figure 2.12., page 31. Oxford University Press. Oxford. 2016 by permission of Oxford University Press.

8. A ★★   OHCD 6th ed. → p. 334

Sodium hypochlorite is considered the gold standard endodontic irrigant. It is relatively cheap and bactericidal and dissolves organic material. Some practitioners prefer to use alternatives (e.g. chlorhexidine), as they do not produce the side effects associated with apical extrusion of sodium hypochlorite. Additionally, chlorhexidine also has fungicidal properties and demonstrates substantivity for up to 12 weeks. It is important to note that concentrations of chlorhexidine below 2% are only bacterio-static (most over-the-counter mouthwashes have concentrations of 0.2%). In certain situations, clinicians may wish to use multiple irrigants by using paper points or saline solutions to prevent cross-contamination. However, concurrent use of chlorhexidine and sodium hypochlorite produces a brown precipitate (parachloroaniline), which is thought to be carcinogenic. Furthermore, although the precipitate may not cause phys-ical blockage or prevention of instruments from reaching the working length, its presence can occlude dentinal tubules, preventing penetration by further irrigants or sealers.

The other answers are incorrect; the by-product is not known to influ-ence gutta percha stability or act as a growth factor, and the two solu-tions do not case selective decontamination. Sodium hypochlorite may also have clinical benefits beyond that of chlorhexidine alone.

Keywords: irrigants, chlorhexidine, sodium hypochlorite, not in conjunction.

→ Darcey J, Jawad S, Taylor C, Roudsari RV, Hunter M. Modern endodontic principles Part 4: irrigation. *Dental Update*. 2016;**43**:20–33.

9. B ★★   OHCD 6th ed. → p. 110

Endodontic management of immature apices can be challenging, mainly due to the wide apical foramina. Thin walls, potential inverse wall tapers, and a lack of apical stop make mechanical debridement and ob-turation fraught with difficulty and at greater risk of clinical complica-tions. Previously, repeated changes of non-setting calcium hydroxide were required to try and induce a hard tissue barrier (apexification). However, this takes considerable time (between 5 and 20 months), and evidence suggests prolonged exposure to calcium hydroxide can weaken dentine, predisposing to root fracture. Although an accept-able technique, newer materials, like mineral trioxide aggregate (MTA), allow the formation of an apical barrier in one visit, facilitating backfilling with thermoplasticized gutta percha. This technique reduces the risk of root fracture and clinical time, alongside improving patient compli-ance as fewer appointments are required. Conversely, MTA can cause discoloration of the tooth over time and some form of bleaching may be required. Alternative bioceramics with reduced risk of discoloration are also available.

Current research is exploring regenerative endodontic procedures with early results reporting similar healing outcomes to apical plug tech-niques. However, whilst research does demonstrate continued root development with this treatment strategy, it remains experimental and is currently not the treatment of choice in a tooth with sufficient root length.

Keywords: immature apex, comparable root length.

→ Bakland LK, Andreasen JO. Will mineral trioxide aggregate replace calcium hydroxide in treating pulpal and periodontal healing complications subsequent to dental trauma? A review. *Dental Traumatology*. 2012;**28**:25–32.

→ Simon S, Smith AJ. Regenerative endodontics. *British Dental Journal*. 2014;**216**:E13.

10. E ★★   OHCD 6th ed. → p. 342

A variety of techniques exist for obturation. The aim of obturation is to produce a three-dimensional hermetic seal of the root canal system, without voids, extending to the apex. The most commonly used material is gutta percha (GP), a rubber-based material, although alternative plastic-based materials are available (e.g. Resilon®). Cold lateral condensation, which involves using a finger spread to compact a master point sideways and allow space for accessory points, was traditionally favoured.

In modern dentistry, more people are using matched-point single cone obturation or plasticized GP obturation techniques. During warm vertical compaction, a heated plugger is inserted through the master GP cone into the canal to within 5 mm of the working length, creating an apical plug. Following this, either further segments of GP are compressed down under heat or, alternatively, plasticized GP is injected in to 'backfill' the remaining space.

Carrier-based systems have a central core (plastic or cross-linked GP) with a GP coating. The point is heated in a special oven and inserted into the canal. In theory, thermoplastic techniques should produce better three-dimensional obturation. However, literature to support improved outcomes is lacking.

Keywords: heated plugger, down-pack, obturation.

→ Darcey J, Roudsari RV, Jawad S, Taylor C, Hunter M. Modern endodontic principles Part 5: obturation. *Dental Update*. 2016;**43**:114–29.

→ Peng L, Ye L, Tan H, Zhou X. Outcome of root canal obturation by warm gutta-percha versus cold lateral condensation: a meta-analysis. *Journal of Endodontics*. 2007;**33**:106–9.

11. D ★★

Mechanical preparation aims to shape the canal to facilitate irrigant exchange and obturation. Adequate preparation should enable the irrigant to penetrate to the apical third of the canal and will secondarily remove some infected dentine. Techniques focus on tapering either from the 'crown-down' or apico-coronally in a 'stepback' approach. The modified double flare technique is used with 2% ISO hand files and combines both approaches. Firstly, the coronal two-thirds are prepared in a crown-down fashion. This has the benefits of removing infected coronal dentine and greater irrigant access. Subsequently, the apical third is prepared in a stepback fashion. The first file to bind at the working length 'gauges' the size of the apical constriction. Next, the file size is increased, most commonly by two sizes, to create a stop at the working length. From here, the apical portion is flared backwards by increasing the file size and reducing the length reached by 1 mm each time, until it meets the coronal two-thirds. The largest-size file to reach working length is known as the master apical file (MAF). In this instance, as a 25 K file binds at length, the MAF would be a 35 K file. It is important to understand the MAF principle, as successful obturation relies upon selecting the correct master apical cone to correspond with the MAF.

Keywords: modified double flare technique, master apical file.

12. C ★★   OHCD 6th ed. → p. 338

The debate on the apical limit of root canal preparation is contentious. The minor apical foramen (apical constriction) is generally considered to be the apical limit. On average, it lies 0.5 mm short of the major apical foramen, but there is considerable variation in the relationship of the radiographical apex to the major apical foramen. This is particularly true in posterior teeth where discrepancies of up to 4 mm have been reported. Modern EALs measure changes in impedance ratios and can accurately identify contact with the apical tissues; they have been shown to identify the major apical foramen more reliably than radiographs. Therefore, in this instance, since the reading is reliable, reproducible, and within an acceptable distance from the estimated length, the EAL reading should be used. If there were concern regarding the measurement given by the EAL, then this can be evaluated against a working length radiograph to make a definitive decision. It is advisable to assess the working length in some form with at least one radiograph at some stage prior to obturation.

Keywords: electronic apex locator, reproducible reading.

→ Gordon M, Chandler N. Electronic apex locators. *International Endodontic Journal*. 2004;**37**:425–37.

→ Martins JN, Marques D, Mata A, Caramês J. Clinical efficacy of electronic apex locators: systematic review. *Journal of Endodontics*. 2014;**40**:759–77.

13. B ★★   OHCD 6th ed. → p. 348

Endodontic failures are common. The European Society of Endodontics have classified success as the 'absence of pain, swelling, and other symptoms, no sinus tract, no loss of function and radiological evidence of a normal periodontal ligament space'. Success rates vary, depending on a number of variables, but the key factors linked with success are homogenous root filling without voids, obturation to within 2 mm of the apex, absence of periapical lesion preoperatively, and a satisfactory coronal restoration. Mandibular incisors most commonly have one canal. However, studies have suggested up to 45% of cases may have more canals in some form, the anatomy of which is often complex and can frequently coalesce, making debridement and obturation challenging; Vertucci's classification is commonly quoted. Parallax views or CBCT can be utilized to help identify missed anatomy. Management of these situations requires good access, good visualization, and patience!

Keywords: lower central incisor, asymmetric distribution of obturation.

→ Kartal N, Yanikoglu FC. Root canal morphology of mandibular incisors. *Journal of Endodontics*. 1992;**34**:1401–5.

→ Ng Y, Mann V, Rahbaran S, Lewsey J, Gulabivala K. Outcome of primary root canal treatment: systematic review of the literature— Part 2. Influence of clinical factors. *International Endodontic Journal*. 2008;**41**:6–31.

→ Vertucci FJ. Root canal anatomy of the human permanent teeth. *Oral Surgery, Oral Medicine, Oral Pathology*. 1984;**58**:589–99.

14. B ★★

Multiple bacteria have been isolated in failed endodontic treatment. However, *E. faecalis* is most frequently isolated in asymptomatic teeth with long-standing periapical infections. Its small size allows it to reside within dentinal tubules, and it can survive long periods of starvation. Furthermore, its ability to maintain and regulate its intracellular pH enables it to withstand prolonged periods in strong alkali conditions (e.g. those created by calcium hydroxide).

Numerous studies have looked into the irrigant effect on *E. faecalis* eradication. Sodium hypochlorite above 3% is effective if used in adequate quantities and furthermore can penetrate biofilms. Chlorhexidine at 2% concentrations is also effective and has the added benefit of substantivity. A newer irrigant MTAD [a Mixture of a Tetracycline (doxycycline), citric Acid, and a Detergent) also shows promise in being effective against a wide number of endodontic pathogens. It is, however, important to ensure suitable apical enlargement and adequate smear layer removal prior to final irrigation regimes, so irrigants can access dentinal tubules where the bacteria reside.

Additionally, as calcium hydroxide is ineffective in eliminating *E. faecalis*, iodine or iodoform-based intracanal medicaments are often recommended.

Aa is commonly associated with aggressive periodontal disease; *P. intermedia* is again more commonly associated with periodontal disease but does have a role in endodontic infections. *S. mutans* is associated with caries, and *N. gonorrhoeae* is the infective agent in gonorrhoea.

Keywords: harsh environments, failed root canal treatments.

→ Stuart C, Schwartz SA, Beeson TJ, Owatz CB. *Enterococcus faecalis*: its role in root canal treatment failure and current concepts in retreatment. *Journal of Endodontics*. 2006;**32**:93–8.

15. B ★★★ OHCD 6th ed. → p. 110

When classified simplistically, root resorption is classified by site (internal or external) and type (surface, inflammatory, or replacement). Additionally, resorption at the cervical margin is known as external cervical resorption. Resorption occurs as a result of stimulation of osteoclasts/odontoclasts, either via an inflammatory pathway or dysregulation of normal homeostatic bone turnover. The protective mechanisms in healthy teeth are thought to be: a vital periodontal ligament, an intact cementum layer, and an extracellular pre-dentine layer internally.

Internal resorption is rare and usually inflammatory in nature. Well-defined ballooning of the canal system occurs, which may be visible as a pink hue if it occurs in the coronal aspect.

Surface resorption results from localized damage to the root surface; frequently, it is subclinical and self-limiting. Prolonged inflammatory stimuli, around a damaged root surface, can lead to external inflammatory resorption and is common after trauma. The root is gradually destroyed, which can occur surprisingly quickly. Alternatively, if union occurs between bone and dentine, normal bony remodelling can occur, leading to replacement resorption.

In this case, the moth-eaten appearance, periapical lesion, and history should lead you to the diagnosis of external inflammatory resorption; root canal treatment should be instigated immediately.

Keywords: fallen, 2 years ago, moth-eaten, periapical radiolucency.

→ Darcey J, Qualthrough A. Resorption: part 1. Pathology, classification and aetiology. *British Dental Journal*. 2013;**214**:439–51.

16. D ★★★

The development of NiTi rotary file systems has improved the efficiency and ability to prepare the root canal system, even in the most challenging of cases. In traditional rotary motors, the file motion is a continuous 360° rotation. If the file binds to the walls of the root canal, then torsional stress can occur within the file, causing deformation along the long axis. Should this deformation exceed the elastic limit of the material, then the instrument will fracture. In torsional fatigue, the file will fracture at the junction between where the file is bound and not bound, as the force will concentrate here. Conversely, cyclical fatigue fractures occur at the point of maximum canal curvature. Safeguards, such as torque limits and auto-reverse within endodontic motors, are designed to stop torsional fatigue. However, fractures can still occur, as average settings do not conform to the environment of each canal.

Asymmetric reciprocation is effectively a mechanized version of the balanced force technique (rotating approximately 150° clockwise, followed by 30° anticlockwise). This repeated disengagement limits the build-up of torsional stress and reduces the number of rotations, thus reducing instrument fracture. This design feature allows the development of a single file system.

Additional benefits of the single file system include: improved cost-effectiveness (due to fewer files used), simplified protocols (again fewer files), and reduced cyclical fatigue because of the lower rotational speeds required of the files.

Keywords: fractured high up, reciprocating file system.

→ Grande NM, Ahmed HM, Cohen S, Bukiet F, Plotino G. Current assessment of feciprocation in endodontic preparation: a comprehensive review—Part I: historic perspectives and current applications. *Journal of Endodontics.* 2015;**41**:1778–83.

17. C ★★★   OHCD 6th ed. → p. 336

Commonly, mandibular molars have two roots with three canals: two mesial canals—mesiobuccal and mesio-lingual—and one distal canal. However, it is not uncommon to have two or three distal canals (approximately 35% have two).

Canal identification is often feared most by junior practitioners, and the use of magnification and appropriate lighting cannot be underestimated. There are several rules for assisting in the identification of canals. Firstly, the cemento-enamel junction (CEJ) is considered to be the most reliable anatomical predictor for the positioning of the pulp chamber and pulpal floor. The CEJ is often protected from coronal restorations and, as such, can assist greatly when teeth are heavily restored.

Canals often display a high degree of symmetry (excluding the maxillary molars), and the mesiodistal midline (running through the mid point of the pulp chamber, from mesial to distal) can often be used to assist in canal identification. A distal canal 2 mm buccally to the mesiodistal midline is highly suggestive of a fourth distolingual canal. See Figure 5.3 which

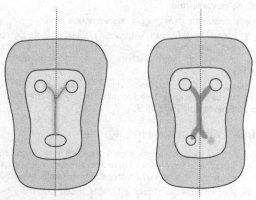

Figure 5.3

shows a diagrammatic representation of the law of symmetry in canal location. The image on the left shows the distal canal to be in the midline, whereas the image on the right shows one distal canal off to the left, indicating the likelihood of a second canal in the hazed region.

Keywords: buccally positioned, mesiodistal midline.

→ de Pablo OV, Estevez R, Péix Sánchez M, Heilborn C, Cohenca N. Root anatomy and canal configuration of the permanent mandibular first molar: a systematic review. *Journal of Endodontics*. 2010;**36**:1919–31.

→ Krasner P, Rankow H. Anatomy of the pulp-chamber floor. *Journal of Endodontics*. 2004;**30**:5–16.

---

18. E ★★★   OHCD 6th ed. → p. 348

The long-term management of any endodontic infection should be with local treatment, and not antibiotics. Given the patient is in pain and wishes to save the tooth, then treatment is required and only options B, D, and E are viable.

Coronal leakage plays a significant part in the success of endodontic treatment, with nearly twice the chance of failure in the presence of an unsatisfactory restoration. Furthermore, a meta-analysis suggested that retreatment provides a better long-term outcome than surgical endodontics. Therefore, in these situations, endodontic retreatment is preferred in the first instance. The decision becomes more complicated when the original root filling appears satisfactory. If the clinician is confident that all the intraoperative components have been optimized (i.e. thorough chemo-mechanical disinfection, use of dental dam) or the coronal restoration would be challenging to remove, then apical surgery may be warranted. In the above scenario, the treatment is suboptimal and the coronal seal has been lost; therefore, retreatment is recommended with replacement coronal restoration. Solely obturating the missed canal would not be advised in this situation, as the buccal canal is likely to be contaminated.

Keywords: deficient crown margin, missed palatal canal.

→ Ng YL, Mann V, Rahbaran S, Lewsey J, Gulabivala K. Outcome of primary root canal treatment: systematic review of the literature—Part 2. Influence of clinical factors. *International Endodontic Journal*. 2008;**41**:6–31.

→ Torabinejad M, Corr R, Handysides R, Shabahang S. Outcomes of nonsurgical retreatment and endodontic surgery: a systematic review. *Journal of Endodontics*. 2009;**35**:930–7.

---

19. B ★★★   OHCD 6th ed. → p. 346

Definitive restoration of teeth should be considered prior to commencing endodontic treatment. There is no merit in root-treating an unrestorable tooth, and, as such, restorability should be assessed first.

The decision on how to retain a core is based upon the clinician's judgement of the clinical scenario. Post-preparation within molar teeth is feasible and can provide adequate retention for core materials. However, complications from post-preparations can occur, including root fracture and perforation, making them less retrievable long term. Furthermore, potentially damaging stress accumulation can occur with dentine pin use. The Nayyar core utilizes inherent undercuts and divergences within the root canal system for retention, although a certain volume of coronal dentine is still considered necessary. The coronal 2–4 mm of gutta percha is removed from each canal, and an appropriate restorative material placed to create a monoblock corono-radicular core. Amalgam is traditionally used, but composite is a suitable alternative. The authors would advocate avoiding post-retained cores in molar teeth where possible—sufficient retention with an adhesive Nayyar core can be gained in most scenarios.

Adhesive dentistry has added an additional treatment approach through the use of endo-crowns and bonded onlays. However, Nayyar core-style restorations continue to be the most widely accepted treatment modality in this scenario.

Keywords: reduced coronal tooth tissue, root-treated molar tooth.

→ Nayyar A, Walton RE, Leonard LA. An amalgam coronal-radicular dowel and core technique for endodontically treated posterior teeth. *Journal of Prosthetic Dentistry*. 1980;**43**:511–15.

20. D ★★★★ OHCD 6th ed. → p. 102

The diagnosis of a vertical root fracture can be challenging. Symptoms tend to be vague and inconsistent with descriptions of sharp pain on biting and 'on/off' dull pains are frequently reported. Careful correlation of symptoms to the clinical signs is important, especially in the context of the biology. Clinically, after excluding other obvious causes of pathology, investigation for indicators, such as obvious fracture lines (with or without flexion), isolated deep probing depths, or pain on release of biting with a tooth sleuth, should be conducted. Crack identification with plaque-disclosing dye or transillumination has been suggested.

Radiographically, the presence of 'j'-shaped lesions, vertical bony defects, or lateral/furcal radiolucencies may indicate some form of longitudinal tooth fracture. Fractures confined to the root can be diagnosed as 'vertical root fractures', whilst fractures including the root and the crown are diagnosed as a 'split tooth'. Additionally, in this case, loss of the restoration without loss of the cusps is unusual, and thought should be given to the reason for loss of retention—potentially from flexion of the cusps. The furcal radiolucency and deep probing depth help differentiate in this scenario.

Keywords: pain on biting, endodontically treated, isolated probing depth, lost restoration.

→ Banerji S, Mehta SB, Millar BJ. Cracked tooth syndrome. Part 1: aetiology and diagnosis. *British Dental Journal*. 2010;**208**:459–63.

21. B ★★★★   OHCD 6th ed. → p. 334

NaOCl is a strongly antibacterial irrigant with organic tissue-dissolving qualities. EDTA is a weakly antibacterial, chelating agent that facilitates smear layer removal. The synergistic effects of combining these two irrigants have been widely researched. However, prolonged or repeated use of EDTA has been shown to cause dentine erosion (through chelation of the mineral component; NaOCl will dissolve the organic component), and this practice should be avoided. Additionally, the mixing of EDTA with NaOCl reduces the availability of free chloride (Cl^-) ions, and *in vitro* studies have demonstrated reduced bactericidal properties. For this reason, a single application of EDTA 17% solution for approximately 1 minute, after mechanical preparation has been completed, has been advocated. Many endodontists choose to follow this with one final rinse with NaOCl in an attempt to penetrate into the patent dentinal tubules. However, this remains controversial, as many argue the final rinse with NaOCl will have a more profound effect upon the degree of dentine erosion that occurs. Dentine erosion may have profound effects upon the strength of the remaining root canal wall.

Some clinicians suggest the use of alternative mild chelators such as 1-hydroxyethylidene-1,1-bisphosphonate [HEBP (7%)] to avoid such problems, but smear layer removal is reduced and less clinical outcome data are available to support their efficacy.

Keywords: irrigation, cycling between, NaOCl, EDTA.

→ Bystrom A, Sundqvist G. The antibacterial action of sodium hypochlorite and EDTA in 60 cases of endodontic therapy. *International Endodontic Journal*. 1985;**18**:35–40.

→ Haapasalo M, Qian W, Shen Y. Irrigation: beyond the smear layer. *Endodontic Topics*. 2012;**27**:35–53.

→ Zehnder M, Schmidlin P, Sener B, Waltimo T. Chelation in root canal therapy reconsidered. *Journal of Endodontics*. 2005;**31**:817–20.

22. B ★★★★   OHCD 6th ed. → p. 248

In October 2012, the law relating to tooth whitening was amended, following changes to European Union law (EU Council Directive 2011/84/EU). As a result, bleaching products that contain or release up to 6% hydrogen peroxide can be prescribed.

Whilst concentrations in excess of 6% hydrogen peroxide are utilized worldwide, in the United Kingdom, concentrations in excess of 6% are not allowed for cosmetic purposes only. Further advice should be sought if concentrations in excess of 6% are deemed necessary to manage disease, but this is rarely the case, as the literature does not report superior outcomes with higher concentrations. Standards of safety must be complied with, and patients must be 18 years or above for cosmetic whitening procedures.

It is important that close attention is paid to the type of product contained within each bleach, as carbamide peroxide is frequently encountered. Carbamide peroxide 16% would release <6% if hydrogen peroxide and is therefore safe for use.

Keywords: United Kingdom, tooth whitening, hydrogen peroxide.

→ Sulieman M, Addy M, MacDonald E, Rees JS. The effect of hydrogen peroxide concentration on the outcome of tooth whitening: an *in vitro* study. *Journal of Dentistry*. 2004;**32**:295–9.

Prosthodontics

Peter Clarke

'I want one of them screw in ones!'

Prosthodontics comprises most of the routine restorative treatments that practitioners perform on a daily basis. Much restorative work results from the impact of caries and periodontal disease. However, the prevalence of toothwear is dramatically increasing and can be expected to form a more prominent feature of the modern practitioner's workload. There is a considerable theory base in prosthodontics, covering all aspects of fixed and removable treatments, both conventional and contemporary.

Although the individual management of teeth can be tricky, a challenge many new practitioners struggle with is treatment planning on a patient level. Treatment planning is rarely black and white, with considerable variations in opinion among clinicians, even for more simple cases. The staging of treatment planning is fairly consistent across the profession (e.g. relief of pain first, then investigatory phase, etc.), but in complex cases, a second opinion may be warranted. Not only is treatment planning a difficult skill, but so is the execution. It takes practice to become adept at the variety of clinical skills in prosthodontics and the staging of treatment, but this makes for a rewarding and fascinating discipline.

Modern dentistry has a much greater focus on minimal invasive treatment, relying on dentine bonding and adhesive dentistry to limit the need for aggressive preparations of teeth and protect the vitality of the pulp. Moreover, the progression in digital dentistry is exponential, with newer production methods and clinical techniques becoming increasingly accurate and ever more accessible. As such, the modern practitioner needs to have a good understanding of both conventional concepts and modern alternatives in order to be able to apply the material and technique of choice to achieve an optimal outcome.

The questions in the chapter aim to cover a wide range of topics, testing conventional concepts in both fixed and removable prosthodontics, whilst touching on contemporary materials and production methods. It is hoped that the reader will be challenged and the more difficult questions will promote wider reading.

Key topics include:

- Diagnosis and treatment planning
- Occlusion
- Toothwear
- Complete dentures
- Removable dentures (including denture design principles)

- Direct restorations
- Crown and bridge
- Implant restorations
- Laboratory processes
- Digital dentistry.

QUESTIONS

1. A 47-year-old woman is undergoing planning for a full mouth rehabilitation. Before taking the interocclusal record, the clinician manipulates her into retruded contact position (RCP). Which is the single most appropriate description of this position? ★

A The initial tooth contact following the rotational movement of the mandible

B The initial tooth contact whilst closing around the terminal hinge axis

C The only clinically reproducible initial tooth contacts

D The position of the condyle whilst closing in the habitual position

E The position of the condyle whilst in its most relaxed functional position during closure

2. A 79-year-old edentulous man has a loose upper complete denture. After the primary impressions are taken, the dentist explains that more impressions will be taken at the next appointment. The patient asks why this is necessary. What is the single main reason for the second impression? ★

A To accurately record soft tissue detail to improve the denture's adaption

B To correct faults in the primary impression

C To identify the path of insertion of the dentures

D To outline to the technician the neutral zone for tooth placement

E To record and define the full functional limits of the denture-bearing area

3. A 64-year-old woman is treatment-planned to have an immediate maxillary complete denture following a full clearance. Prior to the clearance, she is warned that the dentures will need remaking in 6 months to 1 year. Which is the single most appropriate rationale for this warning? ★

A Bony remodelling will result in occlusal irregularities

B Bony remodelling will result in overextended dentures

C Bony remodelling will result in poor denture adaptation

D Bony remodelling will result in poor tooth positioning

E The patient might complain if they are unaware they will have to pay again

4. An 87-year-old edentulous woman has worn dentures and is requesting a new set. As she has no complaints with her current set
and has worn them for 15 years, it is decided to provide a new set via
the copy technique. Which surfaces of the dentures can be changed
easily using this technique? (Select one answer from the options listed
below.) ★

A Fitting and occlusal surfaces

B Fitting and polished surfaces

C Occlusal and polished surfaces

D Occlusal surfaces only

E Polished surfaces only

5. An 80-year-old man attends his jaw registration appointment. He
is happy with the appearance and position of the anterior teeth on
his old maxillary denture, so it is decided to copy this to the new denture.
Which is the single most appropriate device to aid the clinician in doing
this at the chair side? ★

A Alma gauge

B Fox's occlusal plane guide

C Iwanson gauge

D Steel ruler

E Willis bite gauge

6. A 45-year-old woman is having a new cobalt-chrome partial denture made. The primary models have been surveyed and returned
with the special trays. She has a lone-standing upper right second molar
that would make a useful tooth for direct retention with a cast cobalt-
chrome clasp. What is the single most appropriate clasp length and
undercut required for this type of clasp? ★

A 0.25 mm and 8 mm

B 0.25 mm and 15 mm

C 0.5 mm and 8 mm

D 0.5 mm and 12 mm

E 0.5 mm and 14 mm

7. A 19-year-old woman is referred, following completion of her orthodontic treatment for the replacement of her missing lateral incisors. Medically she is fit and well and has a minimally restored dentition. There is insufficient interradicular space for dental implants, and the patient is advised to have adhesive bridgework over conventional bridgework. What is the single main reason for this advice? ★

A Aesthetic

B Cheap to produce

C Ease of construction

D Low biological cost

E Reduced clinical time

8. A 36-year-old man attends an emergency appointment with a decoronated upper right second premolar. The tooth has been previously root-treated, but only 1 mm of supra-gingival tooth tissue remains. It is decided that a post crown is required, but before continuing, the patient is warned the prognosis is guarded and that there is a risk of root fracture long term. What single prognostic feature may increase the risk of root fracture in this scenario? ★

A Limited ferrule

B Long post length

C Narrow post width

D Shallow retention grooves

E Unfavourable crown–root ratio

9. A 35-year-old man attends the practice for the first time. A number of diagnoses are noted. Which single diagnosis should be addressed first? (Select one answer from the options listed below.) ★

A Acute periapical periodontitis LR5

B Chronic periapical abscess LL6

C Clasp fracture of lower denture

D Generalized plaque-induced gingivitis

E Occlusal caries UR67 and UL6

10. A 18-year-old man attends with an enamel dentine fracture of his upper right maxillary central incisor. He is treatment-planned to have a composite restoration placed to restore the tooth, and a rubber dam is going to be used. When is the single most appropriate time to take the shade of the composite? ★

A After bonding the tooth

B After etching the tooth

C After tooth preparation, e.g. bevelling

D At the beginning of the appointment

E Immediately after isolation with a rubber dam

11. A 50-year-old man has recently had his maxillary incisors extracted following blunt trauma to the face. The rest of his dentition is present and sound. The treatment plan includes a cobalt-chrome denture to restore the space until implants can be considered. Which single Kennedy classification does this situation represent? ★

A Class II

B Class II mod 2

C Class III mod 2

D Class IV

E Class IV mod 2

12. A 72-year-old man has just had a set of complete dentures delivered. The articulation is checked, and adjustments are made to ensure bilateral balanced articulation. Which cusps should be adjusted to prevent unwanted change to the occlusal vertical dimension (OVD)? (Select one option from the options below.) ★★

A Buccal upper, lingual lower

B Distal upper, mesial lower

C Lingual upper, buccal lower

D Mesial upper, distal lower

E Palatal upper, buccal lower

13. A 68-year-old woman attends for the try-in of her cobalt-chrome denture framework. At the appointment, it does not fit. Having spoken to the laboratory technician, it is discovered that the wrong type of refractory model was used. What is the single main reason this type of model is required in the production of cobalt-chrome dentures? ★ ★

A To assist in the flow of the molten metal over the cast, preventing air blows

B To block out unwanted undercut

C To facilitate the placement of an investing sprue onto the wax pattern

D To maintain the registration previously recorded, as the original model is often damaged during the casting process

E To withstand casting temperatures and expand/contract in a similar manner to the alloy

14. A 74-year-old man is having a new complete lower denture constructed. He has worn an upper complete denture for 25 years but has never worn a lower one. His resting face height (RFH) is 78 mm. What is the single most appropriate occlusal vertical dimension (OVD) to use during the jaw registration process? ★ ★

A 73 mm

B 75 mm

C 76 mm

D 81 mm

E 83 mm

15. A 72-year-old man is booked for the fit of his new upper complete denture. Upon assessment of the denture, prior to the appointment, a defect within the right buccal flange is noted. The defect has a bubbly-type appearance within the acrylic structure. What is the single most likely manufacturing fault? ★ ★

A Contraction porosity

B Dilation porosity

C Gaseous porosity

D Granular porosity

E Moisture inclusion porosity

16. A 74-year-old woman attends, following the fit of a new set of conventional complete dentures. She complains of generalized aching pain from her cheeks bilaterally, which started a few days after getting the new dentures. She also feels that her teeth 'clatter together' when she is speaking. What is the single most likely cause of the problem? ★★

A An overcontoured base plate in the canine regions

B Inadequate freeway space (FWS)

C Increased overjet (OJ)

D Overextension of both the upper and lower dentures

E Unilateral, unbalanced contact in intercuspal position (ICP)

17. A 37-year-old man is having his four maxillary incisor metallo-ceramic crowns replaced. He has a Class II div 2 incisal relationship, and the anterior guidance is deemed satisfactory. The guidance is planned to be copied from the preoperative mounted study models. Which single element of a semi-adjustable articulator can be used for this purpose? ★★

A Condylar guidance angle

B Incisal guidance table

C Intercondylar width

D Occlusal table

E Progressive side shift

18. A 68-year-old woman attends for a routine check-up. It is noticed that her bridge replacing the upper right canine, which is of a double abutment design, has failed. The upper right second premolar has caries under the retainer. She is advised that the bridge will need to be removed but that a new bridge design will be used because double abutting retainers is no longer considered an appropriate design. What is the single most important reason why this design is not considered appropriate? ★★

A Excessive costs

B Increased occlusal forces increase the risk of crown fracture

C Link retainers have a negative impact on periodontal health

D No mechanical benefit is gained over a cantilever design

E Partial debonding of the distal retainer frequently goes unnoticed

19. A 29-year-old woman has severe localized anterior toothwear affecting her mandibular incisors, with no inter-occlusal space present. Direct composite restorations have been placed, and posterior teeth are no longer in contact. The patient is advised that her 'bite' will feel different for a while, but It will eventually re-establish. What single movement is most likely to occur in the posterior teeth? ★ ★

A Eruption

B Intrusion

C No movement—restoration at new occlusal vertical dimension (OVD) required

D Rotation

E Tipping

20. An 18-year-old woman has a failed single cantilever resin-bonded bridge (RBB) replacing her upper right lateral incisor. What is the single most likely reason for failure of her bridge? ★ ★

A Abutment failure

B Debonding

C Emergence profile

D Shade match

E Pulp necrosis

21. A 25-year-old woman is having a routine examination. Dental caries is suspected buccally on the lower right first permanent molar. The tooth is dried with air, and a white spot lesion becomes more evident. What is the single main explanation for this? ★ ★

A Change in caries assessment Index

B Change in desiccation index

C Change in index of treatment need

D Change in light index

E Change in refractive index

22. A 51-year-old woman is having a gold shell crown placed on her upper right first permanent molar (UR6). Following occlusal reduction of 1 mm, a further 0.5 mm of height is reduced over the palatal cusp. What is the single main reason for doing this? ★ ★

A Aids retention and resistance form

B Better structural durability

C Improved marginal integrity

D Maintains cleansability

E Preserves tooth structure

23. A 59-year-old man is undergoing treatment for his failing dentition. In the maxillary arch, he requires a number of new crowns and a new cobalt-chrome partial denture. Before he had any extracoronal restorations placed, study models were surveyed and a preliminary denture design was created. What is the single most important reason for this? ★★

A So dissimilar metals are not placed in contact, leading to galvanic pain

B To allow incorporation of retentive/supportive features into the restoration

C To assess the amount of tooth reduction needed

D To ensure naturally occurring undercut is maintained

E To give the technician a reference point for the new occlusal table

24. A 38-year-old woman with post-eruptive breakdown subsequent to amelogenesis imperfecta is undergoing full mouth rehabilitation. Following planning on articulated models, the subsequent restorations are provided at an increased occlusal vertical dimension (OVD) in the retruded axis position (RAP). What is the single main reason for using RAP in this scenario? ★★★

A It is the most reproducible position, allowing accurate information transfer to the laboratory

B It reduces chair side time at cementation appointments

C Less damaging forces are transmitted to restorations where premature contacts exist

D RAP provides more space for the restorative material without the need for preparation

E Rehabilitation in RAP is more comfortable for the patient in the long term

25. A 68-year-old woman attends, complaining of a loose upper denture. Clinically, she has an edentulous maxilla and retained lower incisor teeth. She is not currently wearing a lower denture and does not take her upper denture out at night. The upper denture is loose, and the premaxilla is mobile and 'flabby'. What is the single most appropriate diagnosis? ★★★

A Apertognathia

B Bezold–Brucke effect

C Bonwill triad

D Combination syndrome

E Kelly's sign

26. An 82-year-old man attends, wishing to have new dentures made. He only has his mandibular incisor teeth remaining, which are severely proclined, and the residual alveolar ridge is grossly resorbed. It is decided to construct a swing-lock denture to try and provide a satisfactory lower partial denture. When designing the connectors, which single combination would be the most appropriate? ★ ★ ★

A Fixed labial bar and hinged lingual plate

B Hinged labial bar and lingual plate

C Hinged labial bar and sublingual bar

D Lingual plate and coronally approaching clasps

E Lingual plate and gingivally approaching clasps

27. A 58-year-old patient attends with generalized tooth wear. His teeth are vital and have previously been treated with composite restorations, but these have repeatedly failed by wearing down and he now requests an alternative. He is aware that he grinds his teeth at night, and clinically he has very hypertrophic masseters. It is decided to provide full-coverage crowns to restore his teeth. What would be the single most appropriate choice of crown in this situation? ★ ★ ★

A Dentine-bonded crown (feldspathic porcelain)

B Lithium disilicate all ceramic crown

C Metallo-ceramic crown with metal palatal surface

D Monolithic zirconia crown with full coverage glaze

E Veneered alumina oxide all ceramic crown

28. A 53-year-old man has a deep disto-occlusal-lingual amalgam restoration incorporating the cusp on his vital lower right first permanent molar. It is due to be replaced. The tooth has historically been affected by attachment loss, and the restoration margin is supra-gingival but extends below the cemento–enamel junction. He returns after 2 weeks, complaining of food packing. Given that it was very challenging initially to restore the contact point, what would be the single most appropriate course of action? ★ ★ ★

A Addition of amalgam to the contact point

B Provide additional oral hygiene instruction

C Provide new direct composite resin restoration

D Replace the amalgam using a wedge

E Restore with an indirect extra-coronal restoration

29. A 56-year-old woman is having her single implant crown restored. It is opposing a natural tooth. The static occlusal contact is left 'light' (i.e. roughly 20–30 µm of space between the prosthesis and the opposing natural tooth during gentle occlusion). What is the single main reason for doing so? ★ ★ ★ ★

A Account for periodontal ligament compression around the natural teeth

B Compensate for the wear of the natural dentition over time

C Minimize the risk of potential excursive interferences

D Reduce stress accumulation in, and prevent fracture of, the abutment screw

E Reduce the time taken to fit the crown

30. A 34-year-old woman is having a single implant crown provided to replace a congenitally missing lower left second premolar. The implant is well aligned, but there is limited inter-occlusal space present. A screw-retained restoration is provided, and the patient is advised that it will be more retrievable in the long term. What is the other single main benefit of a screw-retained restoration in this scenario? ★ ★ ★ ★

A Better aesthetics

B Improved retention

C Less time-consuming

D Lower costs

E Reduced marginal leakage

31. A local colleague is overheard recommending a local personal trainer who is offering tooth whitening with 10% carbamide peroxide. This person's name is not on the General Dental Council (GDC) register. Which single UK law does this contravene, and how would you manage the scenario? ★ ★ ★ ★

A Dentists Act 1984—contact the GDC

B Dentists Act 1984—contact Trading Standards

C Health and Medicines Act 1988—contact the GDC

D Health and Medicines Act 1988—contact the Medicines and Healthcare Products Regulatory Agency (MHRA)

E The Cosmetic Products Enforcement Regulations 2013—contact the MHRA

ANSWERS

1. B ★ OHCD 6th ed. → p. 226

During opening and closing, the mandible goes through two phases of movement. Initially, it undergoes a rotational movement through the first 20–25 mm of mandibular opening; this is then followed by a translation of the condyle down the articular eminence, as the individual opens wider. The terminal hinge axis or retruded axis position is the fixed axis of rotation joining the condyles, whilst they rotate in centric relation. Centric relation has multiple definitions but generally would be considered to amount to the maxillomandibular relationship when the condyles are in the glenoid fossa, in their most retruded, unstrained position.

When most people close, they come together into a position of maximum intercuspation that is habitually learnt (the intercuspal position—ICP). Alternatively, if the teeth contact with the condyle in centric relation, it is known as the RCP. In 90% of the population, the teeth and condylar head are located more posteriorly in the RCP, compared with the ICP, hence retruded contact position. Convention dictates that when planning a reorganized approach to treatment, the RCP is used, as it is considered to be the only reproducible position to transfer information to the laboratory.

Keywords: retruded contact position.

→ The Academy of Prosthodontics. The glossary of prosthodontic terms: ninth edition. *Journal of Prosthetic Dentistry*. 2017;**117**(5S):e1–105.

→ Wassell R, Naru A, Steele J, Nohn F. *Applied Occlusion*. Quintessence Publishing, London; 2008.

2. E ★ OHCD 6th ed. → p. 296

The master (working) impression aims to not only record the full extent of the denture-bearing area, but also to record the width and depth of the sulci in function. This provides a border seal and ensures the denture contours correctly to the movements of the sulci and frenula, thus preventing displacement of the denture by the soft tissues. Theoretically, it also means that a minimal distance is kept between the denture and soft tissues during function. This ensures the greatest pressure gradient/salivary surface tension (the pressure gradient is related to the thickness of the salivary film thickness) is present, which improves retention and optimizes the border seal. Generally, a special tray is required to accurately modify and border mould the impression to the individual, as stock trays frequently do not 'fit'. However, with modern materials and techniques, master impressions can be recorded using a stock tray with sufficient time and skill. Naturally, some faults from the primary impression will be corrected as the impression is refined. The surface detail may also increase, depending on the material used for each impression, improving the adaptation, but this is a property of material choice, and not the fundamental purpose of the second impression.

The neutral zone can be recorded with a special impression technique at the try-in stage.

The path of insertion for complete dentures is not greatly relevant, unless there are significant areas of bony undercut to be engaged.

Keywords: complete denture, second impression.

→ Jacobson TE, Krol AJ. A contemporary review of the factors involved in complete denture retention, stability, and support. Part I: retention. *Journal of Prosthetic Dentistry*. 1983;**49**:5–15.

→ Massad JJ, Cagna DR. Vinyl polysiloxane impression material in removable prosthodontics. Part 1: edentulous impressions. *Compendium of Continuing Education in Dentistry*. 2007;**28**:452–9.

3. C ★   OHCD 6th ed. → p. 292

Bone is an active structure, constantly being broken down and reformed throughout life. Stimulation from occlusal forces and the connecting periodontium around the teeth is required in order to maintain bone height. When teeth are lost, the alveolar ridge resorbs over time down to the basal bone. Work by Tallgren in 1972 demonstrated that reduction is greatest in the first 6–12 months, after which the rate slows. The amount of bone loss is up to four times greater in the mandible than in the maxilla.

Although the denture may potentially become overextended, the most likely complication to negatively affect retention is poor adaptation of the fitting surface, with loss of the border seal. Therefore, a reline, rebase, or remake is likely to be required for immediate dentures 6–12 months post-extraction. If a significant number of teeth are to be replaced, it is likely to be a poor fit from the outset and need relining promptly. It is wise to ask patients to consider immediate dentures as 'temporary dentures', as significant alteration is likely to be required.

Keywords: full clearance, immediate, denture, bony remodelling.

→ Tallgren A. The continuing reduction of the residual alveolar ridges in complete denture wearers: a mixed-longitudinal study covering 25 years. *Journal of Prosthetic Dentistry*. 2003;**89**:427–35.

4. A ★   OHCD 6th ed. → p. 312

A vital part of successful denture wearing is down to muscular control of the prosthesis by the patient. The polished surfaces of the denture (i.e. all of the denture surface that is not the teeth or impression surface) are controlled by the surrounding soft tissue and musculature. The copy technique aims to transfer this shape to the new denture to aid habituation.

From the impression of the original denture that the clinician takes, the technician will produce a 'copy' with wax teeth and an acrylic base. If required, the occlusal vertical dimension (OVD) is corrected at the registration appointment, before new teeth will be added by the technician at the correct height. A closed mouth wash impression is taken at the try-in appointment, which the technician will use to reline and produce the final product. As the denture base is produced in acrylic from the start, modification of the polished surfaces is much more difficult than the wax teeth (occlusal surface) or the fitting surface (impression surface), which is corrected similarly to a reline. The closed mouth impression minimizes unwanted increases in the OVD. Small modifications to the shape of the polished surface, or correcting the extensions, may be possible. Unfortunately, bodily movements of the denture base are not possible, and as such, significant alterations in tooth position would be easier with a complete remake.

Keywords: worn dentures, copy technique.

5. **A** ★   OHCD 6th ed. → p. 312

The Alma gauge has a vertical spring ruler and horizontal scale. It is used to measure the vertical and horizontal positions of the maxillary anterior teeth of the old prosthesis, using the incisive papilla as a reference point. These measurements can then be transferred to the new registration block to help the clinician maintain the lip support and incisal level, if it was deemed appropriate at the outset (see Figure 6.1 which shows an alma gauge used for transferring the incisal position of old dentures to the new registration rim). A Fox's occlusal plane guide is used to assess the angulation of the occlusal plane to the horizontal and antero-posterior planes; the reference lines are the interpupillary and alar-tragal lines, respectively. A Willis bite gauge measures the resting face height (RFH) and occlusal vertical dimension (OVD), allowing assessment of the freeway space; an alternative would be the two-dot technique. The thickness of material can be checked with an Iwanson gauge, similar to calipers. This instrument is generally used in fixed prosthodontics for

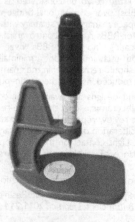

Figure 6.1

measuring small measurement changes and ensuring that indirect restorations are of adequate thickness; the thickness of chrome frameworks can also be checked. A small steel ruler is a multipurpose tool used for measuring distances clinically.

Keywords: position, upper anterior teeth, copy, chair side.

6. B ★   OHCD 6th ed. → p. 284

The high modulus of elasticity and lack of ductility of cobalt-chrome mean that the material is rigid, which is good for denture construction because the denture base can be kept thin for comfort and yet maintaining sufficient strength. However, the design of the clasp needs to consider the amount of distortion the clasp undergoes when engaging the undercut. This needs to be less than the proportional limit of the material to prevent permanent distortion and subsequent lack of retention. Changing the cross-dimensional shape, length, or material of the clasp can increase the flexibility. Alternatively, reducing the depth of undercut the clasp has to engage reduces the amount of flexibility needed. In general, cast chrome should engage undercuts of 0.25 mm and a clasp length of 15 mm is recommended to allow sufficient flexibility (some clinicians consider 14 mm to be an absolute minimum). Additionally, only the final third of the clasp should engage the undercut.

Keywords: cobalt-chrome clasp, length, undercut.

→ Bates JF. Retention of partial dentures. *British Dental Journal*. 1980;**149**:171–4.

→ Davenport JC, Basker RM, Heath JR, *et al*. Prosthetics: clasp design. *British Dental Journal*. 2001;**190**:71–81.

7. D ★   OHCD 6th ed. → p. 278

All of the answers listed could be considered as advantages of resin-bonded bridges (RBBs) over conventional bridge work. Fundamentally, RBBs are a reliable space management strategy with a low biological cost. Tooth preparation for RBBs remains controversial, with a large number of clinicians advocating 'no-prep' RBBs over minimal-preparation RBBs. However, both techniques adopt a minimally invasive approach. Preparation, if any, should remain within the enamel to provide greater bond strengths and reduced insult to the dentin–pulp complex.

Several materials and designs are available for construction of RBBs, including metal, all-ceramic, and glass fibre-reinforced composite. A recent systematic review reported the 5-year survival of RBBs to be 91.4%. Careful consideration of occlusal issues can help to improve the prognosis of RBBs. Light contact on the RBB pontic in the intercuspal position and avoidance of involvement in excursions are thought to be ideal.

Keywords: 19-year old, minimally restored dentition.

→ Durey KA, Nixon PJ, Robinson S, Chan MF. Resin bonded bridges: techniques for success. *British Dental Journal*. 2011;**211**:113–18.

→ Thoma DS, Sailer I, Ioannidis A, Zwahlen M, Makarov N, Pjetursson BE. A systematic review of the survival and complication rates of resin-bonded fixed dental prostheses after a mean observation period of at least 5 years. *Clinical Oral Implants Research.* 2017;**28**:1421–32.

8. A ★

The concept of incorporating a ferrule in post crown design is widely accepted within dentistry. A ferrule is defined as any ring or bushing used for making a tight joint. In dentistry, by having the margins of a crown below the margins of the remaining tooth core, a ferrule is produced—the idea being to reduce the force concentration at the apex of the post by distributing the lateral forces placed on the prosthetic tooth, theoretically reducing the risk of root fracture. A ferrule height of 2 mm and a width of 1 mm are desirable. Additionally, maintaining as much dentine as possible is also very important in reducing root fracture.

A long post length and an unfavourable crown-to-root ratio may increase the risk of fracture, because a greater volume of tooth tissue is removed and greater leverage forces will be applied to the root, respectively. However, a suitable ferrule is a more recognized prognostic factor. A narrow post width will help retain dentine volume and help minimize the risk of root fracture, but this needs to be balanced against having sufficient material thickness to prevent a fracture of the post itself. Shallow retention grooves will have little influence on root fracture outcomes.

Keywords: 1 mm supra-gingival tooth tissue, post crown, root fracture.

→ Eliyas S, Jalili J, Martin N. Restoration of the root canal treated tooth. *British Dental Journal.* 2015;**218**:53–62.

→ Jotkowitz A, Samet N. Rethinking ferrule—a new approach to an old dilemma. *British Dental Journal.* 2010;**209**:25–33.

9. A ★

Despite numerous approaches to treatment planning, it is universally accepted that pain management should be the first item to be addressed within any treatment plan. After the pain has been addressed, the patient should then be stabilized with regard to the primary disease. This will inevitably involve prevention advice, including oral hygiene advice, dietary advice, and fluoride supplements, etc. Following on from this, a provisional treatment planning stage will be undertaken to deconstruct failing restorations and assess for restorability. There also needs to be a period of reassessment of the patient's compliance and motivation with treatment. From here, a definitive treatment plan can be constructed, taking into account the remaining tooth structure, the underlying periodontal status, and the likely prognosis of the remaining dentition. After treatment is completed, patients must be placed on an appropriate recall interval. This will be based on the National Institute for Health and Care Excellence (NICE) guidelines for recall and professional opinion. Treatment planning can often be challenging, particularly when there are multiple diagnoses to consider. Time should be taken to construct a definitive treatment plan and advice sought where required.

→ National Institute for Health and Care Excellence. *Dental checks: intervals between oral health reviews*. Clinical guideline [CG19]. 2004. Available at: https://www.nice.org.uk/guidance/cg19

10. D ★

Anterior composite restorations are considered a reversible and aesthetic management strategy for fractured anterior teeth, with low biological cost and excellent patient satisfaction. Shade matching is crucial to achieve a desirable outcome, and this should be carried out at the start of the appointment, ideally under natural light.

Tooth preparation, etching, and placement of a dental dam can all interfere with shade matching, as well as drying the tooth. Drying or desiccating creates a greater discrepancy in the refractive index of the tooth and can lead to inaccuracies in shade matching. It is considered appropriate and good practice to place a small amount of composite onto the tooth to be restored prior to beginning treatment. This can be cured and aesthetics can be assessed, with the shade being altered, if necessary. This composite can be removed easily, without damaging the tooth.

Dental dam placement can influence the light passing through the tooth, and the colour of the rubber dam can influence shade selection. For this reason, shade matching should be recorded at the beginning of the appointment.

Keywords: shade.

→ Beddis H, Nixon P. Layering composites for ultimate aesthetics in direct restorations. *Dental Update*. 2012;**39**:630–6.

11. D ★

The Kennedy classification system is used to categorize edentulous areas in partially dentate patients. The classes are:

• Class I—bilateral free end saddle
• Class II—unilateral free end saddle
• Class III—unilateral bounded saddle
• Class IV—bounded saddle crossing the midline

The following rules aid identifying to which classification a patient belongs if multiple saddle areas are present:

1. You should classify according to the most posteriorly positioned saddle. A free end saddle is considered more posterior than a bounded saddle.
2. Once the classification has been decided, any additional saddles should be denoted by 'modifications'. The modification should represent the number of additional saddles only, regardless of their size or position.

3. Class IV saddles cannot be modified. They would come under a
modification.

Third molars are not considered when deciding upon a classification.

Keywords: maxillary incisors, extracted, Kennedy classification.

12. A ★★   OHCD 6th ed. → p. 302

The BULL rule (Buccal Upper, Lingual Lower) is a simple acronym to
help remember which cusp to adjust to remove interferences in dynamic
lateral excursions. However, understanding the concept sometimes
takes more thought. When adjusting complete dentures to provide
balanced articulation, thought needs to be given to the function of each
cusp. The supporting or functional cusps (palatal maxillary cusp, buccal
mandibular cusp) maintain the OVD, and they should not be adjusted
when trying to gain balanced articulation, as alteration of the OVD
may result. Therefore, should these cusps cause an interference on
lateral excursions, then the balancing (non-functional) cusp inclines of
the opposing arch (buccal upper, lingual lower) should be adjusted until
balanced working side contacts are achieved. It may not be possible to
apply this rule to the non-working side, as the supporting cusps could
interfere during this movement. In this situation, it is usually possible to
remove the interference without completely removing the supporting
contact point.

Despite this concept being widely recognized and accepted, some
research has questioned the benefit of this occlusal scheme with regard
to masticatory efficiency, function, and patient experience. Results concluded no difference between complete dentures setup with bilateral
balanced articulation and those in canine guidance. The authors consider
this plausible, because as soon as food is introduced between the dentures, the teeth will no longer be in contact and therefore, the role of
balanced articulation may become insignificant.

Keywords: balanced articulation, unwanted change, OVD.

→ Basker RM, Davenport JC, Thomason JM. *Prosthetic Treatment of the
Edentulous Patient* (5th ed.). Wiley-Blackwell, Oxford; 2012.

→ Farias-Neto A, Carreiro A. Bilateral balanced articulation: science or
dogma. *Dental Update.* 2014;**41**:428–30.

13. E ★★   OHCD 6th ed. → p. 652

Casting of metal alloys needs to be conducted on special models for
a variety of reasons. The casting process needs to reach very high
temperatures—up to 1000°C for cobalt-chrome. These extreme
temperatures produce challenges for the model, which needs to be
able to adapt by demonstrating various mechanical properties. Firstly,
the material needs to be able to withstand high casting temperatures
(thermal stability). Secondly, the material must be sufficiently porous
to vent gases produced during the casting process (porous). Finally, the
material needs to demonstrate a similar coefficient of expansion to the

alloy, so as the metal cools, it will be of the correct size (expansion). Refractory models are made of derivatives of silica that are bound to gypsum or silica or phosphate. Phosphate-bonded refractory models are commonly used as adjustment of the colloidal silica component, which means the setting expansion can be varied for the desired alloy.

The other answers are not related to the type of cast material, but rather to other laboratory or clinical procedures.

Keywords: cobalt-chrome, refractory model.

14. A ★★

This question requires good knowledge of the measurements used during jaw registration. A Willis bite gauge is often used during this process. The RFH, or resting vertical dimension, measures the physiological rest position of the lower face. This is the position adopted by the teeth and mandible when the muscles of mastication are at rest. Ideally, the lips should be in contact and the head should be in an upright position.

Freeway space (or inter-occlusal rest space) is the difference between the RFH and the OVD (when opposing arches are in contact). Appropriate freeway space is fundamental for chewing, speech, and comfort.

In the majority of complete denture cases, 2–4 mm of freeway space is deemed acceptable. However, in patients who have not worn a prosthesis before, or in a long time, increased freeway space has been reported to improve habituation and, as such, a measurement of 5–6 mm is considered appropriate. However, it must be remembered that these measurements are somewhat arbitrary and are unlikely to be accurately measured clinically.

Moreover, these measurements are dynamic and change throughout time. This includes the RFH, which is influenced by changes in the stomatognathic system. For this reason, the RFH is often the starting point for calculating the OVD.

Keywords: 74-year old, never worn a lower denture.

→ McCord J, Grant A. Registration: stage 2—intermaxillary relations. *British Dental Journal*. 2000;**188**:601–6.

15. C ★★ OHCD 6th ed. → p. 660

During the processing of acrylic dentures, three main faults can be seen within the acrylic. These are contraction, gaseous, and granular porosities. They result from errors with either the ratio of the acrylic components or as a result of incorrect heating processes. A polymer (powder) to monomer (liquid) ratio of 3.5:1 is required. However, if insufficient monomer saturation occurs, then a dry, spongy/crumbly appearance of the acrylic results. Excess liquid may lead to unreacted monomer present in the denture base, potentially causing irritation of the mucosa. If too little volume of acrylic is packed into the flask, then contraction porosities can occur, resulting in incomplete flange areas of short gingival margins/papilla. There may also be streaks seen within the material. Gaseous porosities occur when the temperature of the resin exceeds its boiling point (100.3°C) before polymerization has completed, resulting in bubbles being included within the cured material. This bubbly appearance should lead you to the answer of gaseous porosity. Inclusion of moisture may lead to pale, cloudy areas within the acrylic, and insufficient tightening would produce an excessively thick denture base, increasing the occlusal vertical dimension from that prescribed.

Keywords: bubbly, appearance, manufacturing faults.

→ Van Noort R. *Introduction to Dental Materials* (4th ed.). Mosby Elsevier, London; 2013.

16. B ★★   OHCD 6th ed. → p. 308

A lack of FWS can produce an array of presenting complaints. However, when combined with an increase in the patient's occlusal vertical dimension (OVD), generalized aching around the mouth is often reported. The pain is often non-specific and vague. A complaint of 'too many teeth' or a 'full mouth' is highly likely to indicate errors within the OVD. Complaints of teeth 'clacking' together are likely to relate to unretentive dentures or inadequate FWS.

With an increased bulk of the baseplate in the canine regions, patients may develop whistling sounds or difficulty with the 'th' or 'ch' sounds when speaking. This is because the phonetic position of the tongue is inhibited laterally by the denture base.

An increased OJ can affect speech, frequently fricatives (e.g. 'f' sounds) and 's' sounds (sibilants). Additionally, some patients complain of difficulty incising foods, which may be corrected with the prescription of a flat anterior bite plane, depending on the situation. Overextension or unbalanced occlusion are common faults that tend to produce localized sores or localized/unilateral aching, respectively; they are less commonly associated with the generalized aching typically seen in OVD issues.

Keywords: generalized aching pain, clatter.

→ Basker R, Davenport J, Thomason J. *Prosthetic Treatment of the Edentulous Patient* (5th ed.). Wiley-Blackwell, Chichester; 2011.

17. B ★★

When providing multiple indirect restorations, use of a semi-adjustable articulator and facebow transfer is recommended. The facebow allows the maxillary cast to be related to the terminal hinge axis and also provides a horizontal plane of reference for future mountings of additional casts. The horizontal reference point varies with each articulator used, and the reader should refer to the manufacturer's guidance. The semi-adjustable articulator has the benefit over an average-value articulator in that the condylar guidance angle, immediate side shift, and progressive side shift can be adjusted (depending on the articulator model). These can be set with the use of excursive check records. Greater freedom on the articulator allows more accurate replication of the mandibular movements and, hopefully, the need for less intraoral adjustments.

Anterior restorations with adequate shared protrusive guidance can be replicated, using a custom incisal guidance table, which is then used to fabricate the palatal contours on the new restorations. Where inadequate or inappropriate guidance is identified, it would be prudent to restore the anterior teeth with provisional restorations, which can be modified chairside until an ideal anterior guidance is achieved and copied. An alternative method of coping the anterior guidance is the 'every other tooth method', whereby definitive restorations are placed on three alternating teeth at a time (e.g. UR3, UR1, UL2). In this way, the guidance in the definitive crowns can conform to the remaining temporary restorations.

Keywords: guidance, copied, semi-adjustable articulator.

→ Wassell R, Naru A, Steele J, Nohn F. *Applied Occlusion*. Quintessence Publishing, London; 2008.

18. E ★ ★

In the past, double abutment was considered a sensible design for fixed bridgework when the adjacent teeth were of poor quality or small in size, in order for the bridge to have better mechanical properties. Unfortunately, it was noticed that debonding of the distal retainer frequently occurred without loss of the bridge, with subsequent caries development in the abutment. This is because flexure of the superstructure during loading leads to the mesial abutment acting as a fulcrum, with the result being the breakdown of the lute under the distal retainer. These days, efforts are made to avoid this type of design, as it is a recognized complication. Careful assessment should be made of the abutments if this type of bridge is seen. The presence of air bubbles developing at the crown margin of the retainers whilst pressing on the pontic can be an indicator of debonding having occurred. See Figure 6.2a (see Colour Plate section) which shows a full-arch fixed bridge that debonded, leading to gross caries underneath the distal abutment. The presence of bubbles under loading is indicative of the retainer having partially debonded at the prosthesis at rest. Figure 6.2b (see Colour Plate section) shows underloading air is displaced, forming bubbles at the mesial aspect.

Keywords: bridge, double abutment, caries.

→ Hemmings K, Harrington Z. Replacement of missing teeth with fixed prostheses. *Dental Update*. 2004:**31**:137–41.

19. A ★ ★

The Dahl principle is a method for creating inter-occlusal space, either for restoring or for moving teeth. Traditionally, it utilized either a removable prosthesis or a cast metal plate bonded to the back of the upper teeth. These removable prostheses historically had issues with patient compliance, affecting outcomes. Original work was conducted by Dahl and colleagues back in 1975 on axial tooth movement to create space for restoring worn anterior teeth. They demonstrated that this occurred by intrusion of the anterior teeth (40%) and eruption of the posterior teeth (60%). There may also be an element of condylar remodelling in some cases. Re-establishment of the posterior occlusion takes on average up to 7 months but can take as long as 18 months. In modern dentistry, bonding direct composite at an increased OVD to manage localized anterior toothwear is a well-accepted technique. Some clinicians also utilize the Dahl principle when cementing resin-bonded bridges to allow a no-preparation technique.

Keywords: posterior teeth, no longer in contact, re-establish.

→ Ahmed KE, Murbay S. Survival rates of anterior composites in managing toothwear: systematic review. *Journal of Oral Rehabilitation*. 2016;**43**:145–53.

→ Poyser N, Porter RW, Briggs PF, Chana HS, Kelleher MG. The Dahl concept: past, present and future. *British Dental Journal*. 2005;**198**:669–76.

20. B ★★

RBBs have been shown to display higher failure rates than conventional full-coverage coronal restorations. However, recent literature reports a 10-year survival of around 80%. Furthermore, most failures tended to occur within the first 4 years. Whilst conventional bridge designs may offer greater mechanical properties for retention, the conservation of tooth tissue associated with RBBs has made them a popular treatment modality, especially for congenitally absent upper lateral or lower incisors where space and a poorly developed alveolar process may complicate implant placement.

Debonding of the retainer is the most common cause of failure, and posterior teeth are more likely to fail than anterior teeth. Careful consideration of the occlusion is fundamental to success. Pulp necrosis is extremely unlikely, given the limited preparation.

Keywords: cantilever, RBB, failure.

→ King P, Foster LV, Yates RJ, Newcombe RG, Garrett MJ. Survival characteristics of 771 resin retained bridges provided at a UK dental teaching hospital. *British Dental Journal*. 2015;**218**:423–8.

→ Pjetursson BE, Tan WC, Tan K, Brägger U, Zwahlen M, Lang NP. A systematic review of the survival and complication rates of resin-bonded bridges after an observation period of at least 5 years. *Clinical Oral Implants Research*. 2008;**19**:131–41.

21. E ★★

The carious process results in porosities developing within the enamel, which is usually filled with water. The refractive index describes how light propagates through a medium. It is a ratio of how light passes through a medium, compared to light travelling through a vacuum. The refraction of light can affect how we interpret the colour of an object. In carious enamel, subsurface porosities are normally filled with water, through which light travels more slowly than in air, and also more dispersion occurs. When the tooth is air-dried, water is expelled from the porosities and replaced with air. This lowers the refractive index in this area, giving a white appearance to the surface. Figure 6.3 (see Colour Plate section) shows a white spot lesion upon air-drying. A lesion visible without drying represents more advanced disease. As the carious process develops to dentine, exogenous staining, bacterial pigments, and denaturing of proteins result in brown discoloration.

The caries assessment index is not a real index. Most epidemiological studies examining caries will use diseased, missing, filled teeth (DMFT) or the international caries detection and assessment system (ICDAS II). There are multiple desiccation indexes in biology, but not one in dentistry. The Light index is used to assess the size of a pneumothorax. The index of treatment need should be known as the index of orthodontic treatment need (IOTN).

Keywords: dried, air, white spot, more evident.

→ Kidd E, Fejerskov O. *Essentials of Dental Caries* (4th ed.). Oxford University Press, Oxford; 2016.

22. B ★★

Shillingburg outlined five main principles of tooth preparation in his textbook of fixed prosthodontics: preservation of tooth structure, retention and resistance form, structural durability, marginal integrity, and maintenance of periodontal health. The functional cusp should be beveled to allow for an adequate bulk of material to be placed in an area of high loading. If insufficient reduction is given, then two outcomes may occur. Firstly, the restoration will be too thin in this region and will be at risk of fracture or an increased wear rate. Alternatively, the technician may overbuild the restoration, resulting in occlusal interference.

Although this concept is well accepted throughout the dental community, there are some who debate the need for this added bulk of material. However, generally, most practitioners will provide the extra room in their preparations over the functional cusp.

Keywords: UR6, 0.5 mm, reduced, palatal cusp.

→ Shillingburg HT Jr, Sather DA, Wilson EL, *et al. Fundamentals of Fixed Prosthodontics* (3rd ed.). Quintessence Publishing, Hanover Park, IL; 1997.

23. B ★★

A vital part of treatment planning for removable prosthodontics is to include features to improve retention and support. Retention can be gained from clasps to engage undercut, a path of insertion that differs to the path of displacement, or the use of precision attachments. If a removable partial denture (RPD) is planned and single or multiple indirect restorations are required, then retentive/supportive features, such as rest seats, guide planes, and desirable undercuts, can be incorporated. Furthermore, use of intra- and -extracoronal precision attachments, such as the FR system® (intracoronal) or Preci Clix^c (extra-coronal), can be integrated into the casting. Therefore, a provisional denture design should be developed prior to providing the indirect restoration.

It is important to remember that when preparing teeth where guide planes or rest seats are planned, extra reduction in the preparation is required to allow for sufficient material thickness and to prevent overcontouring of the crown.

Keywords: new crowns, new cobalt-chrome partial denture, preliminary, design.

→ Burns D; Ward J. Review of attachments for removable partial denture designs: 1. classification and selection. *International Journal of Prosthodontics*. 1990;**3**:98–102.

→ Devlin H. Integrating posterior crowns with partial dentures. *British Dental Journal*. 2001;**191**:120–3.

---

24. A ★★★   OHCD 6th ed. → p. 228

Over the years, various theories on occlusion have appeared in the literature. Although opinion varies, little firm scientific evidence is available to confirm whether one occlusal scheme is better than another. However, convention dictates the use of the RAP when reorganizing the occlusion. In function, mandibular movements are guided by the condyles posteriorly and the teeth anteriorly. The retruded contact position (RCP) is the first tooth contact on the RAP and is guided by the condyles and surrounding musculature/soft tissues. Recording a location on the RAP primarily provides a reproducible position that is defined by anatomical constraints, rather than muscular habituation. Therefore, it allows more accurate transfer of information and changes in the OVD between the patient and the laboratory. The literature also argues that use of the RAP will provide a more harmonious muscular position, with no damaging slides from premature contacts, reducing the risk of temporomandibular disorders and restoration failure. However, the evidence is inconclusive and contradictory evidence exists. Moreover, it is known that a new RCP will re-establish over time in patients reorganized in RCP.

Reduction in chair time at cementation will come from the production of accurate laboratory work, and more space maybe created by distalizing the mandible into the RAP, but these are not the primary reasons for its use.

Keywords: increased OVD, full mouth rehabilitation, RAP.

→ Becker C, Kaiser D. Evolution of occlusion and occlusal instruments. *Journal of Prosthodontics*. 1993;**2**:33–43.

→ Davies SJ, Gray RM, Whitehead SA. Good occlusal practice in advanced restorative dentistry. *British Dental Journal*. 2001;**191**:421–4, 427–30, and 433–4.

25. D ★★★   OHCD 6th ed. → p. 296

Combination syndrome was initially described by Ellsworth Kelly in 1972, and Kelly's syndrome (not sign) is a synonym. However, combination syndrome is the most commonly used name. The original features described were: an edentulous maxilla associated with natural mandibular anterior teeth, including bone loss from the anterior maxillary ridge; overgrowth of the tuberosities; papillary hyperplasia of the palatal mucosa; extrusion of the mandibular anterior teeth; and loss of alveolar bone height below the mandibular removable prosthesis [removable partial denture (RPD)].

Further characteristics were added later by Saunders *et al.* There is debate as to whether combination syndrome exists, as observed scientific evidence of the condition is limited. However, the terminology remains well grounded. It is well recognized that bone resorbs following extractions and that a removable prosthesis can negatively impact upon the rate.

Apertognathia is a synonym for open bite. The Bezold–Brucke effect is the apparent change in colour, depending on the intensity (brightness) of the light source. The Bonwill triad should actually be the Bonwill's triangle, a 4-inch equilateral triangle between the mandibular incisor tips and the condyles—a geometry that Bonwill used when designing his early articulator.

Keywords: edentulous maxilla, retained lower incisors, flabby opposed by natural dentition.

→ Palmqvist S, Carlsson GE, Öwall B. The combination syndrome: a literature review. *Journal of Prosthetic Dentistry.* 2003;**90**:270–5.

→ The Academy of Prosthodontics. The glossary of prosthodontic terms. *Journal of Prosthetic Dentistry.* 2005;**94**:10–92.

26. B ★★★

The swing-lock removable partial denture has been proposed as a cobalt-chrome denture design in patients with a mandibular Kennedy class I. The cobalt-chromium framework consists of a lingual plate opposed by a hinged labial bar. This design utilizes labial alveolar undercut with a swinging labial bar that closes following denture insertion. Moreover, a lingual plate is used over a bar connector, as it will provide indirect retention. The labial component was traditionally constructed with anterior struts that contacted the labial surface of the lower incisors. However, a more aesthetic approach utilizes polymethylmethacrylate in the form of gingival veneers. Disadvantages include: potential wear of the swing-lock components with extended use and possible negative consequences on the remaining abutment teeth, which is usually the remaining mandibular incisors.

Keywords: severely proclined, swing-lock.

→ Lynch CD, Allen PF. The swing-lock denture: its use in conventional removable partial denture prosthodontics. *Dental Update*. 2004;**31**:506–8.

27. C ★★★

Choosing the most appropriate type of crown material can sometimes be confusing, given the number of materials and production methods available today; often there is not a correct answer. Judgement needs to be made on what is best, given the presenting scenario. Consideration needs to be given to the biological cost, aesthetic demands, and mechanical properties required in the given environment. In this situation, the tooth is vital, visible, and needing to withstand high functional forces, and a metallo-ceramic crown is generally considered the most appropriate. This gives the best compromise on aesthetics and durability, whilst minimizing the tooth reduction required.

All ceramic crowns and fully veneered metallo-ceramic crowns require significantly more reduction that metallo-ceramic crowns with palatal metal alone. Although feldspathic porcelain gains strength from bonding to the tooth structure, it is less resistant to fracture under excessive parafunctional loads. Monolithic zirconia, although being strong in thin section, has compromised aesthetics. Alumina oxide cores are also very strong, but the bond to the veneering ceramic is the weak link. Not only will they require greater tooth reduction to provide adequate space for the material, but under parafunctional loads, there is a risk that the veneering ceramic will chip. Additionally, certain forms of porcelain can be abrasive to enamel and cause wear of the opposing dentition when the surface glaze is lost.

Keywords: vital, failed, wearing, grinds, hypertrophic masseters.

→ Shenoy A, Shenoy N, Dental ceramics: an update. *Journal of Conservative Dentistry*. 2010;**13**:195–203.

→ Wassell R, Walls A, Steele J. Crowns and extra-coronal restorations: materials selection. *British Dental Journal*. 2002;**192**:199–202, 205–11.

28. E ★★★

This scenario describes a large direct restoration which has failed due to inadequate contouring of the distal restoration surface. This has left a deficient contact point which has resulted in food packing. This creates an increased risk of caries or periodontal disease if left untreated, and oral hygiene instruction alone is unlikely to be sufficient, especially where previous attachment loss has been identified. Contact points are often difficult to restore, using direct placement of restorative material, particularly where an adjacent cusp has been lost or where the restoration depth is considerable. Contouring the matrix band can be challenging in these situations and, as such, indirect extra-coronal restorations should be considered. Direct composite placement is likely to be equally as challenging as amalgam, with the added difficulty of moisture control and rubber dam placement with a deep margin. The use of wedges helps to avoid ledges and assists in contact point formation by compressing the periodontal ligament to compensate for the thickness of the matrix band; particularly if pre-wedging is performed.

By comparison, indirect restorations can be appropriately contoured in the laboratory and can be constructed in a wide range of materials, including gold, ceramic, and resin composite. Whilst a dental dam may still be required for bonding of the restoration, the length of time required for isolation is often shorter.

Keywords: deep restoration, food packing, challenging, contact point.

29. A ★★★★

Implant-retained restorations are becoming increasingly common amongst the population. Osseointegration of the fixture rigidly secures the implant to the bone. Implants differ from natural teeth in that they do not have a periodontal ligament (PDL) surrounding them. With regard to occlusion, this causes three main problems. Firstly, when the patient occludes, the PDL of the natural dentition has the ability to compress; implants only displace minimally (the distance bone flexes, approximately 3–5 μm vertically and 10–50 μm laterally).

Secondly, proprioception is provided predominantly by the PDL, which is significantly greater than osseoperception around implants, limiting the sensory feedback. Finally, the PDL has the ability to adapt to increased occlusal loads, therefore limiting permanent damaging effects of occlusal overload on natural teeth. If the space for PDL compression of surrounding natural teeth is not accounted for, then there is a risk of occlusal overload, which can lead to bone loss around the implant, screw loosening, or implant component fracture.

These concepts vary slightly, depending on the opposing contact (e.g. natural tooth, another implant, full arch implant restoration, etc.). The clinician therefore needs to consider what the opposing contact is and how this will impact on the occlusal design.

Keywords: single implant crown, natural tooth, static, contact, light.

→ Davies S, Gray R, Young M. Good occlusal practice in provision of implant borne prostheses. *British Dental Journal*. 2002;**192**:79–88.

→ Gross M. Occlusion in implant dentistry. A review of the literature of prosthetic determinants and current concepts. *Australian Dental Journal*. 2008;**53**:S60–8.

30. B ★★★★   OHCD 6th ed. → p. 316

One of the main benefits of screw-retained, compared to cement-retained, restorations is retrievability. If there are problems with the crown or the underlying abutment, it can be difficult to remove a cement-retained restoration intact. The accurate fit of implant restorations and parallelism of the abutment mean retention is excellent, even if weak luting cement is used. However, as in conventional crown preparations, adequate height is still required in order to produce suffi-cient retention and resistance form with cement-retained restorations. Unfortunately, due to fixture angulations, screw-retained restorations are not always possible, as the access hole could emerge on the labial surface (upper anterior incisors particularly). The recent development of co-axial implants and angled screw abutments is helping to resolve this issue, although there are still drawbacks to these solutions. Marginal leakage is less concerning at the crown abutment interface, as there is no susceptibility to caries, but peri-implant disease remains of concern. There are advantages and disadvantages for both methods, and the clin-ician should be aware of these to select the most appropriate one.

The difference in cost is unlikely to be a major consideration in this scenario.

Keywords: cell aligned, reduced inter-occlusal space, screw-retained.

→ Michalakis K, Hirayama H, Garefis P. Cement-retained versus screw-retained implant restorations: a critical review. *International Journal of Oral and Maxillofacial Implants*. 2003;**18**:719–28.

31. A ★★★★

In the UK, the practice of dentistry is protected for GDC-registered dentists and dental care professionals (DCPs) under the Dentists Act 1984. Concentrations that release >0.1% hydrogen peroxide must be prescribed by a dental practitioner. This includes tooth whitening, which has led to a large number of criminal prosecutions in recent years. The Dentists Act also restricts the use of titles associated with practising den-tistry, which could lead to prosecution, should a member of the public claim they were a registered dentist or a DCP. These practices are re-served for dentists. However, appropriately trained therapists, hygien-ists, and clinical dental technicians can provide bleaching if prescribed by a dentist. It is the dentist's responsibility to conduct the initial clinical appointment, which should routinely include photographs and a clearly recorded shade. Reports regarding conduct of this nature should be re-ported to the GDC, which follows up on the practice of illegal dentistry within the UK.

Other laws and European Union regulations may be contravened by practising dentistry illegally, and each case is assessed individually by the GDC. Offering whitening gels that had concentrations in excess of 6% hydrogen peroxide would also be deemed unlawful in the UK under the Cosmetic Products Enforcement Regulations 2013.

Keywords: personal trainer, tooth whitening, law.

→ General Dental Council. *Position statement on tooth whitening*. 2016. Available at: https://www.gdc-uk.org/api/files/Tooth-Whitening-Position-Statement.pdf

Oral and maxillofacial surgery

Tariq Ali

'All bleeding stops eventually.'

Oral and facial surgery has been practised in some form for millennia. Hippocrates himself has described reducing jaw dislocations, and Sushtra was performing reconstructive local facial flaps in India as early as sixth century BC. The modern practice of oral and maxillofacial surgery (OMFS) can be traced back to the battlefields of northern Europe in the early twentieth century. Industrialized warfare produced horrific facial injuries that were treated by frontline oral surgeons, and so the specialty of OMFS, as a crossover between medicine and dentistry, developed. It became evident that both medical and dental education was necessary in order to manage increasingly complex facial surgery that was being undertaken.

It can be argued that OMFS has evolved to be a truly general surgical specialty, manipulating the hard and soft tissues of the head and neck and having the skills to operate on neurovascular, glandular, and airway structures. There is variable exposure to OMFS during dental undergraduate education and scarce exposure during medical undergraduate training. Opportunities for postgraduate training in OMFS for dentists who are not entertaining a career in the discipline are also limited. Knowledge of the scope of OMFS practice is a bare minimum for any practising dentist, as this can inform the limits of their individual competency, as well as ensure a safe transfer of care for their patients.

The questions in this section are there to target the most commonly tested and encountered aspects of OMFS for most junior dentists, focusing on oral surgery, oral pathology, management of the medically compromised patient, and trauma of the facial skeleton.

OMFS is an enormously satisfying endeavour and is recommended to all junior dentists. It can form a granite-like foundation of skills upon which to build a career in clinical dentistry.

Key topics include:

- Trauma
- Oral surgery and exodontia
- Oral pathology
- Orthognathic surgery
- Temporomandibular joint surgery
- Cleft lip/palate repair
- Craniofacial surgery
- Salivary disease
- Head and neck oncology and microvascular reconstruction
- Skin cancer
- Facial aesthetics.

QUESTIONS

1. A 74-year-old man requires the extraction of his upper right second premolar (UR5). He is currently taking warfarin for a recent deep vein thrombosis. His international normalized ratio (INR) was recorded as 2.6 when it was last assessed and has been stable over the last 3 months. What is the maximum time recommended between the extraction and the last INR reading? (Select one answer from the options below.) ★

A 12 hours

B 24 hours

C 36 hours

D 48 hours

E 72 hours

2. A 24-year-old man with an 8-pack year smoking history attends in pain, following a routine extraction of his lower left first permanent molar (LL6) 3 days ago. He has deep-seated, severe pain around the extraction site. Medically, he is fit and well. Which is the single most likely cause of his pain? ★

A Alveolar osteitis

B Fractured jaw

C Osteomyelitis

D Osteonecrosis of the jaw

E Retained root

3. A 64-year-old woman requires the extraction of her lower right first molar. She previously received intravenous (IV) zoledronic acid for breast cancer 6 years ago. Although no longer receiving zoledronic acid, she is now taking denosumab. Which is the single most appropriate management? ★

A Extract the tooth atraumatically

B Extract the tooth under antibiotic prophylaxis

C Maintain the roots as an overdenture abutment

D Perform surgical removal of the tooth

E Refer to your local Oral Surgery/Oral Maxillofacial Department

4. A 21-year-old man has been referred with recurrent bouts of pericoronitis associated with his lower left third molar (LL8). A dental panoramic tomogram (DPT) is taken, and incidentally, a large unilocular lesion surrounding the crown of the unerupted lower right third molar (LR8) is identified. What is the single most likely diagnosis of this lesion? ★

A Calcifying epithelial odontogenic tumour (Pindborg tumour)

B Dentigerous cyst

C Odontogenic keratocyst

D Odontogenic myxoma

E Paradental cyst

5. A 23-year-old woman is having the extraction of an asymptomatic upper right wisdom tooth. During the procedure, a large palatal mucosal tear appears adjacent to the tooth, and the segment is now mobile. Which single complication is most likely to have occurred? (Select one answer from the options below.) ★★

A Crown fracture

B Oro-antral communication

C Oro-antral fistula

D Root fracture

E Tuberosity fracture

6. A 28-year-old man has received a blow to his right jaw. He reports being unable to open his mouth wide or bite his teeth together. He has no problems with his eyes and did not lose consciousness. He has marked tenderness at the right angle of the mandible and over the left parasymphysis. A right angle fracture and a left parasymphyseal fracture are suspected. Which two plain film radiographs should be requested? (Select one answer from the options below.) ★★

A Dental panoramic tomogram (DPT) and occipitomental 30 (OM30O)

B DPT and posteroanterior (PA) mandible

C Occipitomental 10 (OM10O) and OM30O

D OM30O and PA mandible

E Submentovertex and PA mandible

7. A 46-year-old woman is reviewed following the extraction of an upper right first molar (UR6). She says that she has been unable to smoke properly since the extraction and has noticed a salty discharge. A diagnosis of oroantral communication is made, and surgical correction planned. Which is the single most appropriate surgical management in this situation? ★★★

A Buccal advancement flap

B Modified three-sided flap

C Palatal rotation flap

D Semi-lunar flap

E Two-sided flap

8. A 31-year-old woman is seen by the junior oral and maxillofacial doctor in the Emergency Department with a large facial swelling near the angle of her right mandible. Her temperature is 38.9°C. She has 10-mm mouth opening and is struggling to swallow her own saliva. A grossly carious lower right second molar (LR7) is noted, and her floor of mouth is raised and firm. The patient is asked to rest with her head elevated above the level of her heart, and intravenous (IV) steroids and antibiotics are commenced. The senior maxillofacial doctor asks that the patient is discussed with another specialty. Which is the single most appropriate specialty to call? ★★★

A Anaesthetics

B Ear, nose, and throat (ENT)

C Emergency medicine

D Haematology

E Intensive care medicine

9. A 27-year-old man received a blow to the right side of his head during a rugby match and has blurry vision, which is corrected by tilting his head. On ocular examination, his right eye appears elevated and he reports double vision when he attempts to look straight down to read. Which single cranial nerve is most likely to have been traumatized? ★★★★

A Abducens

B Infraorbital

C Oculomotor

D Optic

E Trochlear

10. A 13-year-old boy attends the Emergency Department (ED), following a blow to the face during a recent cricket match. A ball struck him directly on the left eye. He now has double vision on upward gaze, with difficulty tracking objects with this eye. He feels unwell and has vomited multiple times since the injury. There is no subconjunctival haemorrhage or epistaxis, and his visual acuity is normal. What is the single most likely diagnosis? (Select one answer from the options below.) ★★★★

A Acute myospasm of the superior rectus

B Orbital floor fracture

C Retrobulbar haemorrhage

D Transection of the abducens nerve

E Traumatic brain injury

11. A 35-year-old woman has pain behind their right eye, following repair of an orbital floor fracture. The right eye is proptosed and displays a fixed, dilated pupil. What is the single most likely cause of these findings? ★★★★

A Dislodged fixation screw

B Retrobulbar haemorrhage

C Subconjunctival bleed

D Traumatic optic neuropathy

E White-eyed blowout

12. A 36-year-old woman with a large submandibular abscess is scheduled for extra-oral drainage. An incision is made approximately 2 cm below, and parallel with, the body of the mandible on the right-hand side. Which single nerve is at greatest risk when carrying out this procedure? ★★★★

A Cervical branch of the facial nerve

B Lingual branch of the mandibular nerve

C Mandibular branch of the facial nerve

D Mental branch of the mandibular nerve

E Transverse cervical of the cervical plexus

13. A 26-year-old man attends the local Emergency Department, following an alleged assault. The maxillofacial dental core trainee is called to suture his 2-cm lip laceration. The tissue forceps used display the following symbol (see Figure 7.1), and the new healthcare assistant asks what the symbol means and what they should do with the item after use. (Select one answer from the options listed below.) ★★★★

A Class II medical device—wipe the surface and store for later use

B Class II medical device—report to management that this item is not suitable for use in this manner

C Do not reuse—dispose in a sharps bin

D Do not reuse—dispose in a clinical waste bin

E Send to the Central Sterilization Department for sterilization

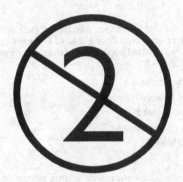

Figure 7.1
Permission to reproduce extracts from British Standards is granted by BSI Standards Limited (BSI). No other use of this material is permitted. British Standards can be obtained in PDF or hard copy formats from the BSI online shop: www.bsigroup.com/Shop

14. A 28-year-old woman had her lower left third molar extracted 6 months ago. The practice subsequently received a letter from her solicitor requesting access to the patient's clinical records, using a subject access request. Under which single law is this request legally valid? ★★★★

A Access to Health Records Act 1990

B Access to Medical Reports Act 1988

C Data Protection Act 2018

D Dentists Act 1984

E Freedom of Information Act 2000

ANSWERS

1. E ★   OHCD 6th ed. → p. 357

The INR should be checked ideally within 24 hours of the extraction. However, this is often difficult to arrange, and in patients with stable INR readings, up to 72 hours is deemed acceptable. Always check the local working environment policy, as variations may exist.

Like all extractions, local haemostatic methods are fundamental in controlling haemorrhage. The timing of the extraction and the day of the week should also be considered. Appointments early in the morning and towards the beginning of the week enable complications to be managed more effectively.

A therapeutic range of 2–4 is considered acceptable for patients undergoing routine dental surgery in primary care. Unstable INR, liver/renal impairment, significant alcohol intake, or the presence of a bleeding diathesis should prompt referral to secondary care, as should combinations of warfarin and antifibrinolytic drugs like aspirin and clopidogrel.

New oral anticoagulants (NOACs) are now available and patients require careful management, as monitoring is still being developed and immediate reversal is not currently possible. The cited recommended reading contains a flow chart for the management of patients requiring extractions who are taking NOACs.

Keywords: extraction, INR, maximum time.

→ Scottish Dental Clinical Effectiveness Programme. *Management of dental patients taking anticoagulants or antiplatelet drugs.* 2015. Available at: http://www.sdcep.org.uk/published-guidance/anticoagulants-and-antiplatelets/

2. A ★

A dry socket is thought to be caused when a blood clot fails to form over a socket; this can lead to bacterial ingress. Severe pain follows 2–4 days after an extraction. Predispositions include: smoking (vasoconstriction and neutrophil dysfunction affect healing), traumatic extractions, poor post-operative care (poor care can dislodge a blood clot), local anaesthetic (vasoconstriction), bone diseases, and use of the oral contraceptive pill in females. It is commonly treated with irrigation and placement of a sedative dressing such as Alveogyl® (iodine-free).

Osteomyelitis is an infection of the bone. It is associated with local infection (dental abscess) or trauma (fracture or extraction). Osteomyelitis can present radiographically with a moth-eaten appearance, after roughly 3 weeks of infection. As the extraction in the question was uncomplicated, it is unlikely to be the cause of the pain.

Small retained roots do not usually cause a problem, unless they are infected, but again in this case, the extraction went as planned, with no fractured apices.

Osteonecrosis of the jaw can have a variety of causes (medication-related and radiotherapy-induced). Patients at risk of this often have underlying medical conditions (bone disease or cancer). The patient in the question is fit and well.

Keywords: smoking, extraction, 3 days ago, lower molar.

3. E ★

Bisphosphonates are a group of drugs used in the management of several diseases, including the skeletal manifestations of malignancy. These agents serve to reduce osteoclastic activity and, as such, influence bone healing following dental procedures, most notably dental extractions. This can result in exposed necrotic bone that is difficult to manage—medication-related osteonecrosis of the jaw (MRONJ).

Intravenous (IV) bisphosphonates would generally be classified as high risk for MRONJ, whilst oral bisphosphonates used for <3 years are generally classified as low risk. Bisphosphonates have been shown to remain inactive within bone for many years following cessation of treatment and, as such, drug holidays confer no apparent benefit.

National guidance regarding bisphosphonate use is limited, and local policies may vary. However, a general consensus regarding high-risk patients would indicate referral to, or advice from, a specialist department to be the most pragmatic management strategy. It would not be unreasonable for a competent practitioner to atraumatically extract the tooth in practice, assuming they have fully informed consent and are able to manage complications appropriately. Denosumab (monoclonal antibody) is an alternative drug used to treat osteoporosis, which has also been implicated in MRONJ.

Despite no high-quality evidence, prophylactic antibiotic cover is often given to high-risk patients to reduce the risk of infection; no current consensus is universally agreed upon.

Keywords: extraction, IV zoledronic acid, denosumab.

→ Ruggiero SL, Dodson TB, Fantasia J, et al. American Association of Oral and Maxillofacial Surgeons position paper on medication-related osteonecrosis of the jaw—2014 update. *Journal of Oral and Maxillofacial Surgery.* 2014;**72**:1938–56.

4. B ★   OHCD 6th ed. → p. 392

These account for approximately 20% of all cysts and are common in the posterior mandible of adolescents. Developing from the reduced enamel epithelium, they are associated with the amelodentinal junction of unerupted teeth. These cysts are typically lined by thin, non-keratinized squamous epithelium. All of the answers can be associated with unerupted or partially erupted teeth but are less common. Pindborg tumours contain amyloid matrix that can calcify and are described as having a driven snow appearance. Odontogenic keratocysts are benign odontogenic tumours that are often multilocular and develop from the rests of Serres. They generally present in the posterior mandible and show marked anteroposterior expansion. Odontogenic myxoma are rare and benign neoplasms containing abundant myxoid extracellular matrix. They are described as soap bubble/honeycomb appearance when visualized radiographically. Paradental cysts usually occur in the mandible but are associated with partially erupted wisdom teeth.

Keywords: unilocular lesion, surrounding the crown, unerupted, third molar.

5. E ★★

Tearing of the palatal mucosa adjacent to an upper wisdom tooth during an extraction is commonly associated with fracture of the maxillary tuberosity. As such, this should be factored into any discussion when obtaining informed consent.

Mobility of the tuberosity or an audible crack are additional signs frequently detected, as mucosal tears can occur independently. Careful assessment of the preoperative radiograph can help reduce the risk of a tuberosity fracture occurring. Loss of the lamina dura, dense trabeculation, or unfavourable root morphology could all predispose to tuberosity fractures. Lone-standing molars often pose the greatest risk.

Management of the fracture is variable and can depend upon the status of the tooth being extracted. Asymptomatic molars with no associated pathology could be splinted to adjacent teeth prior to rearranging surgical removal following bony healing. Small tuberosity fractures or unrestorable teeth with evident pathology would likely still warrant removal. However, assessment of the size of the bone fragment and soft tissue defect is important.

A crown fracture or root fracture can be ruled out because the tooth is intact. An oroantral communication can result from a tuberosity fracture, but this diagnosis usually would not be made unless a hole is visualized following extraction or the patient returns with symptoms. If a communication is long-standing and becomes epithelialized, then it would be classified as a fistula.

Keywords: upper wisdom tooth, palatal tear, segment, mobile.

6. B ★★   OHCD 6th ed. → p. 470

The clinical history and examination suggest a mandibular fracture may have occurred. DPTs provide excellent views of the majority of the mandible and are likely to be the first radiograph indicated. It is possible for a fracture to be missed using a single film only, as the image is a two-dimensional representation of a three-dimensional structure. Therefore, a second parallax view (from a different position—ideally perpendicular) can identify fractures missed on single radiographs or yield more information about them.

A PA mandible (PA jaws) enables good visualization of the mandible, from the condylar head to the body. Generally, these are the second radiographs to be taken.

A standard occipitomental view is sometimes taken when fractures of the coronoid process are suspected, and high condylar neck fractures are often better visualized using a reverse Towne's radiograph.

Note: oral pantomogram (OPG) is a term that can be used interchangeably with dental panoramic tomogram (DPT).

Keywords: mandible, fractures, radiographs.

7. A ★★★

The symptoms would indicate an oroantral communication or a fistula is present. These can often resolve, following careful non-surgical management and antibiotic use. However, should surgical treatment be required, the buccally advanced flap would be the most appropriate.

This involves creating a parallel or near parallel three-sided flap that is advanced across the defect, following excision of any epithelium lining within the fistula. Scoring the periosteal surface of the flap enables greater flexibility, although great care must be exercised when making these incisions. Vertical mattress sutures are recommended for primary closure. A reduction in sulcus depth is one disadvantage of this approach, which can pose problems with denture provision in the future. Buccal fat pad can also be used to repair larger defects.

Palatal rotation flaps are an acceptable alternative [see Figure 7.2 which shows a schematic of a buccal advancement flap (right) and a schematic of palatal rotation flap (left)]. However, a large area of palate remains exposed to heal by secondary intention, which often contraindicates its use, especially in smokers. Smoking cessation is a fundamental component to promoting wound healing with this complication.

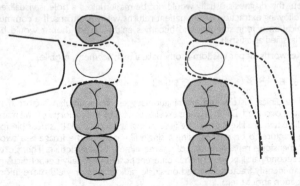

Figure 7.2

The remaining three options are flap techniques generally used for small dento-alveolar procedures.

Keywords: extraction, UR6, unable to smoke, salty discharge.

→ Scott P, Fabbroni G, Mitchell D. The buccal fat pad in the closure of oro-antral communications: an illustrated guide. *Dental Update*. 2004;**31**:363–6.

8. A ★★★

The clinical situation above requires immediate emergency management. Inability to swallow saliva with marked trismus represents an airway risk, and an anaesthetist is required to assess the patient prior to surgical management. This is a time-critical emergency, as severe swellings of this kind can progress quickly, with loss of airway patency. An anaesthetist can provide significant information regarding the severity of symptoms and the urgency of treatment. They can also assess the patient prior to general anaesthesia. Intravenous steroids and antibiotics can be given to reduce the swelling and bacterial load, but the effects are delayed. Awake, fibre-optic intubation may be required if the swelling is extensive and conventional intubation methods are unachievable.

Keywords: large facial swelling, struggling to swallow, floor of the mouth raised and firm.

9. E ★★★★

The trochlear nerve (CN IV) carries efferent nerve fibres to the superior oblique muscle. The muscle serves to depress and abduct the eyeball and is the only extra-ocular muscle supplied by the trochlear nerve. CN IV is generally the most sensitive nerve to any insult, as it is the only cranial nerve to emerge from the dorsal aspect of the brainstem and has the longest intracranial course.

On examination, the patient would likely report blurred vision when looking straight down and would have difficulty looking down and out on the affected side. At rest, the eye may appear elevated and intorted, as the stabilizing action of the superior oblique muscle against the superior rectus is missing. These patients would often compensate with a head tilt or chin tuck to the contralateral side to improve vision.

Damage to the abducens nerve would result in loss of function of the lateral rectus muscle, and patients would be unable to look laterally from the affected eye. Optic nerve damage would create visual field disturbances, amongst other potential problems.

Damage to the oculomotor nerve, which supplies the remaining four extra-ocular muscles and the levator palpebrae superioris, would result in drooping of the eyelid and a fixed, dilated pupil which would fail to accommodate normally, with the eye gazing 'down and out'. Parasympathetic fibres from the ciliary ganglion control dilation of the pupils and accommodation and can be an early sign of oculomotor nerve damage. A good mnemonic is SO4 (superior oblique CN IV) LR6 (lateral rectus CN VI).

Keywords: corrected by tilting head ('head tilt/chin tuck'), elevated, double vision on looking straight down.

10. B ★★★★   OHCD 6th ed. → p. 472

This clinical presentation in a young patient is likely to indicate an orbital floor fracture and is commonly referred to as a 'white-eyed blowout'. This occurs when soft tissue and muscle of the inferior rectus become trapped within the orbital floor fracture, following a direct blow to the eye.

Orbital floor fractures in children can often be more difficult to diagnose due to the apparent absence of symptoms. The elastic nature of bone in young patients can result in the orbital floor acting as a 'trap door', essentially trapping the inferior rectus muscle following injury. This can result in limitation of upward and downward gaze in the affected eye. Oculocardiac/oculovagal reflex can often obfuscate the diagnosis and lead to a delay in treatment.

Ophthalmological assessment and CT scanning are appropriate investigations prior to surgical correction of the fracture, with release of the entrapped soft tissues. Delay in treatment can have serious ramifications for the patient, and it is suggested that surgical treatment occurs within 48 hours of injury to avoid muscle ischaemia. All eye and facial trauma in children should be approached with a high index of suspicion due to the severity of complications.

Acute myospasm of the superior rectus is an unlikely diagnosis but might cause difficulties looking up. Nausea and vomiting would discount this diagnosis, unless combined with a traumatic brain injury. A traumatic brain injury on its own would generally not present with these specific eye signs. The abducens nerve controls the lateral rectus and so would present with problems affecting the lateral movements of the eye.

Keywords: 13 years old, direct blow to the eye, double vision on upward gaze, no subconjunctival haemorrhage.

→ Mehanna P, Mehanna D, Cronin A. White-eyed blowout fracture: another look. *Emergency Medicine Australasia.* 2009;**21**:229–32.

11. B ★★★★   OHCD 6th ed. → p. 472

The signs and symptoms described most likely indicate a retrobulbar haemorrhage, which is one of the few true maxillofacial emergencies. Immediate surgical management with a lateral canthotomy is the treatment of choice. However, these can often take a short amount of time to arrange. As a junior dentist, immediate escalation to senior colleagues and arrangement of medical management using mannitol, acetazolamide, and a steroid (such as dexamethasone) will reduce the swelling in the region and delay the progression of symptoms, thus improving the prognosis. These drugs serve to decrease intravascular and intraocular pressure, thus 'buying time' prior to surgery and improving the prognosis post-surgery. The protocol for medical management can vary by region, and the clinician should familiarize themselves with local trust policy early on in a placement.

A dislodged fixation screw is unlikely at this time point if there was good stability at placement and would not cause these symptoms.

Subconjunctival haemorrhage is a clinical finding indicative of trauma and is not a diagnosis. If the posterior border cannot be seen, then it is suggestive of a fracture, with bleeding coming from the ruptured periosteum.

A traumatic optic neuropathy (TON) is where there is direct or indirect damage to the optic nerve. The patient would have loss of vision and pain, but the eye would not be tense and proptosed. A retrobulbar haemorrhage should be ruled out if a TON is suspected.

A white-eyed blowout is where the orbital floor has fractured and recoiled, trapping the avulsed contents of the eye. This is generally more of a concern in younger patients where the bone is more flexible. If not managed rapidly, the trapped tissue and muscle can become ischaemic, leading to long-term diplopia. Patients would present with diplopia, restricted upward gaze, and potentially a sunken eye. Patients can also have an oculocardiac/oculovagal reflex, in which upward gaze causes nausea, bradycardia, and potentially asystole!

Keywords: pain, behind, eye, proptosed, fixed and dilated pupil.

→ Timlin H, Manisali M, Verity D, Uddin J, Osborne S. *Traumatic orbital emergencies*. Focus—Royal College of Ophthalmologists. 2015. Available at: http://www.rcophth.ac.uk/standards-publications-research/ focus-articles/

12. C ★★★★

Following a superficial incision, blunt dissection through the platysma is carried out prior to navigating superiorly up to the abscess cavity. The lingual border of the mandible is a useful surgical landmark to help locate the abscess.

The mandibular branch of the facial nerve is most at risk with this approach. Stimulation of the nerve during the procedure would often result, with visible contraction of the muscles surrounding the chin. The cervical branch of the facial nerve runs lower down and should not be near the incision site.

The mental nerve usually emerges between the roots of the mandibular first and second premolar teeth, in line with the infraorbital nerve, the supra-orbital nerve, and the pupils and would not be at risk.

The lingual nerve branches off the posterior trunk of the mandibular nerve. It is located medial to the ramus of the mandible, splitting from the main trunk of the mandibular nerve just before it enters the mandible. It runs along the lingual aspect of the body of the mandible but should not be at risk of damage, as the abscess cavity will be explored by blunt subperiosteal dissection, and the nerve should be superficial to this.

The transverse cervical plexus arises deep to the sternocleidomastoid muscle and supplies sensation to the skin on the front of the neck. They are too far posterior from where the surgical incision is made to be harmed. Figure 7.3a shows the facial nerve and its branches in the face. The position of the parotid gland is indicated. Figure 7.3b shows cutaneous innervation of the head and neck and the cutaneous branches of the nerves.

Keywords: extra-oral, submandibular.

13. C ★★★★   OHCD 6th ed. → p. 744

The symbol in Figure 7.1 indicates that the medical device is 'single use' and not fit to be reused on subsequent patients. Additionally, as the instrument has sharp tips, it should be disposed of in the sharps bin, and not the clinical waste. Guidance from the Medicines and Healthcare Products Regulatory Agency in 2013 highlights the important legal and regulatory implications surrounding items of single use, which refers to a number of key legal documents, including the *Medical Devices regulations 2002, Health and safety at work Act etc. 1974*, and the *Consumer Protection Act 1987*, to name a few.

Patient safety is paramount in all dental surgeries and hospitals. Throughout the past century, advances in medical and biological research have highlighted a potential risk of persistent contamination from a number of dental devices. As a result, in the United Kingdom, a wide array of instruments and devices are no longer fit to be reused on different patients, e.g. matrix bands, endodontic files, etc. Severe consequences for both patients and practitioners can result if these regulations are not adhered to. It would also be unethical and unprofessional to knowingly put patients at risk and bring the profession into disrepute with poor infection control standards.

There are three classes of medical devices, and this relates to the complexity of the device and the stringency of regulation the device needs. This is unrelated to the symbol shown.

Keywords: forceps, (symbol shown).

→ Medicines and Healthcare Products Regulatory Agency (MHRA). *Single-use medical devices: implications and consequences of reuse.* 2018. Available at: https://www.gov.uk/government/uploads/system/uploads/attachment_data/file/403442/Single-use_medical_devices__implications_and_consequences_of_reuse.pdf

14. C ★★★★   OHCD 6th ed. → p. 732

Patients are able to access their own medical records under the Data Protection Act 2018. A 'Subject Access Request' can be submitted to request health records. Third-party data or data that may cause harm to the patient on release could be redacted, if deemed necessary. Small administration fees used to be able to be charged under the old Data Protection Act of 1998, but with the updated General Data Protection

(a)

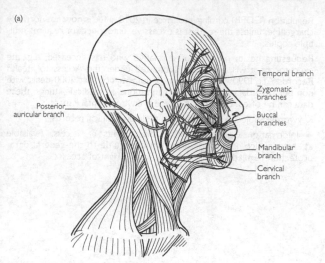

Figure 7.3a The facial nerve and its branches in the face. The position of the parotid gland is indicated.

Reproduced from Atkinson Martin E, *Anatomy for dental students*, figure 23.12, page 236, Copyright (2013) by permission of Oxford University Press.

(b)

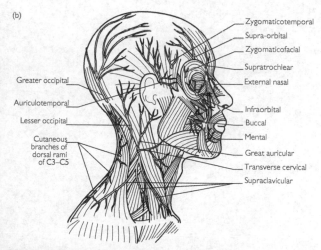

Figure 7.3b Cutaneous innervation of the head and neck and cutaneous branches of the nerves.

Reproduced from Atkinson Martin E, *Anatomy for dental students*, figure 23.13, page 238, Copyright (2013) by permission of Oxford University Press.

Regulation (GDPR) coming into force in 2018, a fee is now not normally chargeable, unless the request is excessive, unfounded, or requires multiple copies.

Requesting health records for a relative who has deceased, e.g. the executor of a will, would be submitted under the Access to Health Records Act 1990. The Freedom of Information Act 2000 deals with non-personal data from public organizations. In medical settings, these data can be of concern to patients, e.g. environmental issues.

Keywords: Subject Access Request, their own clinical records.

→ Information Commissioner's Office. *Rights of access*. Available at: https://ico.org.uk/for-organisations/guide-to-the-general-data-protection-regulation-gdpr/individual-rights/right-of-access/

Oral medicine and oral pathology

Raheel Aftab

'It doesn't look like anything sinister, but we need to take a look under the microscope just to be sure.'

The mouth has often been looked at as a window into the body, and this is no truer than in oral medicine. The oral mucosa is a highly adapted and robust tissue, which, at the same time, can be very susceptible to changes in homeostasis. Dysregulation of the immune system, alterations in cellular signalling pathways, or insult from exogenous stimuli can lead to an array of weird and wonderful oral lesions.

Clinicians today are likely to see changes to the oral mucosa on a regular basis—from common ulcers, bony lumps, or white patches to more exotic pigmented lesions or unusual lumps. It is therefore vital to have good basic knowledge of common conditions and be able to identify lesions that need urgent referral and treatment. It is important to take a thorough medical history, as many oral symptoms can be associated with systemic conditions or changes in medication. A temporal link can be a good indicator of causation from medication changes.

Having a strategic method of constructing a list of differential diagnoses, such as the surgical sieve, can be a great aide-memoire to ensure all the pertinent questions and investigations have been completed. However, it must be noted that many conditions cannot be accurately diagnosed without histological examination, and therefore, referral for specialist input is commonplace.

Oral medicine can be a tricky discipline, fraught with challenging patients to manage, particularly those with chronic conditions. Conversely, the diagnostic challenges make for a thoroughly rewarding and stimulating discipline. The questions in this chapter will test your knowledge of disease symptoms, links to medical conditions, and patient management.

Key topics include:

- Patient assessment and diagnosis
- Investigations
- Basic histology
- Infections (bacterial, viral, and fungal)
- Ulcers
- Soft tissue swelling
- Bony lumps
- Systemic conditions
- White, red, pigmented, and mixed patches
- Oral cancer
- Pharmacology.

QUESTIONS

1. A 45-year-old woman has a sore tongue. She has red atrophic areas on the dorsum and lateral border of the tongue with demarcated white borders (see Figure 8.1) (see Colour Plate section). She says that the appearance has been inconsistent over time. What is the single most likely diagnosis? ★

A Ankyloglossia

B Geographic tongue

C Glossodynia

D Macroglossia

E Median rhomboid glossitis

2. A 33-year-old woman has recent-onset pain from her jaw. She has recently become a new mother. The pain radiates towards her ear and is worse in the mornings. Her temporomandibular joint (TMJ) clicks on opening and closing but is unrestricted and causes no discomfort. Pain is elicited on palpation of the masseter muscles. What is the single most appropriate first-line treatment? ★

A Prescribe non-steroidal anti-inflammatory drugs

B Provide a soft occlusal splint

C Reassure and advise a soft diet with warm compresses

D Refer for acupuncture

E Refer for arthrocentesis

3. A fit and well 14-year-old adolescent girl has a well-circumscribed brown, pigmented area on her lower lip. She says that it is unchanged since she noticed it 2 years ago. Clinically, it is an isolated lesion, flush with the labial mucosa, and measuring 3 × 2 mm in size. What is the single most likely diagnosis? ★

A Amalgam tattoo

B Malignant melanoma

C Melanotic macule

D Pigmentation due to Peutz–Jeghers syndrome

E Pigmented naevus

4. A 60-year-old man attends a primary care dental practice with an ulcer on the ventral surface of his tongue for 4 weeks. The ulcer bleeds and causes discomfort when touched. He has a 35-pack year smoking history. He has sharp, fractured teeth on the same side as the lesion. What is the single most appropriate management? ★

A In-house incisional biopsy

B Non-urgent referral to the local Ear, Nose, and Throat (ENT) Unit

C Smooth the edges of the sharp teeth

D Take clinical photographs and monitor

E Urgent referral to the local Head and Neck Maxillofacial Unit

5. A 44-year-old woman has painless white lesions bilaterally on her buccal mucosa, which have been present for 4 months (see Figure 8.2) (see Colour Plate section). She recently had a patchy rash on her shins, which has resolved. She has multiple amalgam fillings in the upper right and lower right permanent molars. What is the single most likely diagnosis? ★

A Chronic hyperplastic candidiasis (CHC)

B Lichenoid reaction

C Oral lichen planus

D Squamous cell carcinoma

E White sponge naevus (WSN)

6. A medically fit and well 25-year-old woman has recurrent soreness under her tongue. She has approximately 20 ulcers, each of which is a couple of millimetres in diameter on the floor of her mouth. What is the single most likely diagnosis? ★

A Crohn's disease

B Herpetiform recurrent aphthous stomatitis (RAS)

C Major RAS

D Minor RAS

E Traumatic ulcer

7. A 60-year-old man has a red patch limited to the denture-bearing area of his maxilla. His dentures have been recently remade and are well fitting. A provisional diagnosis of chronic erythematous candidiasis is made. However, he has atrial fibrillation and is taking warfarin. What is the single most appropriate management? ★

A Reinforce denture hygiene and prescribe amphotericin tablets

B Reinforce denture hygiene and prescribe chloramphenicol ointment

C Reinforce denture hygiene and prescribe chlorhexidine gel

D Reinforce denture hygiene and prescribe miconazole oral gel

E Reinforce denture hygiene and prescribe nystatin suspension

8. A 3-year-old girl has bloody crusty lips, widespread oral ulceration, and a temperature of 38.5°C. Her mother reports that the condition has lasted for over 3 weeks and says that she is struggling to eat. What is the single most appropriate management? ★ ★

A Prescribe aciclovir tablets

B Prescribe benzydamine hydrochloride mouthwash

C Prescribe chlorhexidine gluconate mouthwash

D Reassure the mother and monitor

E Refer for a specialist's opinion

9. A 28-year-old woman presents with this intraoral appearance (see Figure 8.3) (see Colour Plate section). She says that her previous dentist has suggested avoiding cinnamon in her diet. She has no systemic symptoms, but her lower lip is enlarged. What is the single most likely diagnosis? ★ ★

A Coeliac disease

B Crohn's disease

C Linea alba

D Orofacial granulomatosis (OFG)

E Ulcerative colitis

10. A 79-year-old man has sore, crusted skin lesions at the corner of his mouth. He wears very old complete dentures, which have a freeway space of 12 mm. Swab results indicate mixed *Candida albicans* and *Staphylococcus aureus* infection, and blood tests exclude haematinic deficiencies. Which is the single most appropriate management? ★★

A Prescribe fusidic acid cream, and arrange for new dentures to be made with a decreased occlusal vertical dimension (OVD)

B Prescribe fusidic acid cream, and arrange for new dentures to be made with an increased OVD

C Prescribe miconazole cream, and arrange for new dentures to be made with a decreased OVD

D Prescribe miconazole cream, and arrange for new dentures to be made with an increased OVD

E Prescribe nystatin suspension, and arrange for new dentures to be made with an increased OVD

11. A 57-year-old woman has a dry mouth and dry eyes. Recent blood tests confirm anti-Ro and anti-La autoantibodies, and a labial gland biopsy demonstrates multiple dense foci of lymphocytic infiltrate in a 4 mm² area. She is otherwise fit and well, with no other medical conditions. What is the single most likely diagnosis? ★★

A Chronic bacterial sialadenitis

B Primary Sjögren's syndrome

C Sarcoidosis

D Sicca syndrome

E Systemic lupus erythematosus (SLE)

12. A 39-year-old man attends the Maxillofacial Department with sweating on eating and flushing of the skin. He had a pleomorphic adenoma surgically removed from his right parotid approximately 12 weeks ago. What is the single most likely diagnosis? ★★

A Frey's syndrome

B Graves' disease

C Horner's syndrome

D Melkersson–Rosenthal syndrome

E Sicca syndrome

13. A 50-year-old woman has right-sided jaw pain. She describes it as a recurrent, excruciating shooting 'electric shock'-like pain of rapid onset and short duration. What is the single most likely preliminary diagnosis? ★★

A Atypical facial pain

B Glossopharyngeal neuralgia

C Irreversible pulpitis

D Reversible pulpitis

E Trigeminal neuralgia

14. A 73-year-old man has been suffering with ongoing pain for the past 3 months. He has severe, sudden-onset unilateral head-aches, which becomes worse when chewing. He has a temperature of 38.6°C. The area is tender to touch, and the pulse from the side of the head on the affected side is not detectable. Which is the single most likely diagnosis? ★★★

A Atypical facial pain

B Cluster headache

C Myofascial pain

D Temporal arteritis

E Trigeminal neuralgia

15. A 38-year-old man has diffuse bilateral white lesions on his buccal mucosa and floor of his mouth. The lesions are asymp-tomatic but have a rough texture. He has never smoked and says he has had the lesions since 12 years of age. What is the single most likely diagnosis? ★★★

A Frictional keratosis

B Leukoedema

C Lichen planus

D Stomatitis nicotina

E White sponge naevus

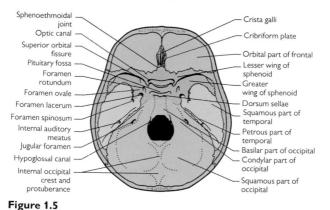

Figure 1.5

Reproduced from Atkinson Martin E, *Anatomy for dental students*, figure 22.5, page 213, Copyright (2013) by permission of Oxford University Press.

(a)

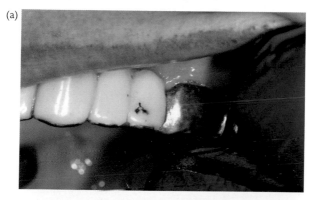

(b)

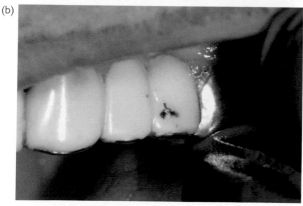

Figure 6.2a

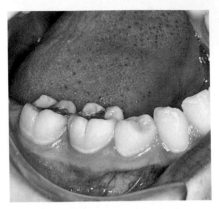

Figure 6.3
Reproduced from Kidd, E. *Essentials of Dental Caries* (3rd Ed). Figure 1.4a, page 6, Oxford University Press. Oxford. 2016 by permission of Oxford University Press.

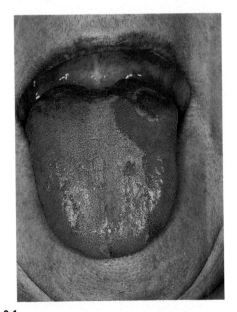

Figure 8.1
Reproduced from Field E.A. & Longman W.R., *Tyldesley's Oral Medicine*, 5th Edition, Figure 6.8, page 70, Copyright (2003), by permission of Oxford University Press.

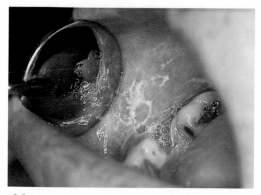

Figure 8.2

Reproduced from Field E.A. & Longman W.R., *Tyldesley's Oral Medicine*, 5th Edition, Figure 11.2, page 127, Copyright (2003), by permission of Oxford University Press.

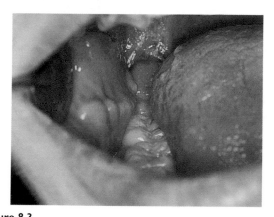

Figure 8.3

Reproduced from Field E.A. & Longman W.R., *Tyldesley's Oral Medicine*, 5th Edition, Figure 12.4, pg 146, Copyright (2003), by permission of Oxford University Press.

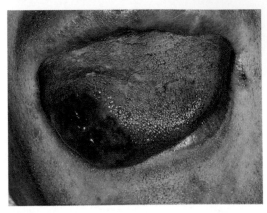

Figure 8.4
Reproduced from Field E.A. & Longman W.R., *Tyldesley's Oral Medicine*, 5th Edition, Figure 4.2, page 33, (2003), Copyright (2003), by permission of Oxford University Press.

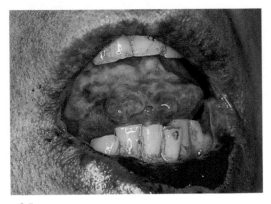

Figure 8.5
Reproduced from Field E.A. & Longman W.R., *Tyldesley's Oral Medicine*, 5th Edition, Figure 11.7, page 131, Copyright (2003), by permission of Oxford University Press.

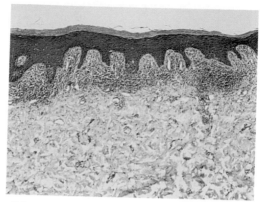

Figure 8.6
Reproduced from Soames J.V. and Southam J.C., *Oral Pathology*, 4th Edition, Figure 9.21, page 129, Copyright (2005), by permission of Oxford University Press.

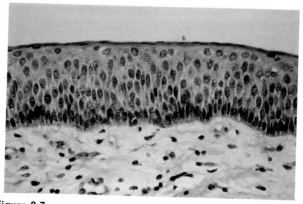

Figure 8.7
Reproduced from Soames J.V. and Southam J.C., *Oral Pathology*, 4th Edition, Figure 6.24, p79 Copyright (2005), by permission of Oxford University Press.

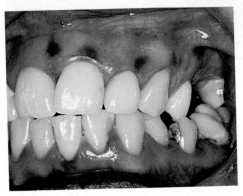

Figure 8.8
Reproduced from Robinson M et al, *Soames' and Southam's Oral Pathology*, Fifth edition, figure 2.58a, page 50, Copyright (2018), by permission of Oxford University Press.

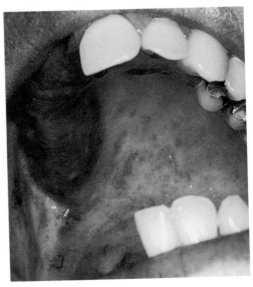

Figure 8.9
Reproduced from Field E.A. & Longman W.R., *Tyldesley's Oral Medicine*, 5th Edition, Figure 4.5, pg 39, Copyright (2003), by permission of Oxford University Press.

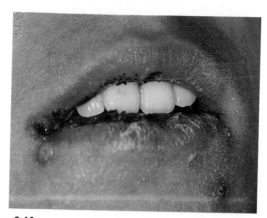

Figure 8.10

Reproduced from Field E.A. & Longman W.R., *Tyldesley's Oral Medicine*, 5th Edition, Figure 4.7, pg 41, Copyright (2003), by permission of Oxford University Press.

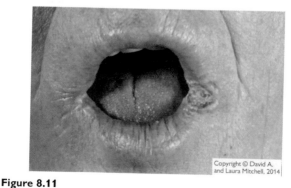

Figure 8.11

Reproduced from Mitchell D, Mitchell L, *Oxford Handbook Clinical Dentistry*, 6th Edition, Figure 10.1, Page 415, (2014) by permission of Oxford University Press.

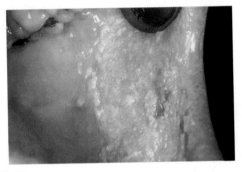

Figure 8.12
Reproduced from Soames J.V. and Southam J.C., *Oral Pathology*, 4th Edition, Figure 9.1, p120 Copyright (2005), by permission of Oxford University Press.

16. A 53-year-old woman re-attends with unilateral, pressure-like pain in the maxilla, radiating towards the ear and associated with an itching sensation. She had a routine extraction of the upper right second premolar 6 weeks ago, followed by root canal treatment of the heavily filled adjacent first molar 3 weeks later. On both occasions, pain initially settled but subsequently returned. What is the single most likely diagnosis? ★ ★ ★

A Atypical facial pain (AFP)

B Atypical odontalgia (AO) (phantom tooth pain)

C Burning mouth syndrome (oral dysaesthesia)

D Temporomandibular dysfunction (TMD)

E Trigeminal neuralgia

17. A fit and healthy 27-year-old man is concerned about a lesion on his tongue (see Figure 8.4) (see Colour Plate section). He does not report any other lesions anywhere else. The lesion is non-tender, and no other oral lesions are seen, but cervical lymphadenopathy is detectable. He is a non-smoker. A blood test is requested to aid diagnosis for the suspected lesion. What is the single most likely provisional diagnosis? ★ ★ ★ ★

A Major recurrent aphthous stomatitis

B Primary syphilitic chancre

C Squamous cell carcinoma

D Traumatic ulcer

E Tuberculosis

18. A 62-year-old woman has a recurrent swelling under her tongue during mealtimes. She has a mobile, unilateral, firm submandibular swelling. She is allergic to iodine. Which is the single most appropriate *definitive* investigation? ★ ★ ★ ★

A Computed tomography of the mandible

B Fine-needle aspiration

C Magnetic resonance imaging of the mandible

D Sialography

E Standard true lower occlusal radiograph

19. A 55-year-old man has very painful, recurrent intraoral ulcerations that have been ongoing for the past 6 months (see Figure 8.5) (see Colour Plate section). He says that the ulceration is preceded by very short-lived blisters. He also has skin lesions and an upper layer of the skin shears with lateral pressure. To complement conventional histology, direct immunofluorescence analysis of a recent biopsy is requested. What is the single most likely result on this biopsy? ★ ★ ★ ★

A negative result

B Granular immunoglobulin A (IgA) deposits and C3 at dermal papillae

C Intercellular immunoglobulin G (IgG) and C3

D Linear IgA and C3 at the basement membrane

E Linear IgG and C3 at the basement membrane

20. A 65-year-old man attends, complaining of a red sore tongue. He also reports backache and ongoing fatigue for the past 3 months. He had radiotherapy for an extramedullary plasmacytoma in his upper respiratory tract 4 years previously. Blood tests from his general medical practitioner confirm hypercalcaemia, normocytic and normochromic anaemia, and elevated immunoglobulins. What is the single most likely diagnosis? ★ ★ ★ ★

A Chondrosarcoma

B Langerhans cell histiocytosis X

C Metastatic squamous cell carcinoma

D Multiple myeloma

E Paget's disease of bone

21. A 51-year-old woman has had a biopsy of a white patch from the buccal gingivae. The pathologist has included the slides visible in Figure 8.6 (see Colour Plate section). What is the single most likely diagnosis? ★ ★ ★ ★

A Chronic hyperplastic candidiasis

B Discoid lupus erythematosus (DLE)

C Frictional keratosis

D Lichen planus

E Mucous membrane pemphigoid (MMP)

22. A 24-year-old man who is diagnosed with moderate autistic spectrum disorder has bleeding swollen gums, which his carers have been unable to brush because they are sore. He appears lethargic and only eats crisps. Early loss of periodontal attachment is present, and generalized hyperplastic gingivae are noted. His full blood count (FBC) shows a white blood cell (WBC) count of 7.4×10^9/L. The patient takes melatonin. What is the single most likely diagnosis? ★ ★ ★ ★

A Acute lymphoblastic leukaemia (ALL)

B Acute necrotizing ulcerative gingivitis (ANUG)

C Drug-induced gingival overgrowth (DIGO)

D Pyogenic granuloma

E Vitamin C deficiency

23. A 19-year-old man recently had his unerupted LR8 surgically extracted. A cyst is also removed that is associated with the lateral aspect of the unerupted crown. Histopathology shows a regular cyst lining, consisting of stratified squamous epithelium. The basal cells are palisaded columnar cells which show high levels of mitotic figures. Parakeratinization is noted on the surface epithelial cells. The cyst contents were pale, with a low protein content consisting mainly of albumin. A copy of the slide is available in Figure 8.7 (see Colour Plate section). What is the single most likely diagnosis? ★ ★ ★ ★

A Dentigerous cyst

B Eruption cyst

C Lateral periodontal cyst

D Odontogenic keratocyst

E Radicular cyst

24. A 62-year-old man attends for a review of his Behçet's disease, following a recent episode of uveitis. Upon arrival, he trips on some torn carpet in the entrance of your practice and is taken by ambulance to Accident and Emergency after losing consciousness briefly. The fall results in a broken jaw, and the patient is admitted to hospital for 2 days and requires 4 weeks off work. To which single organization should this incident be reported? ★ ★ ★ ★

A Care Quality Commission

B Dental Indemnity Firm

C Environment Agency

D General Dental Council

E Health and Safety Executive

ANSWERS

1. B ★ OHCD 6th ed. → p. 430

Geographic tongue (synonyms: benign migratory glossitis or erythema migrans) is an inflammatory condition of unknown aetiology. This scenario is typical of a patient presenting with this condition, with its name explaining the classical clinical appearance of the lesions. The condition can be associated with psoriasis. The condition may be symptomatic, and analgesic mouthwashes may help relieve the pain in some cases.

Ankyloglossia, also known as tongue tie, is a developmental anomaly which may decrease the mobility of the tongue tip and is caused by an unusually short and thick lingual frenulum.

Macroglossia is the term given to an enlarged tongue, which may have a congenital or an acquired component. It has been reported in acromegaly and Down's syndrome.

Glossodynia, also known as burning mouth syndrome/oral dysaesthesia, may be accompanied by glossitis, but classically the tongue appears normal. It can be caused by anaemia, lichen planus, and *Candida* infections. In cases where there is no precipitating factor, the condition may be psychogenic in origin. The history given in this scenario is not typical of glossodynia.

Median rhomboid glossitis is a form of chronic atrophic candidiasis affecting the dorsum of the tongue, commonly anterior to the circumvallate papillae. Clinically, a single and non-migratory area of depapillation is present, and the condition is more common in those using inhaled steroids.

Keywords: sore tongue, atrophic, white borders, inconsistent.

2. C ★ OHCD 6th ed. → pp. 458–60

This presentation is indicative of myofascial pain. The muscles are often tender, and headaches can be an associated factor. Sometimes, limitation of mouth opening may be a problem. Explain the likely pathogenesis (often a parafunctional habit, potentially related to stress—in this case, the patient is a new mother), and provide reassurance that the condition is often self-limiting. Jaw rest, including eating a soft diet, will reduce the workload for the masticatory muscles and should help reduce the symptoms. This can be combined with warm compresses, which promote blood flow to the region. Simple over-the-counter analgesics, such as ibuprofen, may be advised in the short term if safe to do so.

Occlusal splints or appliances can help manage TMDs but are usually only considered if the patient's problems persist.

Arthrocentesis is not required in this case. The TMJ may click in some individuals. However, if there is no discomfort and opening is not significantly limited, then this should only be documented and monitored.

Acupuncture is not a first-line treatment for myofascial pain and is reserved for cases of localized, unresponsive myalgia.

Keywords: new mother, worse in morning, pain on palpation of muscles.

→ Durham J, Aggarwal V, Davies SJ, et al.; Royal College of Surgeons. *Temporomandibular Disorders (TMDs): an update and management guidance for primary care from the UK Specialist Interest Group in Orofacial Pain and TMDs (USOT)*. 2013. Available at: http://www.rcseng.ac.uk

3. C ★   OHCD 6th ed. → p. 424

Melanotic macules are caused by a localized, benign increase in melanin by basal melanocytes. They are commonly found on the lips and are <1 cm in size. See Figure 8.8 (see Colour Plate section) which shows idiopathic oral melanotic macules.

Malignant melanomas are aggressive carcinomas but rarely affect the oral mucosa. Orally, they are most commonly found on the hard palate or the maxillary gingivae. Borders are poorly defined; the lesion generally grows in size, and it can be ulcerated or bleeding. They typically present in patients above the age of 30.

Amalgam tattoos can occur if fractured amalgam is left submucosally during surgical procedures. They are most likely to be found on the gingivae, appearing as blue/grey lesions and sometimes detectable on radiographs.

Mucosal pigmentation around the oral cavity is characteristic of Peutz–Jeghers syndrome; multiple small macules are present circumorally. The condition is hereditary and is associated with intestinal polyps, which have a low chance of malignant change.

Pigmented naevi look very similar to melanotic macules. However, they are more commonly found on the palate or buccal mucosa, with the average age of presentation being around 30. Naevi tend to have a less well-defined border than melanotic macules and are often slightly raised.

It is very difficult to differentiate between melanotic macules, melanomas, and naevi clinically, and a definitive diagnosis can only be made with a biopsy.

Keywords: circumscribed, brown, unchanged, isolated, flush.

4. E ★   OHCD 6th ed. → p. 428

This clinical description suggests a squamous cell carcinoma (SCC). In this scenario, the following should raise suspicion and warrant an urgent referral to the local Head and Neck Unit:

- Use or consumption of cigarettes/betel-nut/alcohol (alcohol and cigarettes have a synergistic relationship)
- Rolled margins of ulcer
- Bleeding ulcer
- Unexplained ulcer persisting for longer than 3 weeks

- Ulcers on the floor of the mouth or ventral or lateral surface of the tongue.

The local Head and Neck Cancer Unit may be run by an ENT and should be referred there if this is the local arrangement. However, a Maxillofacial Unit would be more appropriate, if available.

An incisional biopsy is the first test that would be performed on such a lesion, but it would be inappropriate to do it in practice. It should be performed in a secondary care environment, as part of the cancer care pathway.

Urgent referral and diagnosis are the most important factors affecting the outcome of a suspected cancer. In the United Kingdom, urgent referrals must be seen by the Head and Neck Unit within 2 weeks. Due to the aggressive nature of SCCs, you would not want to monitor this lesion in primary care.

Sharp teeth may cause trauma, but the clinical signs and risk factors present mean histological examination takes precedence.

Keywords: ulcer, ventral surface, 4 weeks, bleeds, smoking.

→ National Institute for Health and Care Excellence. *Suspected cancer: recognition and referral*. NICE guideline [NG12]. 2015. Available at: https://www.nice.org.uk/guidance/ng12

5. C ★   OHCD 6th ed. → p. 422

Lichen planus is an autoimmune disease of the skin and/or mucosa of unknown aetiology. Mild forms are self-limiting, whilst severe forms can be managed with topical corticosteroids. There is, however, no cure. In 0.4–3% of cases, oral lichen planus may undergo malignant change, particularly in patients with erosive lichen planus or associated risk factors. Therefore, most cases are kept under long-term review. Figure 8.2 (see Colour Plate section) shows reticular, non-erosive lichen planus of the buccal mucosa, but other variants are well documented.

Lichenoid reactions are lichen planus-like lesions with a known trigger. Triggers could be any foreign objects (e.g. amalgam), which need to be in direct contact with the mucosa to cause a lesion. Such lesions can also be caused by non-steroidal anti-inflammatory drugs (NSAIDs) and antimalarial, antihypertensive, or diabetic medications. The patient only has unilateral amalgams, which does not correlate with the bilateral presentation.

CHC is a fungal infection of the oral mucosa caused primarily by *Candida albicans*. This type of *Candida* is usually seen at the buccal commissures and is more common in smokers. It presents as a homogenous or speckled white plaque and requires monitoring as it is considered premalignant.

WSN is a relatively rare hereditary condition that presents as a symmetrical, corrugated white plaque.

Squamous cell carcinomas (SCCs) more commonly present on the floor of the mouth or ventral surface of the tongue. SCCs are also exceptionally unlikely to present as multiple bilateral lesions. The patient is also likely to have a history of smoking.

Keywords: bilaterally, buccal mucosa, rash on shins.

6. B ★   OHCD 6th ed. → p. 416

Herpetiform RAS occurs on both keratinized and non-keratinized mucosa, with non-keratinized sites being the most common. The ulcers are usually very small but sometimes may coalesce to form larger ulcers. Numbers vary, but patients may present with ten or more ulcers at a time. Herpetiform RAS responds well to treatment with chlortetracyc-line mouthwash.

Major RAS can affect keratinized and non-keratinized tissue in the oral cavity. Lesions are usually >10 mm in diameter and occur in small numbers (1–3). Lesions take longer to heal (up to 2 months), often leaving behind scar tissue.

Minor RAS usually presents on non-keratinized tissue. Lesions are usually under 10 mm in diameter and occur in small numbers (1–5). Healing takes up to 2 weeks without scarring.

Traumatic ulcers usually present as isolated lesions and may have a readily identifiable cause (sharp or fractured tooth/denture compo-nent). They also tend to have a white keratotic outline. The sulci and palate may be affected in cases where patients hold tablets in their mouth (e.g. aspirin).

Crohn's disease may cause oral ulcers, as malabsorption can lead to defi-ciencies in iron or vitamin B12. However, there is no indication of this in this scenario, as the patient is medically fit and well.

RAS patients often have a family history of the condition. For mild cases, symptomatic relief can be provided with an analgesic mouthwash. Topical steroids can also be prescribed in primary care, whilst more severe cases may require systemic immunomodulators; this is provided in a hospital setting.

Key words: recurrent, under the tongue, 20 ulcers, couple of millimetres.

7. E ★   OHCD 6th ed. → p. 310

Chronic erythematous candidiasis (denture stomatitis) arises from a fungal infection secondary to poor denture hygiene and tissue trauma. Therefore, these factors should be rectified before issuing pharmaco-logical treatment.

Topical antifungal treatment is required, and miconazole gel is the treat-ment of choice, but in this instance, the patient is taking warfarin for atrial fibrillation. Azole antifungals inhibit liver cytochrome P450 enzymes and therefore increase the efficacy of warfarin. To avoid adverse drug interactions, nystatin suspension would be a safer choice. Newer novel oral anticoagulants (NOACs), such as apixaban, are becoming more common and at present are not routinely monitored.

Table 8.1 Common cytochrome P450 inducers and inhibitors

Inducers	Inhibitors
Carbamazepine	Sodium valproate
Rifampicin	Isoniazid
Alcohol (chronic use)	Cimetidine
Phenytoin	Azole antifungals (ketoconazole, miconazole, fluconazole)
	Erythromycin
	Metronidazole

Amphotericin tablets were a traditional alternative but are no longer manufactured. Chlorhexidine has some antifungal properties but is not a conventional antifungal medication. Chloramphenicol ointment is an antibacterial agent typically used in ophthalmology. See Figure 8.9 (see Colour Plate section) which shows *Candida*-associated, denture-induced stomatitis (chronic erythematous candidiasis) affecting the area of mucosa covered by a partial denture. Some of the more common cytochrome P450 inducers/inhibitors are listed in Table 8.1.

Keywords: chronic erythematous candidiasis, warfarin.

8. E ★★   OHCD 6th ed. → p. 410

This is a classic description of primary herpetic gingivostomatitis (PHG). See Figure 8.10 (see Colour Plate section) which shows a patient suffering from PHG of the lips and perioral skin. The causative organism is herpes simplex virus. Along with general malaise and generalized oral ulceration, cervical lymphadenopathy may be present. However, the condition usually resolves itself within 2 weeks. Failure to resolve within this time period warrants a referral to a specialist to exclude underlying blood dyscrasias or other systemic conditions.

Referring to a specialist to search for potential underlying health problems takes priority in this case over the other options, which may be suitable for most other cases of PHG, as described below. In a fit and healthy patient, reassuring and advising the patient to rest and take plenty of fluids is sufficient, as PHG is self-limiting and resolves within 2 weeks.

Aciclovir is ineffective once the infection is clinically detectable (vesicles and pyrexia). However, aciclovir may be helpful for severe infections or for immunocompromised patients.

The antiseptic properties of chlorhexidine gluconate can be helpful in reducing secondary infection.

Benzydamine hydrochloride can help to relieve some discomfort from the oral ulceration.

Keywords: bloody crusty lips, lasted for over 3 weeks, struggling to eat.

→ Nair RG, Salajeghen A, Itthagarun A, Pakneshan S, Brennan MT, Samaranayake LP. Orofacial viral infections--an update for clinicians. *Dental Update.* 2014;**41**:518–24.

9. D ★★   OHCD 6th ed. → p. 444

Figure 8.3 (see Colour Plate section) shows the buccal mucosa with a cobblestoned appearance. This can occur in Crohn's disease or in OFG. OFG is a term used to describe a syndrome, which presents with facial and oral tissue swellings that show non-caseating granulomas on histological examination. The oral presentation is similar to that of Crohn's disease, but without any gastrointestinal problems. In this scenario, the patient does not present with systemic symptoms, and so Crohn's disease can be provisionally eliminated. It is thought that OFG can be exacerbated by certain foods; patients are therefore advised to avoid cinnamon and benzoates in their diets.

Ulcerative colitis does not cause oral swellings. It is more likely to cause aphthous-like ulcers, along with gastrointestinal problems. Pyostomatitis vegetans is an oral condition that is highly specific for ulcerative colitis.

Coeliac disease can present with oral ulcers or other symptoms associated with nutritional deficiencies; these are not noted in this scenario.

Frictional keratosis along the occlusal plane (linea alba) is commonly associated with cheek biting and may indicate a parafunctional habit. Typically, it is less raised in appearance than the image above and is not associated with orofacial swelling.

Keywords: avoid cinnamon, no systemic symptoms, enlarged lip.

10. D ★★   OHCD 6th ed. → p. 414

Sore, erythematous crusted lesions at the corner of the mouth are indicative of angular cheilitis. Management involves excluding haematinic deficiencies and underlying immunosuppression. See Figure 8.11 (see Colour Plate section) for a clinical example of severe angular cheilitis associated with chronic oral candidiasis. Appropriate antimicrobial therapy should be provided, and management of predisposing factors must be addressed.

Dentures with a reduced OVD or excessive freeway space can predispose to the development of angular cheilitis and should be managed by providing new dentures at an increased OVD (approximately 2–6 mm of freeway space).

Extra-oral infections can be managed with application of a suitable cream, whilst intraoral infections will require use of a gel or rinse. Bacterial *Staphylococcus aureus* infection will respond to fusidic acid cream. Mixed infections will respond well to miconazole, which has antifungal and antibacterial properties, although it is mainly an antifungal medication.

Nystatin (polyene class of antifungals) binds to ergosterol in the fungal cell membrane, whilst miconazole (imidazole class of antifungals) blocks ergosterol synthesis.

Keywords: crusted skin, corner of mouth, freeway space of 12 mm, mixed *Candida albicans* and *Staphylococcus aureus* infection.

11. B ★★ OHCD 6th ed. → p. 434

Subjective signs of dry eyes and dry mouth should always be investigated. Sjögren's syndrome results from immune destruction of glandular tissue, which can lead to dry mouth (xerostomia) and dry eyes (keratoconjunctivitis sicca). Commonly, the lacrimal and salivary glands are damaged, but other body sites can be affected. Where a patient has dry eyes and mouth, but no signs of autoimmune destruction, it is known as sicca syndrome, but many use these terms synonymously.

Objective tests for dry eyes and dry mouth can be conducted, including Schirmer's test and salivary flow tests. Anti-Ro and anti-La autoantibodies are extractable nuclear antibodies (ENAs), which can be detected using special blood tests. Patients with primary Sjögren's syndrome are often positive for these tests, which, when combined with lymphocytic infiltrates on a labial gland biopsy, are indicative of Sjögren's syndrome. The absence of an additional autoimmune condition would suggest a diagnosis of primary Sjögren's syndrome. In the presence of additional autoimmune conditions, such as systemic lupus erythematosus (SLE), it is referred to as secondary Sjögren's syndrome.

Other objective tests used to investigate Sjögren's syndrome include sialography and ultrasound. Not all tests are required to be positive for diagnosis, and the American-European consensus Sjögren's classification criteria is cited above. Patients with Sjögren's syndrome should have long-term follow-up due to an increased risk for developing lymphoma.

Sarcoidosis is a granulomatous disease that can affect multiple organs, most commonly the lungs and skin, with pulmonary sarcoidosis reported in 90% of patients with the disease.

Bacterial sialadenitis would not account for the dry eyes or be an indication of labial gland biopsy.

Keywords: dry mouth, dry eyes, anti-Ro, anti-La, labial gland biopsy, multiple dense foci.

→ Vitali CB, Bombardieri S, Jonsson R, et al. Classification criteria for Sjögren's syndrome: a revised version of the European criteria proposed by the American-European Consensus Group. *Annals of the Rheumatic Diseases*. 2002;**61**:554–8.

12. A ★★ OHCD 6th ed. → p. 754

This question is a simple test for matching classical symptoms to a particular condition.

Horner's syndrome consists of constricted pupils, drooping eyelids, unilateral loss of sweating on the face, and the occasional sunken eye.

Melkersson–Rosenthal syndrome consists of facial paralysis, facial oedema, and fissured tongue.

Sicca syndrome is a combination of dry mouth and dry eyes, in the absence of any signs of autoimmune connective tissue disorders.

Graves' disease is characterized by hypothyroidism as a result of the production of autoantibodies to thyroid-stimulating hormone. Classically, there is exophthalmos.

Frey's syndrome is a condition in which gustatory sweating and flushing of the skin occur. It follows trauma to the skin overlying the parotid gland, and it is thought to be the result of post-traumatic crossover of sympathetic and parasympathetic supply to the gland and skin.

Keywords: sweating on eating, flushing of skin, surgical intervention.

13. E ★★   OHCD 6th ed. → p. 438

The history suggests this pain is unlikely to be of dental origin.

Dental pain can be shooting or dull (depending on the stage of disease), but often lasts from minutes to hours.

Reversible pulpitis, although being poorly localized, is not typically described by patients as excruciating or electric shock-like. Commonly, hot, cold, or sweet stimuli induces pain in reversible pulpitis, and it is a sharp pain that lasts as long as the stimulus is present or a few minutes longer.

Irreversible pulpitis presents as a dull, spontaneous ache which tends to be poorly localized, and the involved teeth are usually vital. Very occasionally, it can present in a manner similar to trigeminal neuralgia, and therefore, a thorough dental assessment is required before definitively diagnosing trigeminal neuralgia.

Glossopharyngeal neuralgia presents with a similar history to trigeminal neuralgia, but pain is felt in the back of the throat and is usually triggered by swallowing.

Information on atypical facial pain is available in other questions within this chapter.

Intense, unilateral, shooting pain of very short duration is classic of neuralgic pain. The pain follows the distribution of sensory nerves and is brought on by trigger factors which the patient often self-reports, e.g. shaving or cold wind. Diagnosis is achieved through history, and carbamazepine is effective in treatment and often diagnostic. Gabapentin/pregabalin are alternative medications often prescribed when contraindications to carbamazepine are present (e.g. warfarin).

Keywords: 50-year-old woman, shooting 'electric shock', short duration.

→ Zakrzewska J, Linskey M. Trigeminal neuralgia. *BMJ*. 2014;**348**:g474.

14. D ★★★   OHCD 6th ed. → p. 438

Temporal arteritis is a type of vasculitis, affecting the superficial temporal artery. Pain may be elicited when chewing, as the temporal muscles become ischaemic. The condition usually presents in older patients. If the central retinal artery becomes involved, there is a risk of blindness; therefore, treatment must be provided as soon as possible with high-dose steroids—often prednisolone. Diagnosis can be clinical but can be confirmed by a markedly raised erythrocyte sedimentation rate (ESR) level and the presence of giant cells on arterial biopsy.

Trigeminal neuralgia can be triggered by chewing and is of sudden onset. But the pain is short-lived and classically described as lancinating, not aching. Pyrexia is not associated with trigeminal neuralgia.

Myofascial pain may present in a similar manner, but the patient would not be pyrexial.

Myofascial pain and temporomandibular disorders are also unlikely to be of sudden onset.

Cluster headaches more commonly affect younger males from the age of 20 years. The orbital, rather than the temporal, region is affected more commonly.

Atypical facial pain does not follow the anatomical distribution of nerves and is not associated with pyrexia.

Keywords: unilateral headache, worse on chewing, 38.6°C, pulse, not detectable.

15. E ★★★   OHCD 6th ed. → p. 422

White sponge naevus is a genetic condition with childhood onset. A rough or folded appearance of the mucosa is caused by thickening of the epithelium. The condition often affects the buccal mucosa but can affect any part of the mouth. Only reassurance is required. There is usually a family history with similar lesions in siblings or parents. See Figure 8.12 (see Colour Plate section) which shows oral epithelial naevus affecting the buccal mucosa.

Leukoedema causes a diffuse milky appearance of the oral mucosa. The white patches do not rub off, but the white appearance may reduce when the mucosa is stretched. This is a benign, asymptomatic condition which does not require treatment.

Stomatitis nicotina affects the palate of smokers. The epithelium of the palate thickens to produce a white/grey patch, from which the minor salivary glands protrude as red dots. This is not a premalignant condition and usually resolves when the patient quits smoking. As the patient is a life-long non-smoker, this answer is clearly incorrect.

Lichen planus can be diffuse, but it is unlikely to be present from childhood.

Keywords: diffuse, asymptomatic, rough texture, since 12.

16. B ★★★   OHCD 6th ed. → p. 438

It can be difficult to diagnose vague pain, especially if the patient's pain is not resolved after treatment.

AFP and AO are diagnoses of exclusion, between which it can be difficult to differentiate. Characteristically, they are vague, aching pains distinguished by location and a careful history.

As in the scenario, AO is persistent pain following extraction or root canal treatment, in the absence of clinical or radiographic causes. The pain is thought to be neuropathic, resulting from axonal sprouting and neuroplasticity of localized nerve fibres, and it is therefore more localized than AFP. This confusing presentation may be associated with tingling or itching and can lead to multiple teeth being treated unnecessarily.

AFP is considered psychogenic and often has unusual presentations (e.g. crossing anatomical boundaries) and does not respond to conventional treatment or pain relief. The diagnosis is most common amongst women over the age of 50 years. Associated factors include a history of depression, chronic illness, or irritable bowel syndrome. Treatment is often in the form of cognitive behavioural therapy or antidepressants.

It is important to consider these diagnoses in cases where the pain history is erratic, to avoid unnecessary treatment.

Oral dysaesthesia is a burning sensation from the oral mucosa in the absence of any oral pathology. Almost half of all cases of oral dysaesthesia are idiopathic. Other causes include vitamin B deficiencies, iron deficiency, *Candida* infection (including dentures), and allergies.

Pain from TMD has several overlapping characteristics with atypical pain. However, it is likely to present alongside other features such as clicking, jaw locking, crepitus, trismus, or tenderness of the muscles of mastication.

Trigeminal neuralgia is described as severe pain but is of very short duration and does not cross the midline. Patients are usually able to associate with distinct triggering factors.

Keywords: 53-year-old woman, pressure-like pain, itching sensation, extraction, followed by root canal treatment.

17. B ★★★★ OHCD 6th ed. → p. 408

Although relatively rare, syphilis should be considered in young patients presenting with a solitary, painless ulcer in the mouth when no other cause can be identified. The most recent United Kingdom epidemiology data have shown that peak incidence occurs in men aged between 25 and 35 years and the incidence has been gradually increasing since 2003.

A primary syphilitic lesion caused by infection from *Treponema pallidum* is called a chancre. It presents as a firm, solitary, non-tender ulcer at the site of inoculation. The lesion is highly infectious but resolves within 1–2 months. The *T. pallidum* haemagglutination assay (TPHA) or darkground microscopy can be used to aid diagnosis of a syphilis infection.

Secondary (snail track ulcers) and tertiary (gumma) syphilitic lesions may occur at later stages.

Squamous cell carcinoma is possible but unlikely, as the patient is young and does not have a history of smoking.

Major recurrent aphthous stomatitis may present with a similar appearance. However, the lesion is usually painful and there is usually a history of recurrence. Lymphadenopathy is also unlikely in major recurrent aphthous stomatitis.

Traumatic ulcers are generally painful and would likely be accompanied by a history of localized trauma and frequently have a keratotic outline.

Atrophic glossitis can result in a smooth, erythematous tongue, affecting all or only part of the dorsum of the tongue. However, it would not result in a positive TPHA result.

Keywords: 27-year old, tongue, non-tender, cervical lymphadenopathy, blood test.

18. C ★★★★ OHCD 6th ed. → p. 490

Mealtime syndrome is commonly associated with salivary calculi (sialolith). Recurrent swelling of the salivary gland can be a result of restricted salivary flow. This is generally more common around mealtimes, as saliva flow is stimulated. Sialoliths are more commonly associated with the submandibular gland, due to the convoluted path of Wharton's duct.

Normally, sialography would be the imaging method of choice in non-infected situations, due to the diagnostic and therapeutic information the method provides (with regard to the cause and location). However, sialography involves a radiograph, following injection of an iodine-based radio-opaque medium, to reveal any obstructions or strictures within the salivary gland or duct system.

As the patient is allergic to iodine, contemporary imaging with magnetic resonance would be most appropriate. Magnetic resonance imaging has been reported to have positive and negative predictive values of above 90%. Moreover, it provides accurate three-dimensional information on the location and can be used in cases of gland inflammation. In contrast, resolution of secondary and tertiary branches of the duct is worse than sialography, and therefore, it is not a first-line imaging choice.

Occlusal radiographs alone are useful, with around 80% of salivary calculi detected by this investigation. They are normally taken as a primary diagnostic test, and further imaging may be prescribed afterwards if a calculus cannot be seen. Therefore, in answer to this question, magnetic resonance imaging would be *more* likely to produce a definitive diagnosis.

Computed tomography imaging incurs a relatively high dose of radiation. It also provides limited benefit over the above alternatives and therefore is reserved for select cases.

Fine-needle aspiration is used to biopsy superficial soft tissue swellings.

Keywords: recurrent swelling, mealtime, iodine allergy, definitive.

→ Rzymska-Grala I, Stopa Z, Grala B, *et al*. Salivary gland calculi—contemporary methods of imaging. *Polish Journal of Radiology*. 2010;**75**:25–37.

19. C ★★★★   OHCD 6th ed. → p. 418

This patient presents with pemphigus vulgaris. This is a bullous condition reported to be more common amongst middle-aged people of Ashkenazi Jewish origin. The disease is characterized by autoantibodies that target the intercellular connections of the stratum spinosum layer of the epidermis. This results in fragile, thin-walled intraepidermal bullae that rupture readily. Painful oral mucosal lesions and skin lesions result. These weak cellular junctions can also lead to skin shearing with lateral pressure, known as a positive Nikolsky's sign. Immunofluorescence is used to complement histology in the diagnosis. This would show intercellular IgG and C3 —visually described as a 'chicken wire' or 'basket weave' appearance.

Linear IgG and C3 at the basement membrane can be found by direct immunofluorescence in mucous membrane pemphigoid (MMP) and bullous pemphigoid (BP) disease. Orally, these two conditions both resemble pemphigus vulgaris, but with different pathogenesis. Autoantibodies target hemidesmosomes at the basement membrane, so bullae are more robust and last a few days before rupturing. BP is primarily a skin disorder, with oral lesions in only a third of cases. Nikolsky's sign is absent in BP. In MMP, skin lesions are uncommon, but Nikolsky's sign is present. Ocular involvement can occur, leading to blindness.

Granular IgA deposits and C3 at dermal papillae are found by direct immunofluorescence in dermatitis herpetiformis. Orally, it presents in a similar fashion to lichen planus.

Linear IgA and C3 at the basement membrane are found by direct immunofluorescence in linear IgA disease. This condition is a variant of dermatitis herpetiformis.

Keywords: very short-lived blisters, skin lesions, shear with lateral pressure.

→ Scully C, Challacombe S. Pemphigus vulgaris: update on etiopathogenesis, oral manifestations, and management. *Critical Reviews in Oral Biology and Medicine*. 2002;**13**:397–408.

20. D ★★★★   OHCD 6th ed. → p. 505

Multiple myeloma is cancer of plasma cells, which can present in multiple sites throughout the body. A solitary plasmacytoma affects a single site and may indicate future disease. Malignant plasma cells proliferate, commonly within the bone marrow, and produce a wide variety of symptoms.

Bone pain and osteolytic lesions are common, due to an increase in osteoclastic activity of plasma cells, which can sometimes be identified as 'punched-out' lesions on radiographs, e.g. pepper-pot skull. Anaemia may result, as more bone marrow becomes affected. Calcium levels also rise, as bone is broken down.

Abnormal plasma cells often produce ineffective immunoglobulins (paraproteins). Excretion of these products can be detected in the urine and are often referred to as Bence-Jones proteins (light chains of immunoglobulins). Renal problems can be linked to excessive production of these paraproteins.

'CRAB' is a useful acronym for identifying the key symptoms of multiple myeloma:

- Calcium increase
- Renal failure
- Anaemia
- Bone problems.

Keywords: plasmacytoma, hypercalcaemia, anaemia, elevated immunoglobulins.

21. D ★★★★ OHCD 6th ed. → p. 422

The histology slides presented show classic pathology findings for lichen planus, including a saw-tooth pattern to the rete processes of the epithelium. The epithelium shows hyperkeratosis and can be thicker (acanthotic) or thinner (atrophic). Rete processes are extensions of the epithelium into the underlying connective tissue, which can lengthen and increase in width. Subepithelial band-like lymphocyte infiltration is another pathological finding in lichen planus, largely comprising T lymphocytes. Liquefactive degeneration of basal cells can also be seen, in addition to apoptotic cells. These degenerating cells (Civatte bodies) can also be seen in other keratotic diseases, including lupus erythematosus.

Frictional keratosis would show extremely thickened epithelium and hyperkeratinization, with no subepithelial band-like lymphocytic infiltrate. Acute cases may present with an ulcerated epithelium. This lesion would normally resolve with removal of the source.

DLE shows perivascular lymphocytic infiltration, along with liquefactive degeneration of the basal layer. Immunofluorescence can be used to detect immunoglobulin deposits. MMP has been discussed in other questions within this chapter.

Keywords: gingivae, white patch.

22. E ★★★★

ALL is the most common type of leukaemia in children and young adults. Spontaneously bleeding gums should always raise suspicion. However, this patient's WBC count returned within the normal range.

Pyogenic granuloma produces a hyperplastic lesion on the attached gingivae, which can ulcerate. This lesion is associated with local irritation, and inflammation is exacerbated by the presence of plaque but is localized to one area of the gingivae.

ANUG is a true infection of the gingivae. Presentation can include necrosis of the interdental papillae. It can be painful and associated with marked halitosis, but gingivae are unlikely to appear hyperplastic.

Melatonin is taken to assist with sleeping and has no effect on gingival overgrowth. Common drugs associated with gingival overgrowth are phenytoin, calcium channel blockers, and ciclosporin.

Key clues in the history point to vitamin C deficiency or scurvy. The patient only eats crisps and presents with generalized hyperplastic gingivae that bleed, along with early loss of periodontal attachment. Scurvy is not common in developed countries.

Keywords: lethargic, only eats crisps (poor diet), loss of attachment, hyperplastic gingivae.

23. D ★★★★   OHCD 6th ed. → p. 392

The clinical features given are most likely to represent a dentigerous cyst, which are commonly found enveloping the crowns of unerupted teeth. However, the histopathology described is most likely to indicate an odontogenic keratocyst. It is important to recognize that odontogenic keratocysts can present in a fashion similar to dentigerous cysts (enveloping crowns), and it is therefore important to submit them for histological analysis. The lining of a dentigerous cyst is also thin, but the squamous epithelium is non-keratinizing and often displays mucous metaplasia.

Odontogenic keratocysts show specific growth in an anteroposterior direction along the marrow spaces and can be responsible for resorbing the roots of associated teeth. Small satellite cysts can develop in the cyst wall, and this can account for the high recurrence rates identified.

Eruption cysts are extra-alveolar dentigerous cysts.

Lateral periodontal cysts are thin-walled developmental cysts associated with the lateral aspect of vital teeth. The cyst is non-keratinizing and is more commonly found in the canine and premolar region of the mandible.

Radicular cysts are inflammatory cysts that commonly arise at the apex of non-vital teeth. They are non-keratinizing cysts, which show marked inflammation in the cyst lining. This results in a cyst lining that is much more hyperplastic than that associated with developmental cysts.

Keywords: high levels of mitotic figures, parakeratinization, low protein content (mainly albumin).

24. E ★★★★   OHCD 6th ed. → p. 720

The Health and Safety Executive is responsible for protecting employees, employers, contractors, and the public within the work environment. Employers and those in charge of premises are required to report adverse incidents, including work-related deaths, diseases, and near misses.

Whilst it is common practice for accidents at work to be recorded in an accident log, the 'Reporting of Injuries, Diseases and Dangerous Occurrences Regulations 1995 (RIDDOR)' stipulates that injuries which result in >3 consecutive days off work must legally be recorded.

Incidents which require the injured party to have >7 days off work must be reported to the Health and Safety Executive within 15 days.

Since 1 April 2015, a memorandum of understanding has existed between the Health and Safety Executive and the Care Quality Commission to ensure appropriate information is shared between the two bodies, and it is likely that serious events that occur in the dental setting and reported to the Health and Safety Executive under RIDDOR could be investigated by the Care Quality Commission.

Keywords: trips, admitted to hospital, 4 weeks off work.

→ Care Quality Commission. *Memorandum of Understanding (MoU) between the Care Quality Commission (CQC), Health and Safety Executive (HSE) and local authorities in England.* 2017. Available at: https://www.cqc.org.uk/file/182048

→ Health and Safety Executive. *Reporting accidents and incidents at work.* 2013. Available at: http://www.hse.gov.uk/pubns/indg453.htm

General medicine

Tariq Ali

'Teeth are quite often attached to people.'

The oral cavity is the largest and most used orifice in the human body. It is the opening of the aerodigestive tract, as well as a region of the body that is heavily involved in both sensing the outside world and communicating with it. Simply put, our mouths are complex and deeply intimate structures that can act as windows into the health of the rest of the body. Many disease processes that are systemically invisible may display quite overt oral manifestations.

There are deep associations between bodily diseases and oral disease counterparts, with considerable and mounting evidence to show that oral health may have an impact on systemic wellness. It is therefore important to have an understanding of the wider human anatomy, physiology, and pathology. Understand and treat the patient as a whole, and think about all aspects of their health, whether it be routine preventative treatment for periodontally compromised diabetic patients or polypharmacy patients requiring secondary dental care.

Often at times, patients can be unclear about their own health condition; having a fundamental understanding of general medicine will help to make those difficult choices regarding your patients a little easier and clarify when and whom to refer.

Key topics are not included for this chapter, as it is a vast topic, and not the main focus of the dental undergraduate curriculum. It is, however, important to have a good basic knowledge of general human diseases, how they might interact with dental treatment, and the role that dentists can play in both diagnosis and management

QUESTIONS

1. A 15-year-old girl attends the Emergency Department at the local dental hospital. She suffers from type 1 diabetes mellitus. Damage to which single cell type in the pancreas would lead to the patient's condition? ★

A Alpha cells

B Beta cells

C Delta cells

D Epsilon cells

E Gamma cells

2. A 78-year-old man with poorly controlled type 2 diabetes requires extraction of his lower right first permanent molar (LR6), as he has a periapical abscess on the tooth. He is extremely nervous and, uncommonly for him, did not eat breakfast. During treatment, the patient begins to sweat profusely; he then begins to shake violently and stops responding. What is the single most likely explanation for the presentation? ★

A Brain tumour

B Epileptic seizure

C Hypoglycaemic attack

D Odontogenic sepsis

E Pseudoseizure

3. A 67-year-old man with chronic obstructive pulmonary disease (COPD) attends for a routine restoration. During treatment, he starts to cough and asks if the treatment can be stopped. He sits up and is visibly working hard to breathe. His respiratory rate is 30 breaths per minute. His cough is productive and appears to be clear, but his lips start to develop a blue tinge. Whilst the nurse applies a pulse oximeter, what is the next single most appropriate management? ★

A High-flow oxygen at 10–15 L/minute (through a non-rebreather mask)

B Low-flow oxygen at 2–3 L/minute (through nasal cannulae)

C Medium-flow oxygen at 5–10 L/minute (through a simple face mask)

D Titrate oxygen levels to between 88% and 92% (through a non-rebreather mask)

E Titrate oxygen levels to between 92% and 98% (through a simple face mask)

4. An unaccompanied 79-year-old woman attends her dentist for extraction of her upper right first permanent molar (UR6). She takes warfarin for atrial fibrillation, and her latest international normalized ratio (INR) was 3.1 three days ago. Following the extraction, the socket is packed with a haemostatic agent and sutured; however, after 20 minutes of pressure, the patient is still bleeding. What is the single most appropriate next management strategy? ★

A Ask the patient to continue applying pressure to the area at home and pause the warfarin until the bleeding stops

B Ask the patient to go to the local Emergency Department

C Continue applying pressure over the area and call for an ambulance

D Give high-flow oxygen and suction the blood from the mouth

E Give the patient an intravascular injection of vitamin K

5. A 35-year-old man attends his orthodontist for a review, after completing a course of orthodontic treatment 12 months ago. His retainers no longer fit even, though he has worn them consistently every other night. Clinically, spacing has developed between his anterior teeth, and his facial appearance has changed from his post-operative photos. He now has more prominent supra-orbital ridges and widening of the nose and jaw, and has noticed tingling in both hands. What is the single most likely cause in this scenario? ★ ★

A Addison's syndrome

B Anabolic steroid use

C Conn's syndrome

D Cushing's syndrome

E Pituitary tumour

6. A previously fit and well 55-year-old woman attends her dentist, complaining of recent-onset gingival swelling. She apologizes for being late to the appointment but explains that she has been chronically tired for the past couple of months and slept through her alarm. She is short of breath from walking up the stairs and has multiple bruises visible on her arms as she takes off her coat. Clinically, she has bilateral cervical lymphadenopathy and swollen pale gingivae, which bleed spontaneously. What is the single most likely diagnosis? ★ ★

A Acute myeloblastic leukaemia

B Acute lymphocytic leukaemia

C Beta-thalassaemia

D Chronic myeloblastic leukaemia

E Non-Hodgkin's lymphoma

7. A 70-year-old man attends for a routine examination. He has recently fallen and fractured his foot. He takes time getting up off the chair and shuffles into the surgery. His handwriting on the new patient questionnaire is extremely small and spidery. He is expressionless, whilst recounting the history of his recurrent falls. What is the single most likely cause of the recurrent falls? ★ ★

A Benign paroxysmal positional vertigo (BPPV)

B Cerebellopontine angle (CPA) tumour

C Labyrinthitis

D Parkinson's disease

E Posterior circulation infarct

8. A 37-year-old woman attends for a routine scale and polish. Medically, she is under investigation with her general practitioner for symptoms of excessive thirst, palpitations, excess sweating, and recent weight loss. Clinically, she has a large lump in her neck. The lump moves when she swallows, but not when she sticks her tongue out. What is the single most likely cause for her neck lump? ★ ★ ★

A Diabetes insipidus (DI)

B Graves' disease

C Hashimoto's thyroiditis

D Thyroid cancer

E Tuberculosis (TB)

9. A 65-year-old man presents with a large dental abscess in the lower right quadrant. He suffers from polymyalgia rheumatica (PMR), for which he has recently been taking high-dose prednisolone. He has not taken his medication for the last 2 days, as he knows steroids 'make infections worse'. He is profusely sweaty and looks extremely unwell. His current temperature is 39°C, and his blood pressure is 70/50 mmHg. His blood sugar is 2.9 mmol/L. What is the single most likely underlying cause for his presentation? ★ ★ ★

A Acquired immune deficiency syndrome (AIDS)

B Addison's disease

C Adrenal crisis

D Hyperadrenalism

E Septic shock

10. A 75-year-old man with hypertension attends for the fit of his upper complete denture. During insertion of the denture, he begins slurring his speech, and then the left corner of his mouth droops. When he sees the abnormalities in the mirror, he becomes alarmed and raises both his eyebrows in surprise. At his next review, he reports he went to hospital, but the symptoms resolved after half a day, and he is now under review with his doctor. What was the single most likely diagnosis? ★ ★ ★

A Bell's palsy

B Cerebrovascular accident (CVA)

C Subarachnoid haemorrhage (SAH)

D Transient ischaemic attack (TIA)

E Vertebrobasilar insufficiency

11. A 45-year-old man presents to the dental hospital emergency clinic with toothache. He denies any medical problems but admits to drinking 2 L of cider a day. The sclerae of his eyes are faintly yellow; his abdomen is distended, and he appears to have red, spider-like patterns on the skin of his face and neck. On examination, the lower left second molar (LL7) displays gross subgingival caries and requires extraction. The patient is in severe pain and wants immediate treatment. What is the next single most appropriate course of action? ★ ★ ★

A Decline to extract the tooth and prescribe a course of metronidazole

B Decline to extract the tooth and extirpate to alleviate pain

C Extract the tooth as normal immediately

D Extract the tooth tomorrow, asking the patient not to drink until then

E Request a full blood count, liver function tests, and a clotting screen

12. A 59-year-old woman attends for the first time, complaining of wobbly teeth. She has a smoking history of 40 pack years but has recently quit. She has a chronic cough and is seen to be using a bloodstained handkerchief. Her left eye is sunken in, with a smaller pupil, compared to the right eye, and her left eyelid is also drooping. What is the single most likely underlying diagnosis? ★ ★ ★ ★

A Mesothelioma

B Pancoast tumour

C Pneumothorax

D Pulmonary embolism (PE)

E Tuberculosis (TB)

13. A 32-year-old man attends for a routine appointment. He is a recovering intravenous drug user, has a smoking history of 25 pack years, and drinks six cans of lager every day. He has had a cough and been experiencing night sweats for the past 4 weeks. He says his clothes feel a lot looser in the last 6 months. Clinically, a dark purple, irregular lump is seen on the upper left buccal gingiva, which the patient was unaware of. White plaques are present on his tongue, which can be scraped off. What is the single most likely underlying diagnosis? ★ ★ ★ ★

A Acquired immune deficiency syndrome

B *Candida albicans* infection

C Malignant melanoma

D Oral squamous cell carcinoma

E Tuberculosis

14. An 85-year-old man is brought for a routine appointment in his wheelchair, accompanied by his carer. He appears very drowsy, and his carer states he has been sleeping excessively over the last 2 days. He has been off his food and not drinking much. He wakes up intermittently, complaining of toothache. The only new medication he has started taking is over-the-counter ibuprofen. His other medications include bisoprolol, candesartan, aspirin, glaucoma eye drops, and a morphine patch. His carer explains he has barely woken up over the last 2 days, not even to go to the bathroom. Attempts to rouse him are to no avail. Upon performing a sternal rub, he opens his eyes and moves his hands over the sternal area. He makes an attempt to mumble something, but it is not comprehensible. What is the single correct Glasgow coma scale (GCS) score for this gentleman? ★ ★ ★ ★

A 3

B 6

C 7

D 8

E 9

15. A 65-year-old woman requires an extraction due to advanced periodontal disease. She suffers from stage 5 chronic kidney disease (CKD) and has haemodialysis three times a week. When is the single most appropriate time for the extraction? ★ ★ ★ ★

A Four hours after dialysis

B One day before dialysis

C The day after dialysis

D The morning of dialysis

E Two days prior to dialysis

ANSWERS

1. B ★   OHCD 6th ed. → p. 518

All of the above cells are part of the islets of Langerhans in the pancreas. Beta cells produce insulin and amylin (60–85% of pancreatic anabolic activity). Both are essential for glucose homeostasis. Insulin promotes absorption of glucose from the bloodstream, and subsequent glycogenesis (production of glycogen) in the liver and skeletal muscle and lipogenesis (production of triglycerides) in adipocytes.

Alpha cells produce glucagon (15–20%) used for glycogenolysis (breakdown of glycogen into glucose), gluconeogenesis (formation of glucose from amino acids, lactate, and glycerol), and lipolysis (breakdown of triglycerides into free fatty acids). Amylin inhibits the effects of glucagon.

Delta cells produce somatostatin (3–10%), also known as growth hormone inhibitory hormone (GHIH). This, as the name suggests, inhibits the release of pituitary growth hormone, as well as inhibition of insulin and amylin.

Gamma cells produce pancreatic polypeptide (PP) (3–5%). PP promotes gastric secretion and plays a role in satiety.

Epsilon cells produce ghrelin (<1%). It is a neuropeptide that acts as a hunger stimulator and is usually secreted when the stomach is empty.

Keywords: diabetes mellitus, pancreas.

→ Devlin H, Craven R. *Oxford Handbook of Integrated Dental Biosciences*. Oxford University Press, Oxford; 2018.

2. C ★   OHCD 6th ed. → p. 518

Hypoglycaemia can cause a range of different autonomic and neurological symptoms, including tremors, clamminess, tachycardia, tachypnoea, anxiety, and behavioural changes. If prolonged, hypoglycaemia can lead to seizures and coma. In normal circumstances, patients can recognize the symptoms early and remedy the situation with consumption of a rapidly absorbed carbohydrate.

Diabetics often lose their ability to recognize their own hypoglycaemic symptoms because of their defective autonomic responses and therefore may not treat their hypoglycaemia in time.

Dental infection may place additional metabolic stress on the body, but this on its own would not explain the incident.

Epilepsy cannot be diagnosed from this one incident and would require additional investigations, as would the diagnosis of a brain tumour. A pseudoseizure (conscious attempts by the patient to mimic a seizure, often due to behavioural issues) should only be considered once all other possibilities have been excluded.

A brain tumour may cause seizures but is unlikely to present in this manner and usually would present with other neurological findings.

Keywords: type 2 diabetes, did not eat breakfast, sweat profusely, shake violently.

3. A ★   OHCD 6th ed. → p. 510

COPD is characterized by progressive airway obstruction and worsening breathlessness. It is an umbrella term for chronic bronchitis and emphysema; smoking is the major cause. Chronic airway inflammation results in hypertrophy of the mucus glands and destruction of distal bronchioles, limiting gas exchange in the alveoli and resulting in hypoxaemia [low blood partial pressure of oxygen (PaO_2)] and hypercarbia [high blood partial pressure of carbon dioxide ($PaCO_2$)].

The patient is having difficulty oxygenating, hence the increased respiratory rate, and is hypoxaemic, as evidenced by the cyanosis. In this situation, it is important to provide the greatest concentration of inspired oxygen as possible. Therefore, applying 10–15 L of oxygen via a non-rebreather mask would be the best way to improve the situation immediately.

In normal physiology, respiratory drive is stimulated by hypercarbia. In patients with COPD, chronically high $PaCO_2$ leads to the respiratory drive being converted to hypoxia. Therefore, prolonged exposure to high-concentration oxygen can result in respiratory depression, and ultimately loss of consciousness and death.

For this reason, it is recommended that patients with COPD have their oxygen saturations titrated to 88–92%, once any acute hypoxaemia is alleviated. In normal patients, a target range of 92–98% can be titrated.

Keywords: COPD, 30 breaths per minute, blue tinge.

→ O'Driscoll BR, Howard LS, Earis J, et al. BTS guideline for oxygen use in adults in healthcare and emergency settings. *Thorax*. 2017;**72**(Suppl 1):ii1–90.

4. C ★   OHCD 6th ed. → p. 506

Generally, when a patient is on warfarin, oral surgery procedures can be performed as long as the INR is below 4.0. Some clinicians would suggest an upper limit of 3.5 for block injections. It should also be checked within 72 hours of the procedure, as the INR is very liable to change, particularly if the patient is forgetful with taking tablets or consumes substances that might interact with warfarin (e.g. alcohol, grapefruit).

When a patient on warfarin has a problem with haemorrhage after a minor surgical procedure, it is important to apply pressure for at least 20 minutes. This will allow time for a clot to form and stabilize. Additional local measures could include additional local anaesthetic, placement of a haemostatic agent, and suturing of the wound. In this case, the bleeding was excessive and did not stop; the best option here would be to call an ambulance and send the patient to a secondary care facility—particularly as they do not have anyone to escort them.

Vitamin K can reverse the effect of warfarin, but this can take up to 6 hours to occur. If immediate reversal is required, then prothrombin complex concentrate or fresh frozen plasma can be given in a hospital setting.

Keywords: warfarin, still bleeding.

→ Scottish Dental Clinical Effectiveness Programme (SDCEP). *Management of dental patients taking anticoagulants or antiplatelet drugs*. 2015. Available at: http://www.sdcep.org.uk/published-guidance/anticoagulants-and-antiplatelets/

5. E ★★ OHCD 6th ed. → pp. 518–19

Acromegaly develops as a result of overproduction of growth hormone (GH), commonly caused by a benign tumour of the pituitary gland called an adenoma. All of the signs described in the scenario are indicators of an excess in GH. The classic aide-memoire in dentistry is 'hats and dentures' that have become too small.

Complication include:

- Severe headaches
- Arthritis and carpal tunnel syndrome
- Hypertension
- Diabetes mellitus (excess GH leads to insulin resistance)
- Compression of the optic chiasm leading to loss of vision in the outer visual fields, described as bitemporal hemianopia (tunnel vision).

Addison's syndrome is used to describe hypoadrenalism, and therefore inadequate corticosteroid production, leading to an electrolyte disturbance (hyponatraemia, hypoglycaemia, and hypokalaemia).

Anabolic steroids can lead to iatrogenic hypogonadism and insufficient endogenous production of androgens.

Conn's syndrome, or primary hyperaldosteronism, leads to hypernatraemia and hypokalaemia. This can manifest itself as high blood pressure and muscular weakness or spasms.

Cushing's syndrome is described as an excess of glucocorticoids, which can lead to a number of symptoms such as high blood pressure, abdominal obesity with thin arms and legs, abdominal striae (stretch marks), a 'moon-shaped' face, a hump between the shoulders, weak proximal muscles, osteoporosis, acne, depression, and thin and fragile skin.

Keywords: spacing, prominent supra-orbital ridges, widening of the nose and jaw, tingling, hands.

→ Devlin H, Craven R. *Oxford Handbook of Integrated Dental Biosciences*. Oxford University Press, Oxford; 2018.

6. A ★★ OHCD 6th ed. → p. 504

The symptoms presented here are indicative of an underlying haematological malignancy. The presence of signs suggesting anaemia, coupled with abnormal bleeding, should make the reader consider pathology of

both white and red blood cell lineages. Leukaemia is a neoplastic proliferation of white blood cells in the bone marrow. The symptoms occur
because of bone marrow failure and crowding out of healthy leucocytes,
erythrocytes, and platelets. General manifestations include anaemia,
thrombocytopenia, liability to infections, and lymphadenopathy. There
are four main subtypes of leukaemia: acute and chronic lymphocytic
(ALL and CLL), and acute and chronic myeloblastic leukaemias (AML and
CML). ALL is the most common childhood leukaemia, whereas AML is
the most common acute adult leukaemia. In this scenario, the majority of
symptoms are common to all leukaemias, but the age of the patient and
the presence of gingival swelling are more suggestive of AML. Gingival
swelling from leukaemic infiltration is most commonly seen in AML (subtypes M5 and M4).

Beta-thalassaemia is an inherited anaemia resulting from decreased production of the beta chains of haemoglobin. Although the shortness of
breath and fatigue could suggest this disease, the abnormal bleeding
would not be associated with this condition. Other symptoms of beta-
thalassaemia include skeletal abnormalities, splenomegaly, and cardiac
abnormalities.

Non-Hodgkin's lymphoma could be responsible for these symptoms, as
leukaemia occurs in a small percentage of these patients, but it is usually
associated with immunocompromised patients.

Keywords: 55-year old, tired, short of breath, swollen gingivae, spontaneous bleeding.

→ Wu J, Fantasia J, Kaplan R. Oral manifestations of acute myelomonocytic
leukemia: a case report and review of the classification of leukemias.
Journal of Periodontology. 2002;**73**:664–8.

7. D ★★   OHCD 6th ed. → pp. 526–7

The patient is demonstrating many of the classical features of
Parkinson's disease. They have postural (proximal) muscle weakness,
as evidenced by difficulty getting up from his chair, a shuffling gait,
expressionless (mask-like) facies, micrographia (small handwriting),
and bradykinesia (slow movements). Other features include resting
tremor, very labile mood, and autonomic nervous system dysfunction (commonly presenting as loss of urinary continence or postural
hypotension).

Parkinson's disease sufferers are susceptible to falls. Their shuffling gait
can lead to trips and slips; weak postural muscles limit their ability to
control their centre of gravity, and slowness of movement obtunds their
ability to break a fall.

BPPV and labyrinthitis are both benign conditions that affect the vestibular system and can give the sensation of vertigo (subjective sensation
of the individual or the surroundings rotating). BPPV gives short-lasting
(seconds to minutes) symptoms of vertigo, often precipitated by changes
in posture or movements of the head. Labyrinthitis (vestibular neuritis)
is inflammation of the vestibular apparatus, often secondary to an upper

respiratory tract infection, that can lead to symptoms of vertigo that may last from days to weeks.

CPA tumours can affect the cranial nerves that emerge from the region between the cerebellum and the pons (CN V, CN VI, CN VII, CN VIII). Although rare, CPA tumours should be excluded where there is any persistent vertigo, loss of hearing, or tinnitus.

Posterior circulation infarct describes a stroke in the posterior circulating artery and/or the vertebrobasilar system of the brain. It can lead to vertigo, ataxia, visual field defects, slurred speech, and paralysis.

Keywords: shuffles, handwriting, spidery, expressionless.

8. B ★★★

Graves' disease is caused by an autoantibody that mimics thyroid-stimulating hormone (TSH), and this leads to overproduction of thyroid hormone (hyperthyroidism). Patients can present with palpitations, weight loss, heat intolerance, and irritability, amongst other symptoms. The main sign of Graves' disease is diffuse swelling of the thyroid gland, otherwise known as thyroid goitre.

Hashimoto's thyroiditis is another autoimmune disorder that can also present with swelling of the thyroid gland (goitre). However, in this case, the anti-thyroid antibodies slowly destroy the thyroid tissue, leading to hypofunction of the gland (hypothyroidism). This would present as lethargy, weight gain, slow pulse, feeling cold, and depression.

DI can lead to weight loss and may present with polydipsia (frequent thirst) and polyuria (frequent urination). As opposed to diabetes mellitus, where dehydration is caused by the diuretic effect of having glucose in the urine, DI leads to loss of water in the urine because of a problem with the kidney reabsorbing water from the collecting tubules. Diabetes mellitus and DI are unlikely to cause swelling of the thyroid gland.

Thyroid cancer (there are many different forms) is a possibility with any new presentation of a neck swelling that moves on swallowing and tongue protrusion. However, given the clinical context in this case, it is more readily explained by the answer given.

TB, caused by *Mycobacterium tuberculosis*, can affect any part of the body, most commonly the lungs. Symptoms can include coughing, haemoptysis, fevers, night sweats, and weight loss. TB can also cause painless swelling of the lymph nodes, including those of the neck. These are known as cold abscesses due the absence of inflammatory signs.

Keywords: thirst, palpitations, sweating, weight loss, lump in neck.

9. C ★★★

The patient is suffering from an adrenal crisis, secondary to the withdrawal of his usual steroids. Normal endogenous adrenal glucocorticoid and mineralocorticoid production will diminish as a result of exogenous prednisolone administration (this causes a negative feedback loop, limiting adrenal production). If there is sudden cessation of the exogenous steroids, insufficient endogenous glucocorticoid production will lead to inadequate lipolysis and gluconeogenesis, and therefore a low blood sugar level. Inadequate mineralocorticoid production will lead to less retention of sodium (it is likely that the patient will be hyponatraemic) in the blood, and therefore less retention of water, leading to hypovolaemia and hypotension.

Steroids do have an immunosuppressive effect. However, the overriding concern in this case would be compensating for the loss of exogenous steroids. Anyone taking steroids for longer than a few weeks would require a reducing regime before stopping completely. Patients taking long-term steroids often require increased doses if they develop systemic infections.

Addison's disease may have a similar presentation to this case, but the underlying pathology in this scenario is based on inadequate endogenous production of corticosteroids due to exogenous steroid consumption.

Septic shock is suggested by features of systemic inflammatory response syndrome (SIRS)—in this case, hypotension (low blood pressure) and pyrexia (high temperature)—in the presence of a source of infection. This may be a compounding factor involved in the patient's presentation, but unlikely to be the main cause, given the history.

AIDS can have a varied presentation and is thought of as one of the 'great pretenders' in medicine, along with tuberculosis and syphilis. It should always be thought of when other causes of pathology have been excluded but is unlikely to present with these symptoms.

Keywords: abscess, high-dose prednisolone, not taken, sweaty, 70/50 mmHg, 2.9 mmol/L.

10. **D** ★★★ OHCD 6th ed. → p. 526

A TIA is any vascular insult to the brain that causes a neurological deficit (weakness of limbs, hemisensory loss, slurring of speech, or unusually a reduction in conscious level) that lasts for <24 hours. All that can be said from this scenario is that the patient has just begun to have a central (upper motor neurone) neurological deficit, that has lasted for <24 hours. If the neurological deficit persists beyond 24 hours, it can be categorized as a cerebrovascular accident (CVA), also known as a stroke.

The insult may be as a result of an embolus—a fragment of blood clot occluding the vessel, causing ischaemia—or a haemorrhage where blood supply to certain parts of the brain may be disrupted due to an intracranial bleed. The latter often results in a neurosurgical emergency.

Being able to raise both eyebrows differentiates this central neurological deficit from a peripheral (lower motor neurone) neurological deficit such as Bell's palsy. The forehead is bilaterally innervated from the motor cortex, so an ischaemic event in one hemisphere will not lead to loss of function, as the other hemisphere will still be innervating the forehead muscles.

A subarachnoid haemorrhage is usually a bleed from one of the major intracranial blood vessels and is characterized by a sudden and severe occipital headache (often described as a 'thunderclap' headache), nausea, and vomiting and can lead to confusion and coma. It generally does not lead to unilateral neurological symptoms.

Vertebrobasilar insufficiency usually leads to a very transient loss of consciousness (syncope), due to compression of the vertebral arteries or basilar artery with certain neck positions. It can present as presyncopal symptoms that include fading vision, vertigo, and confusion.

Keywords: slurring, left, droops, raise both eyebrows.

11. E ★★★ OHCD 6th ed. → p. 514

The scenario alludes to a patient who is drinking excessive amounts of alcohol and displaying signs of chronic liver damage. The liver is a robust organ with numerous functions, most importantly detoxification of compounds in blood, bile production, carbohydrate and lipid metabolism, storage of essential vitamins and minerals, and production of proteins essential to life, including coagulation factors. It has a substantial capacity for regeneration; however, prolonged toxic insults can cause hepatocellular necrosis and normal liver architecture to be replaced with fibrous tissue. The result is liver function deterioration and obstruction of blood flow. There are multiple signs and symptoms that develop from portal hypertension and reduced liver function, including jaundice (also evident in palatal gingivae) and pruritus (itching), hepatomegaly, splenomegaly, peripheral and central oedema (ascites), finger clubbing, and hyperdynamic circulation (palmar erythema, spider naevi).

In this scenario, the, patient has signs indicative of severe hepatic impairment, and one should suspect derangement of liver functions and inadequacy of clotting capability even if the patient is trying to push for treatment. Additional consideration should be given to alcohol-induced thrombocytopenia (low platelets), which will also affect the patient's ability to form a primary blood clot.

It is important to be safe, and therefore, a full blood count, liver function tests, and a clotting screen are required before any intervention is performed. It may be possible to extirpate the tooth, but generally local anaesthetic via a block injection will be required for a lower molar and it is unlikely that a dental dam can be placed. In patients with clotting impairment, even injections are contraindicated until the bleeding risk can be assessed. Uncontrolled bleeding in the parapharyngeal area can become a life-threatening situation! Once the blood requests are confirmed, treatment can be planned.

Metronidazole can produce an unpleasant disulfiram-like reaction and is contraindicated in combination with alcohol. Additionally, it is metabolized by the liver and, if prescribed, requires significant dose reduction.

Asking a chronic alcoholic to cease drinking alcohol immediately is not advisable, as it may lead to adverse neurological consequences, coma, and death (delirium tremens).

Keywords: cider, sclera, yellow, distended abdomen, spider-like patterns.

→ Quach S, Brooke AE, Clark A, Ellison SJ. Blood investigations prior to oral surgery for suspected alcohol-induced coagulopathy. Are they necessary? *British Dental Journal.* 2015;**219**:121.

12. B ★★★★

Named after Henry Pancoast, an American radiologist, this is an apical lung tumour located close to the superior ribs. Compression of the superior part of the sympathetic chain causes the examination findings described in the question: miosis (constricted pupil), ptosis (droopy eyelid), and enophthalmos (sunken globe). Anhidrosis (decreased sweating) of the ipsilateral face is also described in this syndrome. This constellation of signs is otherwise known as Horner's syndrome.

Other sequelae of a Pancoast tumour include weakness and wasting of the muscles of the ipsilateral arm and hand (due to compression of the brachial plexus) and alteration of the voice (due to recurrent laryngeal nerve compression).

PE is a reasonable differential diagnosis, as it can produce haemoptysis (coughing up blood) and dyspnoea (in addition to chest pain and cough), but PE would not explain Horner's syndrome.

Pulmonary TB can also cause dyspnoea and haemoptysis. Additionally, TB can cause night sweats, anorexia, weight loss, and fatigue—all of which can be seen in any malignancy. In this case, the strong smoking history and the presence of Horner's syndrome should make you think of cancer.

Mesothelioma is unlikely, as this carcinoma of the pleura almost exclusively occurs in those with asbestos (a common building and insulation material in the pre-1990s) exposure.

A spontaneous pneumothorax is unlikely to lead to haemoptysis.

Keywords: smoking, chronic cough, blood, eye, sunken, smaller pupil, eyelid, drooping.

13. A ★★★★   OHCD 6th ed. → p. 534

AIDS is defined by a CD4+ T cell count of below 200 cells/μL and the presence of an array of different conditions that occur after the immune system is compromised by the human immunodeficiency virus (HIV).

This question alluded to the patient's previous intravenous drug use—a common cause for HIV transmission, along with sexual contact, blood transfusion, and vertical transmission (from mother to child). However, the rest of the signs and symptoms revealed in the question allude to conversion of HIV infection to AIDS. A chest infection is suggestive of either pulmonary tuberculosis (the symbiotic twin of HIV/AIDS) and/or *Pneumocystis jirovecii* pneumonia (PJP), an AIDS-defining condition.

The patient is also a heavy smoker and a drinker—both high risk for oral squamous cell carcinoma. Equally, a dark, irregular lesion in the mouth or anywhere else on the body may also be suggestive of a melanoma. However, in the context of this question, this lesion would fit better with Kaposi's sarcoma—a vascular lesion related to human herpesvirus 8 (HHV 8) that is another AIDS-defining condition.

Keywords: intravenous drug user, cough, dark purple and irregular lump, white plaques, scraped off.

14. E ★★★★

See Table 9.1.

This patient is not drinking fluids and is taking ibuprofen (non-steroidal anti-inflammatory drug) and candesartan (angiotensin II receptor blocker); all three are risk factors for developing pre-renal acute kidney injury (loss of renal function after a drop in blood supply to the kidneys). This is evidenced by a lack of urine production. As morphine is renally excreted, it is likely this opiate has accumulated in the patient's body and is causing his narcosis (drowsiness due to high levels of opiate medication). He would need some naloxone (a μ-opioid receptor antagonist) to reverse his narcosis and monitoring with pulse oximetry, as well as oxygen supplementation.

As a rule of thumb, one should seek anaesthetic assessment once the GCS score is ≤8, as the patient may not be able to protect their airway.

Keywords: opens eyes, hands to sternal area, mumble, incomprehensible, GCS.

Table 9.1 Glasgow coma scale

	1	2	3	4	5	6
Eyes	Not opening eyes	Opening eyes to pain	Opening eyes to voice	Opening eyes spontaneously	N/A	N/A
Verbal	No sound	Incomprehensible sounds	Inappropriate words	Confused	Orientated	N/A
Motor	No movement	Extensor response to pain	Abnormal flexor response to pain	Flexor response/withdrawal from painful stimulus	Localizes to painful stimulus	Able to follow commands

The scores for this patient are: Eyes = 2; Verbal = 2; Motor = 5.

15. C ★★★★ OHCD 6th ed. → p. 516

CKD is classified by a reduction in the estimated glomerular filtration rate. A rate of below 60 mL/minute/1.73 m² is considered abnormal in adults. Below this, there are five stages of CKD, with stage 5 alternatively being known as end-stage renal failure (ESRF). At stage 5, dialysis or a renal transplant is required.

There are two types of dialysis: peritoneal dialysis (PD) where the patient's peritoneal membrane is used as a semi-permeable membrane to filter blood, or haemodialysis where blood is taken out of the body and filtered through a machine.

There are many clinical manifestations of CKD relevant to dentistry, including: increased prevalence of periodontal disease, xerostomia, oral ulcerations, increased bleeding tendency, reduced drug excretion capabilities, etc. In the case of patients on haemodialysis, there is some debate as to when the most appropriate time is to treat, but generally, it is considered that the day after dialysis is best, as any accumulated by-products will have been cleared. However, this is always driven by the degree of volume overload and serum levels of potassium/urea.

Heparin (an anticoagulant used during haemodialysis) has a half-life of 4 hours, and so treatment later in the day after dialysis is feasible, but the so-called 'dialysis hangover' (a collection of unpleasant post-treatment symptoms) may deter patients from undergoing treatment immediately.

Some authors do argue treatment on the day before dialysis is better when major surgery is required, because it will remove post-operative inflammatory mediators or high protein loads from swallowed blood. Either way, preoperative clotting screens, appropriate reduction in any drug used, and a discussion with the renal physician are mandatory.

Keywords: extraction, CKD stage 5, haemodialysis.

→ Greenwood M, Seymour R, Meechan J. *Textbook of Human Disease in Dentistry*. Wiley-Blackwell, Oxford; 2009.

→ Proctor R, Kumar N, Stein A, Moles D, Porter S. Oral and dental aspects of chronic renal failure. *Journal of Dental Research*. 2005;**84**:199–208.

Therapeutics and medical emergencies

Tariq Ali

'*Primum non nocere.*'

Firstly, do no harm. This is held as the first law of clinical practice when considering any intervention to improve the health of our patients. This may at times be a difficult proposition, especially when the approach to treating a condition is fraught with risks and can carry the danger of adverse and unwanted side effects.

Prescribing therapeutics is the time perhaps when this maxim should be most at the forefront of a clinician's mind, as therapeutic interventions may not cause any immediately discernible danger or harm in the same way as operative interventions. It is therefore important for the prescriber to understand the relevant pharmacodynamics (the effects of the agent on the body) and pharmacokinetics (the effects of the body on the agent). To add a further layer of complexity, the reader should understand that pharmacological sciences are possibly the fastest evolving part of medicine. It would be a fair bet to say that, within the course of the reader's undergraduate education, entire new classes of therapeutics will have emerged and established perceptions of other agents would have significantly changed.

Practically speaking, this does not mean that it is necessary to memorize the nuances of all therapeutic agents (although you should have a good grasp of those you prescribe regularly); rather it is more important that a clinician understands how to recognize potential dangers and then be resourceful enough to mitigate against them, given the best knowledge available at the time. Access to an up-to-date formulary and the will to use it are the surest way to navigate any prescribing pitfalls.

'We don't rise to the occasion, we fall to the most basic level of our training'.

Thankfully, medical emergencies occur infrequently in the general practice setting. It is the rarity of such events that often leads to anxieties when dealing with them. This reaction is amplified by the caregiver's natural instinct to do something immediately, but often not knowing exactly what to do because the diagnosis is not immediately clear.

The ABCDE approach, as advocated by the Resuscitation Council, is a safe and methodical way to approach any emergency. ABCDE is not only a hierarchy of importance for systems critical to life, but it also acts as an aide-memoire to undertake examinations and interventions when necessary. Most importantly, it buys time whilst the diagnosis is found or declares itself, without adversely affecting the outcome by inaction.

Key topics include:

- Common drugs for common medical conditions
- Drug interactions
- Oral side effects of medications
- Basic life support
- Medical emergencies in dentistry (including the Resuscitation Council UK guidelines)
- ABCDE approach.

QUESTIONS

1. Prior to the administration of a local anaesthetic, a 25-year-old man with well-controlled epilepsy begins to have a tonic–clonic seizure. The dental chair is laid flat, and high-flow oxygen is delivered through a non-rebreather mask. His blood sugar is checked, whilst your nurse has called for an ambulance; the result is 5.3 mmol/L. After 5 minutes, the seizure has not self-terminated. What is the single best intervention that should be available in dental practices? ★

A Buccal midazolam 10 mg

B Intravenous lorazepam 4 mg

C Intravenous phenytoin infusion 140 mL (10%)

D Oral diazepam 10 mg

E Rectal diazepam 35 mg

2. A 40-year-old insulin-dependent diabetic man becomes very sweaty and tremulous during a dental examination. He thinks his sugars are low and asks whether any sweets are available. As the nurse goes to get some, he rapidly deteriorates, developing speech slurring before losing consciousness. He is still breathing and has a pulse. What would be the single best course of action to take? ★

A Administer 10 mL of oral glucose gel

B Administer high-flow oxygen and 300 mg of soluble aspirin dissolved in water

C Infuse 20 units/mL of insulin intravenously

D Inject glucagon 1 mg intramuscularly

E Use ammonium carbonate 1 puff nasally

3. A nurse raises the alarm as she finds a 77-year-old man unconscious. She has already called for an ambulance, but she wants
help managing him. Following the ABCDE approach, after 10 seconds,
no pulse or respiratory effort is noted. Another nurse has retrieved the
resuscitation trolley. What would be the single best immediate course
of action to take? ★

A Administer a precordial thump, whilst an automated external defibril-
lator (AED) is attached

B Begin chest compressions at a rate of 15:2 (15 compressions and
then 2 breaths), whilst an AED is attached

C Begin chest compressions at a rate of 30:2 (30 compressions and
then 2 rescue breaths), whilst an AED is attached

D Begin continuous chest compressions at a rate of 100–110, whilst an
AED is attached and oxygen is continuously delivered

E Place the patient in the recovery position, and continuously deliver
oxygen until the ambulance arrives

4. A 29-year-old woman attends, concerned about the recent dark
staining of her teeth. She has acne vulgaris, iron deficiency anaemia
associated with heavy periods, hay fever, and gastro-oesophageal disease (GORD). She has also been regularly using 0.2% chlorhexidine
digluconate mouthwash for periodontal disease for the past 3 months,
having seen a television advert. Her most recent prescription is
shown below:

Doxycycline 100 mg once daily (OD)

Diphenhydramine 25 mg four times daily (QDS)

Ferrous fumarate tablets 210 mg twice daily (BD)

Lansoprazole 15 mg OD

Which single medication is most likely responsible for the discoloration
in this scenario? ★★

A Chlorhexidine digluconate

B Diphenhydramine

C Doxycycline

D Ferrous fumarate

E Lansoprazole

5. A 40-year-old woman enters the dental surgery, visibly breathless, coughing, and wheezing. She expresses that her fingers feel tingly but struggles to complete her sentence. She is a known asthmatic, so the nurse exits the room to call for an ambulance. What is the single most appropriate next step? ★ ★

A Administer beclomethasone 10 mg orally

B Administer ten puffs of salbutamol via a spacer

C Administer adrenaline 0.5 mg intramuscularly

D Measure her peak expiratory flow rate (PEFR) before administering any drugs

E Oxygen via a non-rebreather mask at 10–15 L/minute

6. A 68-year-old woman is waiting for a dental appointment. Whilst waiting, they become flushed, clammy, and short of breath. A dental team are called to help, at which point she tells them she has some central crushing chest pain that radiates into her jaw and to her left arm. She has tried her glyceryl trinitrate (GTN) spray, with no effect on her symptoms. What is the single most likely diagnosis? ★ ★

A Acute coronary syndrome (ACS)

B Angina attack

C Aortic aneurysm rupture

D Oesophageal spasm

E Pulmonary embolus

7. A 64-year-old man attends his local dental practice for surgical extraction of his upper right first molar (UR6). He is anxious as he sits in the chair. Medically, he takes insulin for diabetes mellitus, ramipril for hypertension, and atorvastatin for high cholesterol. After administration of the local anaesthetic, he begins to experience crushing central chest pain that radiates to his neck and left arm. He is noticeably clammy and short of breath. Which medications from the emergency kit are the most appropriate for managing this situation? (Select one answer from the options listed below.) ★ ★

A Oxygen and midazolam

B Oxygen, aspirin, glyceryl trinitrate

C Oxygen, aspirin, salbutamol

D Oxygen, glucose, glucagon

E Oxygen, salbutamol, adrenaline

8. A 70-year-old man attends as a new patient. He is being treated for hypertension and ischaemic heart disease by his doctor. He has had a coronary artery stent placed 3 years ago and a renal transplant roughly 20 years ago. He takes bendroflumethiazide, nifedipine, atorvastatin, clopidogrel, and ciclosporin. Clinically, his gingivae are very enlarged, with a lobular shape, and there are deep periodontal pockets. Which single medication is most likely responsible for the signs? ★★★

A Atorvastatin

B Bendroflumethiazide

C Ciclosporin

D Clopidogrel

E Nifedipine

9. A 23-year-old woman presents with severe facial swelling and signs suggestive of systemic involvement. Antibiotics are prescribed and administered at the dental practice, before referring her to the local Maxillofacial Unit. Whilst awaiting the taxi, the receptionist notices a deterioration in her situation. She has developed an urticarial rash, an audible wheeze, cold sweaty hands, and a thready, rapid, pulse. What is the single most appropriate next step to take? ★★★

A Administer five puffs of the Ventolin® inhaler via a spacer

B Administer 10 mg of chlorphenamine orally

C Administer hydrocortisone 200 mg intramuscularly (IM)

D Administer adrenaline 0.5 mg IM

E Administer 0.5 mL of 1:1000 adrenaline intravenously

10. A 58-year-old woman, who has smoked 26 pack years, has a past medical history of breast cancer, rheumatoid arthritis, osteoporosis, and Crohn's disease. She historically received radiotherapy for breast cancer and is currently taking methotrexate, folic acid, prednisolone, and twice-yearly denosumab injections. She had an extraction 3 months ago, but there is no evidence of healing and exposed necrotic bone is present. What is the single most likely causative agent for the pathology? ★★★

A Denosumab

B Methotrexate

C Prednisolone

D Radiotherapy

E Smoking

11. A 24-year-old man attends as a new patient. He has just returned from working as a holiday rep in Ibiza. He has been taking numerous recreational drugs, caffeinated drinks, and his usual antidepressant (citalopram). Clinically, he has scalloping of the lateral borders of the tongue, occlusal wear facets on opposing cusps, and hypertrophic masseters. Which single recreational drug is most likely linked to these findings? ★★★

A Caffeine

B Cocaine

C Ketamine

D Marijuana

E MDMA (3,4-methylenedioxymethamphetamine)

12. A 55-year-old woman attends, complaining of multiple large mouth ulcers over the last 3 months. She sees her cardiologist for severe angina who started a new oral medication 9 weeks ago. She takes this regularly and uses her glycerin trinitrate spray, as necessary. Clinically, the mouth ulcers are similar in appearance to major recurrent aphthous stomatitis (RAS). It is suspected that the new medication is linked to the mouth ulcers. Which single commonly prescribed cardiac medication has the patient most likely been prescribed? ★★★

A Bisoprolol

B Naproxen

C Nicorandil

D Nifedipine

E Ramipril

13. A 34-year-old man attended the Emergency Department 2 days ago, complaining of toothache. He was diagnosed (provisionally) with a dental abscess, prescribed amoxicillin, and advised to see his dentist. Since then, he has been feeling progressively unwell, with fever and sore throat. Numerous painful mouth ulcers have stopped him eating and drinking normally, and he has developed a rash on his abdomen. There are a number of lesions which display a red and white target appearance, some of which have blistered. What is the single most likely diagnosis? ★★★★

A Erythema multiforme minor

B Erythema multiforme major

C Primary herpetic gingivostomatitis

D Staphylococcal scalded skin syndrome

E Steven–Johnson syndrome (SJS)

14. An 82-year-old man with hypertension, angina, and epilepsy presents for a routine examination. He is concerned that his breath has begun to smell in the last 3 weeks. He does not feel he has a dry mouth; his diet is unchanged, and routine dental examination does not appear to offer a cause for his halitosis. His cardiologist has changed one of his medications 2 months ago. Which single commonly prescribed medication for his medical problems could explain his halitosis? ★ ★ ★ ★

A Bendroflumethiazide

B Isosorbide dinitrate

C Lamotrigine

D Ramipril

E Ranitidine

15. An 81-year-old woman presents as an emergency after having had a simple extraction by a colleague earlier that day. Bleeding has still not stopped, but because she was nervous, she forgot to mention before the extraction that she has been started on ticagrelor following a coronary artery stent placement 4 months ago. Clinically, the socket has been packed and sutured but oozes blood every time it is agitated. Her blood pressure is 129/78 mmHg, and her pulse is 72 beats per minute. Which therapeutic intervention may be of benefit in this situation? (Select one answer from the options listed below.) ★ ★ ★ ★

A Intravenous (IV) protamine sulfate

B IV prothrombin complex

C Oral vitamin K

D Topical 15.5% ferrous sulfate

E Tranexamic acid 5% mouthwash

16. A 62-year-old man with hypertension attends for a routine dental examination. He begins to complain of sudden-onset, severe headache at the back of his head 5 minutes after walking into your room. He mentions he has never experienced any headaches in his life and that the pain feels like he was being hit with a cricket bat. The nurse is asked to call for an ambulance. After 10 minutes of onset, the pain becomes unbearable and he develops an aversion to light and says that his neck feels stiff and he wants to vomit. What is the single most likely diagnosis? ★ ★ ★ ★

A Idiopathic intracranial hypertension

B Meningitis

C Migraine

D Subarachnoid haemorrhage

E Trigeminal neuralgia

17. A new dental nurse is unclear on the medical emergency protocols within the practice. She informs the practice manager that she has not carried out any continuing professional development (CPD) during her first 12 months as a registered nurse. What is the single most appropriate action in these circumstances? ★ ★ ★ ★

A Advise the nurse to complete a minimum of 10 hours of CPD in the next 12 months, in line with her current personal development plan

B Advise the nurse to contact the General Dental Council (GDC) about her situation

C Give the nurse the practice's standard development plan for new nurses, for the remaining 4 years of her CPD cycle

D Reassure the nurse and inform her she must complete 150 hours of CPD by the end of her 5-year cycle, of which 50 hours must be verifiable

E Reassure the nurse and inform her she must complete 50 hours of verifiable CPD in each 5-year cycle

18. A 39-year-old woman has just had four dental restorations performed, under intravenous (IV) conscious sedation with midazolam. After completing treatment, there are 2 mL of midazolam left. Which single option is the most appropriate for managing the remaining drug? ★ ★ ★ ★

A All remaining midazolam should be administered

B Decant into a sterile container for storage

C Denature or irretrievably dispose of the remaining midazolam

D Securely store all remaining midazolam in the original packaging

E Sign midazolam back into the local pharmacy/controlled drug store

ANSWERS

1. A ★

Most epileptic seizures self-terminate, without the need for pharmacological intervention and usually in under 5 minutes. Once the initial first-aid steps have been taken to ensure that the patient is lying in a safe position, there is no obstruction to the airway, and high-flow oxygen is being administered, thoughts should turn to interventions that may help terminate the seizure. Before assuming the aetiology is idiopathic epilepsy, one should search for reversible causes such as low blood sugar and electrolyte imbalance—the latter is only practicable in the hospital setting. In this case, the patient was not hypoglycaemic.

The initial agent of choice for seizure termination is a medium- to long-acting benzodiazepine; ideally, this should be given intravenously (IV), e.g. lorazepam 2–4 mg. In the dental practice setting, buccal midazolam should be available as part of the emergency kit, and this is a safe first-line intervention whilst waiting for emergency assistance to arrive. If there is no effect from the first dose, it can be repeated. Oral diazepam, commonly distributed in tablet form, is unlikely to be absorbed and would be a significant aspiration risk.

A seizure lasting 5 minutes or multiple seizures without clear neurological recovery is defined as status epilepticus and is an extreme neurological emergency, as prolonged seizure times are associated with post-seizure neurological deficits and death. Continuous seizure activity carries a risk of hypoxia from inadequate ventilation, which explains the potential complications.

Keywords: epilepsy, seizure, after 5 minutes.

→ Resuscitation Council UK. *Quality standards for cardiopulmonary resuscitation and training*. Available at: https://www.resus.org.uk/quality-standards/

→ The Scottish Government, National Dental Advisory Committee. *Emergency drugs and equipment in primary dental care*. 2015. Available at: http://www.scottishdental.org/wp-content/uploads/2015/01/Emergency-Drugs-and-Equipment-in-Primary-Dental-Care-2015.pdf

2. D ★

It is important to remember that the response to all medical emergencies should follow the ABCDE (Airway, Breathing, Circulation, Disability, Exposure) approach. This patient continues to breathe and have a pulse, and the progression of the scenario clearly points towards a hypoglycaemic attack (defined as a blood sugar level of 3.9 mmol/L or below). Symptoms are as follows:

• Autonomic: sweating, palpitations, hunger, tremor
• General: headache, nausea
• Neurological: confusion, paralysis, seizures, coma.

Glucagon is a hormone that antagonizes insulin and increases glucose levels by glycogenolysis (breakdown of stored hepatic and muscular glycogen into glucose) and gluconeogenesis (production of new glucose from amino acid substrate or lipids) in the liver. Maximal plasma concentrations are achieved within 5 minutes, and the half-life is between 8 and 18 minutes, so it is important to give further simple (sugary foods) and complex (starchy foods) carbohydrates when the patient regains consciousness to prevent rebound hypoglycaemia.

Oral glucose should be used in those with a preserved conscious level. Despite the fact that it can be rubbed into the oral mucosa, there is an aspiration risk and, if possible, other measures should be tried first. It should be noted that prolonged periods of hypoglycaemia may lead to irreversible brain damage.

There appears to be no clear indication for oxygen administration, but it is good practice to give oxygen in emergency situations until a reliable oxygen measurement can be undertaken.

Diabetics can have so-called silent (asymptomatic) myocardial infarctions, due to autonomic neuropathy, and aspirin may be helpful in these acute ischaemic events. However, this patient's symptoms can be better explained by hypoglycaemia, and it may be unsafe to administer oral medication to a patient with variable consciousness.

Ammonium carbonate are used as smelling salts and has previously been used as a stimulus to reverse non-serious causes of syncope (such as orthostatic, vasovagal, or postural hypotension).

Keywords: diabetic, sugars are low, in and out of consciousness.

→ National Institute for Health and Care Excellence, British National Formulary. *Treatment of hypoglycaemia*. Available at: https://bnf.nice.org.uk/treatment-summary/hypoglycaemia.html

3. C ★

This question tests working knowledge of the basic life support algorithm. All General Dental Council (GDC)-registered dentists and dental care professionals should undergo yearly basic life support (BLS) training. The Resuscitation Council (UK) guidelines updated in 2015 stipulate chest compression at a ratio of 30:2 and a rate of 100–110 for those who are trained to do so.

For those who are not trained or not confident, there is increasing emphasis on providing continuous chest compressions until the airway can be secured. The reason for this approach is to improve the quality of bystander chest compressions and this may lead to less neurological morbidity in successful resuscitations. With a full emergency drug kit, a pocket mask would be available and abstaining from breaths due to cross-infection reasons would not be appropriate. The emergency kit in dental practices must comply with the latest GDC and Resuscitation Council (UK) guidelines. The current Resuscitation Council (UK) minimal requirements in a primary dental care setting include an AED.

In situations where a patient is found unconscious, assessing for danger and then following the ABCDE approach is highly recommended and provides a systematic way to assess the patient in a high-stress situation. In cases of cardiac arrest, calling for an ambulance early and applying defibrillation as soon as possible are vital.

Keywords: unconscious, no pulse or respiratory effort.

→ Resuscitation Council (UK). *Adult basic life support and automated external defibrillation.* 2015. Available at: https://www.resus.org.uk/resuscitation-guidelines/adult-basic-life-support-and-automated-external-defibrillation/

4. A ★★

Tetracyclines (which are used for acne vulgaris) and diphenhydramine (the active ingredient of over-the-counter antihistamines like Benadryl®) are known to cause intrinsic staining of the teeth when taken during tooth development. Chlorhexidine mouthwash and liquid iron salts can cause extrinsic tooth discoloration that can be reversed with cessation of treatment and professional cleaning.

Lansoprazole, a proton pump inhibitor used to treat GORD, has been reported to stain the tongue yellow but has no staining effect on teeth.

In this situation, the staining has developed recently and is unlikely to be intrinsic staining from medication. Although the iron salts can cause staining, the patient is taking tablets, not a liquid form, and therefore the chlorhexidine mouthwash is the obvious culprit. Chlorhexidine mouthwash is known to cause staining of the teeth and recommended to be used for periods no longer than 2 weeks at a time. If patients are required to use chlorhexidine mouthwash for longer periods, then they should be warned of the risk of staining and other side effects (e.g. taste disturbances) and should be advised to avoid food and drink immediately after using the mouthrinse. Alternative daily formulations are now available.

Keywords: recent, dark staining, chlorhexidine, 3 months.

5. B ★★

The patient is exhibiting signs and symptoms of a severe asthma attack: shortness of breath, wheeze, inability to complete sentences, high pulse rate, and high respiratory rate. PEFR is extremely important as part of the assessment of asthma exacerbations. A PEFR of <50% of the predicted value for this patient would indicate severe restrictive airway disease. However, it is not the intervention that would improve the patient's condition.

In this situation, salbutamol (a short-acting beta-2 receptor agonist that works to relax smooth muscles in the bronchioles) takes priority. Patients above the age of 5 years can have ten puffs of salbutamol inhaler via a spacer. Salbutamol administration can be repeated every 10 minutes until the ambulance arrives. There is evidence that this has a comparable effect to 5 mg of nebulized salbutamol—the likely first-line treatment this patient would receive from paramedics or at hospital.

Beclomethasone (inhaled steroid) via a spacer in an emergency setting is a suboptimal treatment, as the amount delivered to the patient can be very variable and they are slow-acting. Oral steroids are the preferred choice and may be given by medical practitioners but again are slow-acting in comparison to beta-2 agonists.

High-flow oxygen should be administered until the oxygen level can be measured. Oxygen can be safely withdrawn if oxygen saturations are above 94%. Again, in this scenario, salbutamol takes priority, as bronchoconstriction should be reversed to give the best chance of treating potential hypoxia. If a nebulizer were present, both could have been administered concomitantly. Alternatively, oxygen should be given via a non-rebreather mask, whilst salbutamol is not being inhaled.

Adrenaline, given as an intramuscular injection, is an important treatment for anaphylaxis with cardiovascular compromise. This patient displays no other signs of anaphylaxis, and you have already deduced she has airways disease from her past medical history.

Finally, it is important to state that an ambulance would need to be called and the patient should be reassessed regularly after administering the drugs.

Keywords: visibly breathless, wheezing, struggles to complete her sentence, asthmatic.

6. A ★★

The patient has chest pain at rest, which is radiating to the left arm and jaw. These features can be best described as ACS. Other features include autonomic features (sweating, nausea) and the heart trying to compensate for local hypoxia by increasing the cardiovascular rate (breathing and heart rate).

ACS is the preferred nomenclature for the spectrum of conditions that include:

- Unstable angina—chest pain at rest in someone with known heart disease, due to cardiac muscle ischaemia (inadequate oxygen perfusion)
- Non-ST segment* elevation myocardial infarction (NSTEMI) (death of cardiac muscle)—a minor heart attack that does not lead to electrical changes on the electrocardiogram (ECG)
- ST segment* elevation myocardial infarction (STEMI)—a major heart attack leading to electrical changes on the ECG.

GTN is a vasodilator (widens artery diameter by causing smooth muscle relaxation) and can relieve ischaemic pain associated with angina (coronary ischaemic chest pain which is brought about by activity and relieved by rest or nitrates).

Pulmonary embolism can lead to chest pain. But this is typically pleuritic (worsened by deep inspiration). Other features include haemoptysis,

*ST segment refers to a specific electrical deflection noted on the ECG.

dyspnoea, tachycardia, features of deep vein thrombosis, cough, and syncope.

Oesophageal spasm can present very similarly to ACS. There is normally an absence of autonomic features, and if the patient lives an active lifestyle, there would be an absence of preceding exertion-induced chest pain (this would be difficult to elicit in sedentary patients!).

Thoracic aortic aneurysm rupture presents with acute chest pain. It can lead to chest pain that radiates to the back and is described as 'tearing' in nature. Other clinical features include a difference in blood pressure between both arms.

Keywords: central crushing pain, radiates into jaw and left arm, GTN, no effect.

7. B ★ ★

The scenario clearly alludes to an acute coronary syndrome (ACS)—the umbrella term for conditions that range from unstable angina to acute myocardial infarction (MI). An electrocardiogram (ECG) would be required to differentiate the severity of ischaemic heart disease, the classical signs of which are chest tightness that may radiate into the left arm or jaw, shortness of breath, nausea, vomiting, clamminess, and a 'sense of impending doom'. It should be noted patients may present with atypical chest pain, particularly the elderly and diabetics.

Oxygen is important in ensuring that there is adequate oxygenation of blood perfusing the heart. There is evidence to suggest hyperoxygenation can cause reperfusion injury and that it should only be administered if oxygen saturations are below 96% on room air. In the absence of reliable pulse oximetry, it should always be administered. Oxygen will help correct any hypoxia present and should be given until pulse oximetry can be taken.

The most common cause for coronary ischaemia and infarction is rupture of atherosclerotic (subendothelial calcified fatty plaques) lesions and subsequent formation of a thrombus (blood clot) that occludes blood supply to the cardiac muscle. Aspirin, which has antiplatelet effects and minimizes the formation of a thrombus, must be given promptly at a loading dose of 300 mg.

Glyceryl trinitrate (GTN) releases nitric oxide, a potent smooth muscle relaxant that leads to vasodilatation and increased perfusion. This is the intervention most likely to lead to the fastest symptom relief.

Morphine is also recommended for pain relief in a secondary care environment, but this will not be available in a primary care setting. MONA is a useful acronym to remember the necessary medication in a hospital setting—morphine, oxygen, nitrate, aspirin.

Keywords: diabetes, hypertension, atorvastatin, crushing central chest pain.

8. C ★ ★ ★   OHCD 6th ed. → p. 436

Phenytoin, ciclosporin, and nifedipine (calcium channel blockers) interact with epithelial keratinocytes, fibroblasts, and collagen, leading to an overgrowth of gingival tissue which is exacerbated by gingival inflammation. Gingival hyperplasia can be complicated by bleeding, pain, and periodontal disease, as hyperplastic tissue may lead to plaque trapping. Unfortunately, the presence of plaque may induce further enlargement and lead to a vicious cycle of disease. If plaque control can be optimized, then often gingival inflammation will resolve. However, surgical removal of the enlarged tissue via gingivectomy is required to facilitate effective oral hygiene. Further management may include liaising with the patent's general practitioner (GP) to change medication, where possible.

In this scenario, both ciclosporin and nifedipine are contributing to gingival overgrowth, but the literature would suggest that gingival overgrowth is more common with ciclosporin. Anecdotally, it also tends to be more excessive than with calcium channel blockers [phenytoin (50% incidence) > ciclosporin (30%) > nifedipine (20%)].

Keywords: renal transplant, ciclosporin, gingivae, enlarged.

→ Seymour RA, Thomason JM, Ellis JS. The pathogenesis of drug induced gingival overgrowth. *Journal of Clinical Periodontology*. 1996;**23**:165–75.

9. D ★ ★ ★

The patient is having an anaphylactic shock precipitated by the antibiotics. It is a type I [immunoglobulin E (IgE)-mediated] hypersensitivity reaction. Following an initial ABCDE approach, the most important step, if this is suspected, is to give adrenaline 0.5 mg IM (0.5 mL of 1:1000). It can be repeated if the patient's cardiovascular parameters do not respond every 5 minutes.

Adrenaline can be administered intravenously, but the clinician must be experienced with intravenous administration of adrenaline, and it shoud be undertaken with cardiac monitoring. Therefore, it is not recommended that dental professionals use this route. If you suspect hypotension, then the patient should be nursed supine, with the feet raised.

High-flow oxygen through a non-rebreather mask is also an important part of the patient's management. Clearly, the patient needs to be sent to an Emergency Department via an emergency ambulance.

The other options are worthwhile exploring after adrenaline is given. For instance, antihistamines are important, but the recommended route is intravenous, chlorphenamine (10 mg) being the agent of choice. Salbutamol is reasonable if the patient is wheezy, preferably via a nebulizer (5 mg); otherwise, 5–10 puffs via a spacer can be very effective. Another important treatment is corticosteroids (hydrocortisone 200 mg intravenously). Although corticosteroids take approximately 6 hours to work (independent of the route of administration), it is important to administer this medication in a timely fashion.

Keywords: antibiotics, urticarial rash, wheeze, thready, rapid, pulse.

→ Resuscitation Council (UK). *Emergency treatment of anaphylactic reactions: guidelines for healthcare providers.* 2008. Available at: https://www.resus.org.uk/anaphylaxis/emergency-treatment-of-anaphylactic-reactions/

10. A ★★★   OHCD 6th ed. → p. 364

Medication-related osteonecrosis of the jaw (MRONJ) is defined as exposed or necrotic bone of the maxillofacial skeleton 8 weeks after dental treatment in patients who have a history of using anti-resorptive (bisphosphonates and denosumab) or anti-angiogenic agents and that cannot be attributed to any other cause (i.e. jaw bone necrosis secondary to radiotherapy).

Bisphosphonates are a useful therapy for conditions that include osteoporosis and hypercalcaemia resulting from malignancies like myeloma and breast cancer. It can happen spontaneously but more commonly occurs after instrumentation or local trauma. Risk factors for MRONJ include intravenous bisphosphonates, long-term oral bisphosphonate use, especially with concomitant steroid use (e.g. prednisolone), immunosuppressants (e.g. methotrexate), and a previous history of MRONJ. Secondary risk factors include smoking, poor oral hygiene, pre-existing inflammatory disease (e.g. periodontitis/periapical disease), and denture trauma. These patients should ideally have their oral health optimized prior to commencing bisphosphonate therapy and less traumatic treatments (root canal treatment or coronectomy versus extraction) provided where possible. If extraction cannot be avoided, one should consider the least traumatic method and frequent post-operative reviews, to ensure healing of the patient, or referral to an oral surgeon.

Denosumab [monoclonal antibody inhibiting the receptor activator of nuclear factor kappa-B (RANK) ligand] is an alternative drug used to treat osteoporosis, which has also been implicated in MRONJ. However, as it has no bone-binding affinity, and the actions only last for 6 months. Patients receiving this medication may benefit from drug cessation for 6 months, but there is no consensus on drug holidays as yet and this decision must be made in conjunction with the patient's physician.

Bone turnover markers like C-terminal telopeptide (CTX)/beta crosslaps in serology have been suggested for use to stratify risk where a serum value of >150 pg/mL is suggestive of a safe threshold for invasive bone procedures. However, the evidence for this is less than definitive.

Although radiotherapy can cause osteonecrosis, in this scenario, the primary beam would not have affected the head and neck region; therefore, it is very unlikely to be implicated. A threshold value of 65 Gy of radiation to the facial skeleton confers significant risk of osteoradionecrosis.

Keywords: denosumab, extraction, exposed necrotic bone.

→ Kunchur R, Need A, Hughes T, Goss A. Clinical investigation of C-terminal cross-linking telopeptide test in prevention and management of bisphosphonate-associated osteonecrosis of the jaws. *Journal of Oral and Maxillofacial Surgery.* 2009;**67**:1167–73.

→ Ruggiero SL, Dodson TB, Fantasia J, et al. American Association of Oral and Maxillofacial Surgeons position paper on medication-related osteonecrosis of the jaw—2014 update. *Journal of Oral and Maxillofacial Surgery.* 2014;**72**:1938–56.

11. E ★★★

The findings are consistent with clenching and bruxism, both being parafunctional activities of the jaw joint that can cause tooth wear, tooth fracture, myalgia, joint pain, limited movement of the jaw, and head-aches. Bruxism is a parafunctional process which involves 'clenching or grinding of the teeth and/or bracing or thrusting of the mandible'. Bruxism is considered a centrally mediated process (i.e. controlled by higher processes in the brain). A number of psychotropic stimulants and antidepressants (selective serotonin reuptake inhibitors) can cause bruxism. Other agents which can cause bruxism include alcohol, smoking, and caffeine. Non-pharmacological causes include stress, anxiety, and sleep disorders. The influence of local occlusal factors is still debated but is not widely considered a causative agent. It may, however, be an aggravating factor.

In this case, the most likely causative agent is MDMA, the most potent pharmacological agent to cause clenching and bruxism on the list. Rat models suggest that MDMA inhibits the jaw opening reflex, therefore allowing uninhibited action of the jaw-closing muscles.

Keywords: recreational drugs, scalloping, tongue, occlusal wear facets, hypertrophic masseters.

→ Milosevic A, Agrawal N, Redfearn P, Mair L. The occurrence of toothwear in users of ecstasy (3,4-methylenedioxymethamphetamine). *Community Dentistry and Oral Epidemiology.* 1999;**27**:283–7.

12. C ★★★

Nicorandil is a second-line anti-anginal medication for symptomatic benefit. It has a number of adverse drug reactions, including palpitations, flushing, and toothache. Moreover, it is well known for causing large painful mouth ulcers, similar in appearance to major RAS.

Naproxen belongs to a group of drugs known as non-steroidal anti-inflammatory drugs. These drugs can cause upper gastrointestinal ulceration, including mouth ulcers. NSAIDs have a number of adverse drug reactions, including kidney injury and increased cardiac risk. So it is unlikely the cardiologist prescribed this.

Nifedipine is a calcium channel antagonist used primarily for hypertension, Raynaud's phenomenon, and premature labour. It can cause gum hyperplasia and hypotension.

Bisoprolol is a beta blocker, which is used primarily in arrhythmias and ischaemic heart disease. It can be associated with a number of adverse drug reactions, including hypotension, bronchoconstriction in asthmatics, bradycardia, and lichenoid reactions.

Ramipril is an angiotensin-converting enzyme (ACE) inhibitor. It is used primarily as an antihypertensive and has prognostic benefits in coronary artery disease, cardiac failure, and left ventricular remodelling associated with hypertension. It is associated with a dry cough, angio-oedema, and kidney injury. Some ACE inhibitors have been linked with oral ulceration, but they are not specific anti-anginal drugs and ulceration is less severe than with nicorandil.

Keywords: large mouth ulcers, severe angina, oral medication.

13. E ★★★★ OHCD 6th ed. → p. 420

SJS or toxic epidermal necrolysis (TEN) is an immune complex-mediated (type III) hypersensitivity reaction that classically presents as a mucocutaneous disorder, with febrile erosive stomatitis, severe conjunctivitis, and disseminated cutaneous eruption. An important cause of SJS is medication, along with infections and malignancies. Confusion regarding the nomenclature has existed for some time. The following describes the consensus in the literature:

- Erythema multiforme minor—target lesions or raised, oedematous papules (circumscribed solid, raised lesion) distributed on the extremities
- Erythema multiforme major—typical targets or raised, oedematous papules distributed acrally, with involvement of one or more mucous membranes; epidermal detachment involves <10% of total body surface area (TBSA)
- SJS/TEN syndrome—widespread blisters predominantly on the trunk and face, presenting with erythematous or pruritic macules and one or more mucous membrane erosions. Epidermal detachment of 10–30% of TBSA is described as SJS TEN overlap syndrome, whereas >30% of TBSA is described as TEN syndrome.

Staphylococcal scalded skin syndrome is a blistering eruption that occurs with A and B toxins from disseminated staphylococcal infection. The condition normally affects children but can also affect adults. In addition, with time, the rash typically affects the whole body, and given the duration of this patient's rash, it makes the diagnosis unlikely, but it is a reasonable differential, given the history of abscess.

Keywords: amoxicillin, fever, sore throat, mouth ulcers, red and white, target appearance.

→ Mockenhaupt M. The current understanding of Stevens-Johnson syndrome and toxic epidermal necrolysis. *Expert Review of Clinical Immunology*. 2011;**7**:803–13.

14. B ★★★★

Isosorbide dinitrate, a first-line anti-anginal medication, is associated with halitosis. A number of other drugs are also associated with halitosis, including:

- Chloral hydrate—a sedative that can be misused recreationally
- Calcium channel blockers—used for hypertension

- Ranitidine—a H2 antagonist used for reflux
- Statins—used to treat high cholesterol
- Selective serotonin reuptake inhibitors—used for treating anxiety and depression.

Amitriptyline can cause xerostomia, which can lead to halitosis, but this patient denies symptoms of xerostomia. Amitriptyline can cause ageusia (losing taste).

Ramipril can cause lichenoid reactions in the oral mucosa and dysgeusia (distortion of the correct taste). Phenytoin can cause gum hyperplasia, and aspirin can cause white pigmentation on oral mucosa.

Development of new signs and symptoms after changes in medication should lead you to investigate whether they may be a potential cause. The *British National Formulary* (*BNF*) is an excellent resource and lists common and rare known side effects of medications.

Keywords: angina, halitosis, cardiologist, changed, medications.

15. E ★★★★

Ticagrelor is a highly effective antiplatelet treatment used to minimize any clots that could form as a result of having a coronary artery stent. The medication has a similar mechanism of action to that of clopidogrel. It acts on adenosine diphosphate (ADP) receptors on platelets, leading to their activation as part of the initial stages of clot formation and subsequent cross-linking with fibrin. It has a shorter half-life than other antiplatelet agents like aspirin, clopidogrel, and prasugrel, and therefore, it is the only antiplatelet medication given as a twice-daily dose.

Tranexamic acid is a pro-thrombotic agent that reversibly binds to plasminogen to prevent it from forming active plasmin (fibrin clot-degrading factor), thereby preventing the breakdown of cross-links between aggregated platelets and the resultant fibrin formed during the coagulation cascade. It can be prescribed as a 5% mouthwash to be used up to five times daily to allow for clot stabilization, or orally to provide a more robust and systemic effect. In this case, it would be advisable to treat this patient with a topical preparation, as a systemic agent may lead to adverse coronary outcomes (blockage of the stent and heart attack). Close review would be paramount if the patient was prescribed, and sent home with, tranexamic mouthwash, along with advice on what to do if bleeding does not stop.

Protamine sulfate is the reversal agent used for low-molecular-weight heparins (LMWHs) like Clexane® and dalteparin. LMWH are a class of anticoagulants that activate anti-thrombin III in the coagulation cascade, which inactivates factor Xa (thrombin), which ultimately prevents a fibrin clot from forming.

Vitamin K is a reversal agent used for warfarin. It can be administered orally or intravenously and works to replace vitamin K not reduced from vitamin K epoxide (a by-product of the production of coagulation factors II, VII, IX, and X).

Ferrous sulfate 15.5% is the active ingredient in astringedent. Although it is an effective haemostat, given the medication the patient is taking, tranexamic acid would be more appropriate. Moreover, it produces a precipitate that may impair wound healing.

Keywords: ticagrelor, oozes blood, therapeutic intervention.

16. D ★★★★

This patient has sudden-onset occipital headache, with photophobia, neck stiffness, and nausea. One could be forgiven for thinking this may be meningitis. However, given the rapidity of onset in which the symptoms have progressed, subarachnoid haemorrhage is the leading differential diagnosis. Typically, the pain reaches maximal onset within 30 minutes.

Migraines normally present earlier in life, and this patient denies a previous history of headaches. They are also often associated with an aura. The aura normally comes in the form of flashing lights, unusual smells, or seeing blurred lines.

Idiopathic intracranial hypertension normally affects young, obese females who may be taking an oestrogen-containing contraceptive pill. Symptoms include headache which has features of raised intracranial pressure (such as worse upon waking/stooping), nausea in the morning, papilloedema, and an increased blind spot.

Trigeminal neuralgia presents with severe intense stabbing pain, lasting seconds, in the distribution of the trigeminal nerve. It is often unilateral, affecting either mandibular or maxillary divisions of the trigeminal nerve.

Keywords: sudden-onset severe headache, unbearable, aversion to light, neck feels stiff.

17. A ★★★★

CPD is a mandatory requirement for registration with the GDC. It is imperative that all clinicians remain up-to-date with new developments and technologies. Persistent failure to comply may ultimately result in erasure from the register. Verifiable CPD must have clear learning objectives and outcomes and should be quality-controlled, i.e. continually improved following participant feedback.

Enhanced CPD (commenced on 1 January 2018 for dentists and 1 August 2018 for dental care professionals) instigated a number of changes, including:

- Developing a personal development plan
- Changes in the number of verifiable hours
- Declaration of hours each year
- Formal CPD log
- Reflection for each activity
- An even spread of hours across a 5-year cycle.

These changes follow the 'plan, do, reflect, record' model. In line with these regulations, a minimum of 10 hours of verifiable CPD must be recorded every 2 years. Therefore, in this scenario, despite requiring 50 hours within a 5-year cycle, the nurse must complete 10 hours of verifiable CPD in the next 12 months to comply with the regulations.

Non-verifiable CPD may still be completed and reflected upon, but it is not formally required.

Keywords: CPD, 12 months.

→ General Dental Council. *Enhanced CPD guidance for dental professionals*. 2017. Available at: https://www.gdc-uk.org/professionals/cpd/enhanced-cpd

18. C ★★★★

Midazolam is a Class C controlled drug, as defined by the Misuse of Drugs Act 1971, and comes under Schedule 3 of the Misuse of Drugs Regulations 2001. As such, there are strict rules regarding its disposal, supply, possession, and prescribing, as well as rules regarding record-keeping of midazolam.

Any midazolam that has not been administered (no drug should be unnecessarily administered to a patient), is out-of-date, or is no longer required needs to be either denatured or irretrievably disposed of. Midazolam must not be recognizable once disposed of nor should it be deposited into the sewage system. Ideally, it needs to be incinerated. The denaturing kits are usually a type of binding matrix that means, once reacted with the matrix, the drug cannot be re-extracted for use. This requirement comes under the Misuse of Drugs Regulations 2001.

The remaining answers are incorrect. Midazolam should not be stored for future use and returned to the pharmacy.

Keywords: midazolam, completing treatment, leftover.

→ UK Medicines Information (UKMi) Pharmacists for NHS Healthcare Professionals. *How should dentists prescribe, store, order and dispose of controlled drugs?* 2016. Available at: https://www.sps.nhs.uk/wp-content/uploads/2016/06/NW-QA178.4-Controlled-drugs-for-dentists-.pdf

Analgesia, anaesthesia, and sedation

Thomas Albert Park

'Can you not just put me to sleep?'

The ability to practise dentistry and provide invasive treatments to patients is based on the ability to make such procedures comfortable and acceptable for patients to tolerate, as well as manage post-operative pain. A good working knowledge of the different treatment modalities available, and analgesic agents that can be prescribed, is key to effective management of patients. This must include the indications and limitations of each modality.

The pharmacology of most drugs used in modern-day dentistry has changed very little since their introduction, some as far back as 100 years ago. However, it is important to understand the processes regarding their method of action, their effect on the human body, and their indications and contraindications. All of these factors must be considered to maximize the clinical benefit to the patient. Several guidelines regarding the use of conscious sedation in dentistry have recently been introduced, and it is important that those wishing to provide conscious sedation and refer patients appropriately familiarize themselves with these guidelines.

Key topics include:

- Principles of analgesia, anaesthesia, and conscious sedation
- Pharmacology and pharmacodynamics of commonly used pharmacological agents
- Indications and contraindications of commonly used pharmacological agents
- Conscious sedation with nitrous oxide
- Conscious sedation with midazolam
- General anaesthesia
- Treatment planning for conscious sedation and general anaesthesia
- Managing complications and adverse reactions

QUESTIONS

1. A 27-year-old man has a left inferior alveolar nerve block prior to a dental restoration. After 2 minutes, he reports he has lost feeling along the left side of his face. Clinically, there is ptosis of the left eye, which he cannot close fully, as well as drooping of the left corner of the mouth. Into what single anatomical space has the local anaesthetic most likely been administered? ★

A Buccal space

B Carotid sheath

C Parotid capsule

D Pterygomandibular space

E Submasseteric space

2. A 7-year-old fit and well boy attends with his mother for two dental restorations under inhalation sedation with nitrous oxide. The practice is equipped with a Matrix MDM® Flowmeter machine. What is the maximum percentage of nitrous oxide that can be provided to in this scenario? ★

A 65%

B 70%

C 75%

D 80%

E 85%

3. A 7-year-old fit and well girl is receiving treatment under inhalation sedation. Nitrous oxide has been delivered at a concentration of 50% and a flow rate of 5 L/minute, to achieve adequate sedation. All planned dental treatment has been completed without complication, and the session is about to be finished. What is the single most appropriate action to complete sedation safely? ★

A Decrease the flow rate of the gases incrementally over 2 minutes

B Increase the oxygen concentration to 100% for 2 minutes

C Reduce the nitrous oxide concentration incrementally

D Remove the nasal hood

E Switch off the nitrous oxide delivery system

4. A 50-year-old man is receiving an inferior alveolar nerve block for a composite restoration. The clinician inadvertently needle-sticks his thumb, while withdrawing the needle. When the glove is removed, there is a small puncture wound which is not actively bleeding. What is the single most appropriate first stage of management for this event? ★

A Assess the relevant medical history of the patient involved

B Clean the wound under running water

C Contact your local Occupational Health Department

D Encourage the wound to bleed

E Place a sterile dressing on the wound

5. A 52-year-old woman is undergoing intravenous (IV) conscious sedation for a simple restoration. She is anxious about dental injections. The final dose is titrated, based on her response. At which single point would it be most appropriate to attempt treatment? ★★

A When the patient accepts local anaesthesia

B When the patient becomes motionless

C When the patient no longer responds to pain

D When the patient's breathing rate is <10 breaths per minute

E When the patient's oxygen saturation drops below 90%

6. A 15-year-old fit and well woman suffers with dental anxiety and is offered the option of having her treatment completed under intravenous sedation with midazolam. As part of the informed consent process, the properties of midazolam are discussed. From which single medicinal property will this patient derive the most benefit? ★★

A Amnesic

B Anaesthetic

C Analgesic

D Anticonvulsive

E Antiemetic

7. A 35-year-old woman is under intravenous (IV) sedation with midazolam for extraction of the lower left first premolar (LL4). Before starting the extraction, her eyes have become closed and she fails to respond to verbal commands. Which single pharmacological agent is the most appropriate to administer in this scenario? ★★

A Activated charcoal

B Flumazenil

C Midazolam

D N-acetylcysteine

E Naloxone

8. A 24-year-old fit and well, dentally anxious woman attends for an extraction under intravenous sedation with midazolam. She has recently been diagnosed with an allergy to ester compounds. Which single commonly used dental anaesthetic would be contraindicated for the management of this patient? ★★

A Benzocaine 20% topical gel

B Lidocaine 2% with 1:80,000 adrenaline

C Mepivacaine 3% plain

D Prilocaine 3% with felypressin

E Prilocaine 4% plain

9. A 10-year-old boy is being treated with inhalation sedation which has been titrated to a dose of 60% nitrous oxide. During the treatment, he begins to twitch, his pupils dilate, and his eyes become divergent. When spoken to, he mumbles incomprehensibly. What would be the single most appropriate first-line action? ★★

A Ask the nurse to call for an ambulance

B Ask the patient to take deep breaths

C Continue treatment

D Decrease the flow rate of the nitrous oxide/oxygen mix

E Give 100% oxygen

10. A 21-year-old fit and well man is being prepared for treatment under intravenous sedation with midazolam. Treatment includes extraction of the upper left second premolar (UL5) and ultrasonic scaling. He arrives alone and plans to get public transport back home at the end of his appointment. What is the single most suitable course of action in this scenario? ★ ★

A Carry out the scaling under sedation, but defer the extraction

B Continue as planned, and arrange for your nurse to escort him home

C Do not carry out any sedation until the patient has an escort present

D Provide sedation as planned, but ask the patient to book a taxi first

E Provide sedation as planned, as this patient does not require an escort

11. A 47-year-old woman has been referred for treatment under intravenous conscious sedation. Her medical history includes bipolar disorder, severe chronic obstructive pulmonary disease (COPD), poorly controlled non-insulin-dependent diabetes mellitus (NIDDM), hypertension, and ischaemic heart disease (IHD). She had 'happy gas' a long time ago for dental treatment and requests this instead, as it worked well previously. Which single medical condition is considered a contra-indication for inhalation sedation (IHS) with nitrous oxide? ★ ★ ★

A Bipolar disorder

B Hypertension

C IHD

D Poorly controlled NIDDM

E Severe COPD

12. A 23-year-old woman attends the Emergency Department in the evening. The on-call maxillofacial doctor diagnoses irreversible pulpitis of her upper right first permanent molar (UR6). She has an appointment with her dentist tomorrow. The doctor offers to administer a long-lasting anaesthetic to help with pain relief, as there is no facility to extirpate or extract the tooth. Which commonly available local anaesthetic is the most appropriate for this? (Select one answer from the options listed below.) ★ ★ ★

A Articaine

B Bupivacaine

C Lidocaine

D Mepivacaine

E Prilocaine

13. A 70-year-old man presents to the Oral Surgery Department for consultation regarding the surgical extraction of a grossly carious, partially erupted lower left third molar (LL8). Medically, he suffers from Parkinson's disease and moderate claustrophobia. He reports dental anxiety after a previous bad experience as a child. What is the single most appropriate strategy for anaesthesia? ★★★★

A General anaesthesia with sevoflurane

B Intravenous sedation with midazolam

C Local anaesthesia with prilocaine

D Oral sedation with diazepam

E Relative analgesia with nitrous oxide

14. An 11-year-old girl is referred to the Oral Surgery Department for exposure of a palatally impacted upper right permanent canine (UR3). She is not obviously anxious but has no previous experience of dental treatment and no experience of local anaesthesia. What is the single most suitable treatment modality for this patient? ★★★★

A General anaesthesia

B Intravenous sedation with midazolam

C Local anaesthesia

D Nitrous oxide inhalation sedation

E Oral sedation with diazepam

15. A 19-year-old woman reattends, having had a dental restoration completed an hour ago by a colleague. The notes record the administration of 2.2 mL of 4% Citanest®. She reports to be fit and well, with no known allergies. Clinically, the patient is cyanosed and struggling to breathe. She now reports a similar, less severe occurrence, following her previous restoration 6 weeks ago. From which single blood disorder is she most likely to be suffering? ★★★★

A Haemophilia A

B Methaemoglobinaemia

C Pernicious anaemia

D Sickle-cell anaemia

E Thalassaemia A

16. A 42-year-old woman, who is non-verbal and has severe autism, attends for an examination with her brother, who is her carer. She requires three simple restorations and one dental extraction. She has accepted local anaesthesia in the past. You assess that she lacks capacity to consent for dental treatment. Regarding the treatment required, what is the single most appropriate next step? ★ ★ ★ ★

A As the patient lacks capacity to consent, treatment should be delayed

B Complete the required treatment as planned

C Perform the restorations, and defer the extraction until the patient has capacity

D Discuss the options with the brother, and decide on treatment in her best interests

E Liaise with a colleague before arranging for general anaesthesia; two-doctor approval is required

17. A sedation-trained nurse is 8 weeks pregnant and informs her line manager on the morning of a nitrous oxide sedation list about her change in circumstances. What is the single most appropriate course of action? ★ ★ ★ ★

A Advise the nurse that she is safe to continue normal duties

B Ask the nurse for proof of pregnancy

C Discuss the patient list with the clinical manager and cancel complex treatment

D Ensure active scavenging is used on all patients throughout the list

E Liaise with the clinical manager to reassign your nurse to alternative duties

ANSWERS

1. C ★   OHCD 6th ed. → p. 610

The answer to this question relies upon good knowledge of the anatomy of the motor distribution of the facial nerve (CN VII). Within the parotid gland, the main branch of the nerve divides into five *terminal* branches: temporal, zygomatic, buccal, marginal mandibular, and cervical.

In this case, the needle of the local anaesthetic syringe has gone beyond the ramus of the mandible and entered the medial aspect of the parotid capsule. This allows the local anaesthetic to affect the branches of the facial nerve. Aetiology may be due to patient anatomy (such as a low sigmoid notch) or poor technique.

Local anaesthetic administration into the other listed spaces would not result in facial palsy. However, injection of local anaesthetic into the submasseteric space may lead to trismus, due to the volume of anaesthetic or haematoma formation secondary to trauma.

Management involves reassurance that the symptoms will resolve when the anaesthetic wears off, taping the affected eye shut, as well as prescribing eye drops/ointment to prevent drying of the cornea (which can result in permanent damage to the eye and vision), and providing a protective dressing to prevent physical trauma to the eye. Treatment may be continued or postponed, depending upon the patient's wishes.

Keywords: ptosis, drooping, anatomical space.

2. B ★   OHCD 6th ed. → p. 612

Inhalation sedation with nitrous oxide is widely used, as it is considered very safe, with few contraindications. It has poor solubility in tissues and, as such, reaches peak saturation in blood, and is then subsequently eliminated, very quickly. This means that the vast majority of patients will become adequately sedated relatively quickly and at low concentrations. Moreover, as nitrous oxide gas is expelled via expiration, recovery is usually rapid.

Concentrations of nitrous oxide under 50% are usually sufficient for the vast majority of patients to provide adequate sedation for treatment. Higher concentrations can be given but are likely to result in inadvertent over-sedation, and close observation is required.

As a safety feature, most inhalation sedation machines, including those fitted with a Matrix MDM® Flowmeter (a common machine used in many UK clinics), do not allow the clinician to provide >70% nitrous oxide (i.e. a minimum 30% oxygen). They also have a cut-off feature, should the oxygen supply run out. A 'Pin Index Safety System' ensures oxygen and nitrous oxide cylinders cannot be attached incorrectly. This is to prevent over-sedation and, more dangerously, asphyxiation.

Keywords: inhalation sedation, nitrous oxide, Matrix MDM® Flowmeter.

→ Intercollegiate Advisory Committee on Sedation in Dentistry. *Standards for conscious sedation in the provision of dental care and accreditation.* 2015. Available at: https://www.rcseng.ac.uk/dental-faculties/fds/publications-guidelines/standards-for-conscious-sedation-in-the-provision-of-dental-care-and-accreditation/

3. B ★ OHCD 6th ed. → p. 612

One of the benefits of inhalation sedation with nitrous oxide over other forms of conscious sedation is the rapid recovery from the effects of sedation. This means that the small amount of nitrous oxide that provides sedation is quickly expired once the supply is discontinued.

A *minimum* period of 2 minutes on 100% oxygen is recommended to reverse the effects of nitrous oxide. However, the patient should be observed closely during this time. Any evidence of continuing sedation after 2 minutes should alert the clinician that the patient requires further administration of 100% oxygen.

Any concentration of oxygen of <100%, switching off the delivery system, or removing the nasal hood immediately leaves the patient susceptible to the continued effects of residual nitrous oxide that could make them unfit for discharge or delay recovery. Similarly, nitrous oxide dissolved in tissue fluids could rapidly diffuse back into the alveoli of the lungs, diluting oxygen and carbon dioxide concentrations in the lungs, and prevent adequate reoxygenation of venous blood. This is termed diffusion hypoxia.

Keywords: inhalation sedation, complete sedation safely.

4. D ★ OHCD 6th ed. → p. 354

A needle-stick injury is a type of sharps or percutaneous injury, caused when a medical instrument inadvertently breaks the skin. Unfortunately, they are fairly common events and can potentially expose health professionals to a number of blood-borne viruses, including hepatitis B, hepatitis C, and human immunodeficiency virus (HIV). The risk of transmission for these diseases has been reported as 6–30% (if unvaccinated), 1.8%, and 0.3%, respectively.

Whilst the risk of transmission of these pathogens remains low, sharps injuries remain incredibly emotive episodes for those involved and prevention of these events is paramount. Local policies may vary from region to region, but the following protocol has been suggested by the UK's Health and Safety Executive in their guidance on sharps injuries.

If you suffer an injury from a sharp which may be contaminated:*

- Encourage the wound to gently bleed, ideally holding it under running water.
- Wash the wound using running water and plenty of soap.

---

* Contains public sector information licensed under the Open Government Licence v3.0. [http://www.nationalarchives.gov.uk/doc/open-government-licence/version/3/]

- Do not scrub the wound whilst you are washing it.
- Do not suck the wound.
- Dry the wound, and cover it with a waterproof plaster or dressing.
- Seek urgent medical advice (e.g. from your Occupational Health Service), as effective prophylaxis (medicines to help fight infection) are available.

Your Occupational Health Department may suggest completing a risk assessment form with the patient, with their consent, to assess their risk status. However, the standard procedure is that all patients should be managed as potentially being unknown carriers of a blood-borne virus, regardless of a needle-stick injury or not.

Keywords: needle-sticks, puncture wound, first stage of management.

→ Health and Safety Executive. *Sharps injuries*. Available at: http://www.hse.gov.uk/healthservices/needlesticks/

5. A ★★ OHCD 6th ed. → p. 616

Observing the patient's response to any sedative agent is fundamental to delivering safe and effective conscious sedation. This is achieved by providing the sedative agent in small dose increments and evaluating the patient's objective and subjective responses, *titrating* the dose.

IV administration allows the response to be assessed almost immediately (there is a short delay, as the agent travels through the blood vessels to the brain, a journey approximately 20–30 seconds long). This is different for oral or nasal administration of sedative agents, which can vary considerably in terms of absorption rate and total dose absorbed, and therefore the patient response.

A needle-phobic patient who is willing to accept local anaesthesia is showing signs of adequate sedation. Other signs of effective conscious sedation include:

- An awake, communicative patient
- A calm demeanour
- Slow responses to questions
- Slurred speech
- Heart rate, oxygen saturation, and blood pressure all within normal limits for the patient.

The other answers in this question suggest the patient has become over-sedated, and this should be managed appropriately.

Keywords: conscious sedation, titrated.

6. A ★★ OHCD 6th ed. → p. 614

Midazolam is a member of the benzodiazepine family of drugs. Its pharmacological actions on the central nervous system result in disinhibition, reduced anxiety, amnesia, muscle relaxation, respiratory depression, an anticonvulsant effect, and anaesthesia, amongst others.

In this scenario, the patient will benefit from amnesia regarding her dental treatment. The patient will not benefit from the anticonvulsant properties of midazolam, as she is fit and well, with no previous relevant diagnosis of a condition causing seizures.

Anaesthesia, the result of extreme over-sedation, is the result of higher doses of midazolam and is to be avoided. In contrast to nitrous oxide, midazolam has no analgesic or pain-relieving properties. Midazolam has no proven direct antiemetic effects but can indirectly reduce a patient's gag reflex.

Keywords: anxiety, midazolam, informed consent.

7. B ★★   OHCD 6th ed. → p. 614

Over-sedation can be more common with some patients, compared to others (e.g. patients who have never had IV conscious sedation before, with an unknown response). However, with a good, cautious titration technique, this risk can be minimized. It is important that two sedation-trained members of staff are present during treatment, as the treating clinician cannot continually assess the sedated patient.

When over-sedation occurs, flumazenil is the reversal agent used. It is a member of the benzodiazepine family but has no sedative effects and competitively antagonizes other benzodiazepines. It has a shorter half-life than midazolam, around 40–80 minutes, compared to 1–6 hours for midazolam.

A recommended dosing for flumazenil is 200 µg over 15 seconds, followed by 100 µg every 60 seconds, until the sedation is reversed.

Naloxone is the reversal agent for overdose of opioid analgesics.

N-acetylcysteine is the antidote to paracetamol overdose.

Activated charcoal is used to cause vomiting, thus limiting the absorption of substances without a specific antidote or reversal agent, when overdose occurs.

Additional midazolam would be significantly detrimental in this situation.

Keywords: midazolam, fails to respond to verbal commands

8. A ★★

Local anaesthetics can be classified based on their chemical structure. Ester local anaesthetics have an ester link. Conversely, amide local anaesthetics have an amide link between groups.

Ester local anaesthetics have a much longer history of use but are generally reserved as topical agents, due to a higher frequency of hypersensitivity reactions with these compounds. It is very rare to have a true allergy to amide local anaesthetics, with allergy to preservatives in the amide local anaesthetic formulation being relatively more common.

Benzocaine is a common topical anaesthetic agent used on the mucosa and skin prior to injections or cannulation. As it is an ester anaesthetic, its use is therefore contraindicated in this case. The other agents are amide local anaesthetics and should be safe to use.

Keywords: allergy, ester compounds.

→ Meechan J. Local anaesthesia: risks and controversies. *Dental Update*. 2009;**36**:278–83.

9. E ★★ OHCD 6th ed. → p. 612

These signs are indicative of over-sedation. Verbal contact, one of the defining features of conscious sedation, must be maintained at all times during any form of conscious sedation.

Because of low tissue solubility of nitrous oxide, by giving the patient 100% oxygen, the inhaled nitrous oxide would be expelled rapidly and replaced with oxygen, allowing a rapid recovery.

Asking the patient to breathe more will not help in this situation, as the concentration of nitrous oxide you are delivering is too high and has caused the patient to become over-sedated in the first place. Moreover, they are also unlikely to be able to respond to your requests.

Similarly, decreasing the flow rate will only reduce the *volume* of nitrous oxide and oxygen the patient receives, not the *concentration*. To reverse the sedation, you need to reduce the concentration of nitrous oxide and increase the concentration of inspired oxygen.

You should not continue the treatment as planned because you have lost verbal contact with the patient.

At this stage, the patient's condition does not constitute a medical emergency, and to ask for the assistance of the ambulance service is not a first-line action. Should the patient's recovery be delayed or atypical, or should they develop a concurrent medical emergency, then escalation would be appropriate.

Keywords: 60% nitrous oxide, eyes, divergent, mumbles incomprehensibly.

10. C ★★

Patients who have undergone conscious sedation can have variable responses to the sedation that has been provided. This is especially true with agents such as midazolam that has prolonged effects on patients' cognitive function. As such, it is compulsory that patients attend with an escort on the day of the procedure, who stays in the building throughout the procedure (in the waiting room) and takes the patient home immediately—preferably by car or taxi. The escort must be a competent adult, must stay with the patient for the rest of the day, and overnight, and must not be responsible for the care of anyone else during this period.

Without an escort, the patient is at risk of harm on discharge, and no compromise should be made in this regard. This information should be given to the patient as part of the preoperative information for the procedure, both verbally and in writing.

Keywords: intravenous sedation, alone.

→ Intercollegiate Advisory Committee for Sedation in Dentistry. *Standards for conscious sedation in the provision of dental care and accreditation.* 2015. Available at: https://www.rcseng.ac.uk/dental-faculties/fds/publications-guidelines/standards-for-conscious-sedation-in-the-provision-of-dental-care-and-accreditation/

11. E ★★★   OHCD 6th ed. → p. 612

In severe cases of COPD, respiration is controlled by hypoxic drive, rather than higher concentrations of carbon dioxide. Extreme caution should be exercised with such patients, as prolonged sedation, of any kind, may cause respiratory depression, further reducing oxygen levels in the blood. IHS with nitrous oxide provides relatively higher concentrations of oxygen, compared to inspired air, for prolonged periods and so can 'switch off' the hypoxic drive, further reducing a patient's ability to adequately respire. Short-term administration of oxygen is acceptable, should a medical emergency arise.

Upper respiratory tract obstructions, such as colds or enlarged adenoids, can be considered a relative contraindication to IHS, because they may make inhalation via the nose difficult or impossible.

IHS is beneficial to those with IHD and hypertension. Firstly, it decreases stress and anxiety, which may exacerbate or precipitate acute episodes of angina. Secondly, nitrous oxide is a vasodilator that may help to reduce the risk of an ischaemic episode.

IHS is also beneficial for those with a prominent gag reflex. It acts both as an anxiolytic and alters the functional trigger zone in the oropharynx where the reflex is initiated. IHS makes the trigger zone smaller and less sensitive. A reduction in anxiety, by any sedative means, will also generally reduce the sensitivity of the reflex.

Keywords: COPD, happy gas, contraindication.

12. B ★★★   OHCD 6th ed. → p. 606

The local anaesthetics listed have broadly similar chemical features. They comprise a lipophilic group, a hydrophilic group, and an intermediate chain that connects the two opposing groups. Chemically, the intermediate chain can be an 'ester' or 'amide', and local anaesthetics are categorized as such. The agents listed in the question are amide-linked anaesthetics.

Variations in all three chemical components can influence the solubility, affinity, and elimination of the anaesthetic. This influences the duration of action and potency of the anaesthetic (see Table 11.1). Bupivacaine has the longest duration of action and is often used following surgery where prolonged analgesia is desired.

Keywords: long-lasting anaesthetic, commonly available.

Table 11.1 Duration of action of local anaesthetics

Local anaesthetic	Duration of action (hours)
Articaine	1–3
Bupivacaine	3–7
Lidocaine	0.5–2
Mepivacaine	2–2.5
Prilocaine	0.5–1

Adapted by permission from Springer International Publishing Switzerland: Frankhuijzen A.L. (2017) Pharmacology of Local Anaesthetics. In: Baart J., Brand H. (eds) *Local Anaesthesia in Dentistry*, Second Edition. Copyright © 2017.

→ Baart JA, Brand HS. *Local Anaesthesia in Dentistry*. Wiley-Blackwell, Oxford; 2008.

13. B ★★★★

Parkinson's disease is a progressive disease of the nervous system, marked by tremor, muscular rigidity, and slow and imprecise movement, chiefly presenting in the middle-aged and elderly. Benzodiazepines have a muscle-relaxant effect, reducing muscle tremors and stiffness, potentially improving cooperation for such patients. However, as all benzodiazepines are respiratory depressants, airway control is easily compromised with these patients, so extreme care is required.

Inhalation sedation is of particular value in anxious patients undergoing relatively atraumatic procedures and in children for whom the effects of benzodiazepines are less predictable and can be paradoxically excitatory. In the scenario presented, the patient may find the nasal hood difficult to tolerate, due to his claustrophobia, and the level of sedation may be insufficient for a challenging surgical extraction.

The extraction could be attempted with a local anaesthetic alone, but the patient may find it difficult to tolerate the procedure due to his reported anxiety and the effects of Parkinson's disease.

A general anaesthetic is not appropriate as a *first* line of management in this case, and should only be considered when other management options are contraindicated or are not successful.

Keywords: Parkinson's disease, third molar, anxious.

14. A ★★★★   OHCD 6th ed. → p. 604

Impaction of upper canines are relatively common, and after lower third molars, upper canines are the most common teeth to be impacted. The clinician should be vigilant for this in all examinations of children from the age of 8 onwards, as this tooth should be palpable in the buccal sulcus. If the upper canine cannot be palpated in the buccal sulcus by the age of 10, then referral should be made at the earliest opportunity for an orthodontic assessment.

Exposure of canines on the palate will likely require a palatal flap to be raised. Although this procedure can be done under local anaesthesia, with or without sedation, it can be a long and unpleasant procedure. The patient's relative inexperience at the dentist and how this may affect her compliance during the procedure (particularly given her age) must be considered. A negative experience could further affect her compliance with subsequent orthodontic treatment.

Guidelines for the management of patients under general anaesthesia are quite strict, but few centres in the United Kingdom would not consider this procedure an acceptable indication for general anaesthesia.

Keywords: 11 years old, exposure, palatally impacted upper canine, no previous experience of dental treatment.

15. B ★★★★ OHCD 6th ed. → p. 606

Several therapeutic agents, including local anaesthetics, can cause the conversion of haemoglobin into a non-oxygen-binding form called methaemoglobin. Usually methaemoglobin is converted back to haemoglobin by the enzyme nicotinamide adenine dinucleotide (NADH)-methaemoglobin reductase. Deficiencies in this enzyme, or genetic variants of haemoglobin, may mean this conversion does not happen as readily. This resulting condition is called methaemoglobinaemia where the oxygen-carrying capacity of blood is reduced.

Prilocaine (Citanest®) and benzocaine reportedly carry the highest risks of common dental anaesthetics. O-toluidine, a liver metabolite of prilocaine, can induce methaemoglobin. Signs such as cyanosis and shortness of breath would be cause for concern, and the patient should be referred immediately for medical assessment. Prilocaine use in these patients is contraindicated, and caution should also be exercised with benzocaine.

Haemophilia is an inherited bleeding disorder. Sickle-cell anaemia and thalassaemia A and B are disorders of the structure of the haemoglobin protein, whilst pernicious anaemia involves autoimmune destruction of stomach cells that produce intrinsic factor, which is responsible for the uptake of vitamin B12 from the gastrointestinal tract. These disorders may be associated with cyanosis and breathlessness, but they are unlikely to present immediately following dental injections.

Keywords: Citanest®, cyanosed, struggling to breathe, similar, occurrence.

16. D ★★★★ OHCD 6th ed. → p. 674

The Mental Capacity Act (2005) states that all adults should be assumed to have capacity until proven otherwise. It also states that no other adult can consent for another. When determining capacity, the first question that needs to be answered is 'Does this patient have an impairment or disturbance of the mind or brain?' If the answer is NO, then the patient therefore has the ability to make any decision they wish, even if it is an unwise one, e.g. declining a lifesaving blood transfusion.

If the answer to this question is YES, then the following questions are asked of the person in this order:

- Does the patient understand the information?
- Is the patient able to retain the information for long enough to make the decision?
- Can the patient use or weigh up this information as part of a decision-making process?
- Can the patient communicate the decision by any means?

Should the answer to any one or more of these four questions also be NO, then that patient does not have capacity to make that decision for that *particular* decision. However, a patient may have capacity to make other decisions, e.g. the patient may be able to make the decision to have an examination, but not the extraction recommended from the examination.

This process needs to be clearly written in the patient's notes, including any discussion with the family, carers, or senior staff. The reason for your decision also needs to documented.

Any patient who does not have family or unpaid carers, or where there is conflict over a proposed treatment between clinicians and involved third parties, may benefit from being referred to an Independent Mental Capacity Advocate (IMCA).

The patient's brother is unable to provide consent, but would be involved in decisions regarding her care.

It is not in the patient's best interests to carry out no treatment or to avoid/ignore treatment where it is required. The brother should be consulted as to what he feels is most appropriate, and then a best interest agreement made. Two-doctor agreement is not a fundamental requirement of the MCA but would be wise where radical or restrictive treatment is proposed.

Keywords: Mental Capacity Act, capacity, consent.

→ Burke S, Kwasnicki A, Park T, Macpherson A. Consent and capacity—considerations for the dental team part 1: consent and assessment of capacity. *Dental Update*. 2017;**44**:660–6.

17. E ★★★★

The use of nitrous oxide for conscious sedation is regarded as being safe for patients, and acute exposure has not been demonstrated to present a long-term danger to clinical staff. However, chronic exposure to relatively low levels of nitrous oxide (potentially received when conducting inhalation sedation) can have a number of effects, which include: liver disease, central nervous system toxicity, reduced blood cell production, reduced fertility, and increased risk of miscarriage in females. Exposure to nitrous oxide is managed under the Control of Substances Hazardous to Health 2002, from the Health and Safety Executive.

Because of this, dental staff are in danger of side effects from chronic nitrous oxide exposure. This may arise either due to leakage from poorly maintained equipment or through exhaled gases from the patient. To mitigate these risks, scavenging, ideally active, is advised by many guidelines to help remove waste gas from the environment and limit exposure to staff. Also, equipment should be maintained and serviced, as suggested by the manufacturer.

For the above reasons, it is therefore prudent to find alternative duties for your pregnant nurse in this situation. Cancelling patients on the day is not ideal for either the service provider or the service user, but may be necessary where no safe alternative is feasible.

Keywords: pregnant, nitrous oxide.

→ Donaldson D, Meechan JG. The hazards of chronic exposure to nitrous oxide: an update. *British Dental Journal*. 1995;**178**:95–100.

Dental materials

Raheel Aftab

'How long will this last?'

Dental material science can be a daunting subject for most dentists, given its origins in the pure sciences of physics and chemistry. Combining this with human biology, and trying to see through the fog of material manufacturers' commercial claims, can make it seem like a truly mystifying subject. It is important that any student of material sciences maintains a critical eye and an evidence-based approach when it comes to material selection and use.

Today we are lucky enough to work with the most advanced dental materials we have ever had. But simply having such materials at your disposal does not ensure success. Clinical procedural techniques are often the prime focus in restorative dentistry; however, to achieve optimal aesthetics, function, and longevity from restorations, a clear understanding of material sciences is required.

Ancient Roman engineers clearly understood this concept when constructing Rome. They had to work within the limitations imposed by the materials they had at their disposal. However, the longevity and solidity of the impressive infrastructure we see today can be attributed to their expertise in exploiting the unique properties of the material resources they had available. The Romans perfected concrete production (based on volcanic ash and lime reacting with seawater to form tobermorite crystals) to yield a water-hardening material, so durable and resistant to cracks that modern-day concrete (based on Portland cement) is still considered weaker.

It can be argued whether operator skill or advancements in dental materials have resulted in improvements in restorative dentistry. However, few would disagree that it is the combination of good operator skill and appropriate use of dental materials that is the key for successful long-term dentistry.

Key topics include:

- Adhesive dentistry concepts
- Understanding material physical properties
- Elemental make-up of materials
- Manufacturing processing of materials
- Biocompatibility
- Appreciation of setting reactions and working time
- Appreciation of material aesthetic and optical properties.

QUESTIONS

1. A 22-year-old man attends for restoration of a large posterior class V cavity with glass-ionomer cement (GIC). Which single conditioning agent is the most appropriate to improve bond strength of this material to the tooth structure? ★

A Dentine bonding agent

B Fluorocarbonic acid

C Hydrofluoric acid

D Polyacrylic acid

E Resin-modified GIC

2. A 26-year-old man returns 1 week after having a deep amalgam restoration in his lower right first molar (LR6). The patient experienced shooting pain that lasted for a few seconds when drinking cold drinks. The restoration was removed by an emergency dentist and replaced with zinc oxide eugenol (ZOE). What is the primary benefit of using this material in this situation? ★

A Antimicrobial

B Less microleakage

C Fast setting

D High compressive strength

E Obtundent

3. A 45-year-old man is having his upper left lateral incisor (UL2) crowned. Prior to taking the impression with a monophase addition-cured polyvinylsiloxane (PVS) material, the tooth is thoroughly air-dried. What is the single main reason for this protocol? ★

A Absorption of residual surface moisture will lead to an inaccurate die

B Moisture acts as a separator between the light- and heavy-bodied PVS, leading to folds

C Moisture may cause air blows in the impression, as PVS materials are hydrophobic

D Moisture retards the polymerization of the material, potentially causing drags

E Moisture stops the material being placed in the correct place, as it slips off the teeth

4. A 47-year-old woman has received revision root canal treatment (ReRCT) on an upper central incisor. After chemomechanical preparation, which single irrigant would be the most appropriate for removing the residual inorganic matter from the root canal system? ★

A Acetone

B EDTA (ethylenediaminetetraacetic acid)

C MTAD (mixture of tetracycline, citric acid, and detergent)

D Saline

E Sodium hypochlorite

5. A 15-year-old boy attends for root canal treatment on a recently traumatized upper central incisor. Following root canal treatment, a significant proportion of the crown is missing and a glass-fibre post is used to retain the restoration. Which single type of cement should be used when placing the post? ★

A Dual cured resin cement

B Flowable resin cement

C Light cured resin cement

D Resin-modified glass-ionomer cement

E Zinc phosphate cement

6. A 56-year-old man attends for construction of an upper partial cobalt-chromium (CoCr) denture. He has previously struggled to tolerate a full palatal coverage acrylic denture because of his gag reflex. The patient is a chemical engineer by trade and wishes to know what property of CoCr allows provision of a thinner and less extensive major connector. Which single property of CoCr can facilitate this design? ★

A Good corrosion resistance

B High fatigue resistance

C High yield strength

D Low mobility

E Low thermal resistance

7. A 21-year-old woman attends the Emergency Department, following lateral luxation of her upper right central incisor. A self-etch adhesive bonding system is used for composite splint placement, as no dental chair or water line is available. What single component of the bonding agent has been modified to avoid the need for a separate etching stage? ★

A Bond

B Cement

C Conditioner

D Phosphoric acid

E Primer

8. A 40-year-old woman attends for another amalgam filling with her new dentist. The dentist is a new graduate and, on a number of occasions, has been struggling to pack the amalgam sufficiently before it sets. Having spoken to their trainer, it is decided to order a lathe-cut amalgam instead—for which primary reason? ★

A Easier to condense

B Hardens slowly

C Has more shrinkage

D Less difficult to achieve tight contact points

E Smoother finish after polish

9. A 46-year-old man has had four permanent lower molars prepared for gold onlays to manage his generalized moderate toothwear. The preparations have minimal retention or resistance form. What single material is the most appropriate for cementation? ★

A Glass-ionomer cement

B Polycarboxylate cement

C Resin cement

D Resin-modified glass-ionomer cement

E Zinc phosphate

10. A 44-year-old woman requires a mesio-occlusal composite restoration in a lower first premolar. The supervising consultant recommends a 'wet bonding' approach, and the assisting dental care professional asks what this refers to. ★ ★

A Bonding in low humidity conditions

B Isolating without a rubber dam

C Irrigating with saline prior to surface priming

D Not excessively drying the dentine

E Not setting the bonding agent prior to composite placement

11. A 26-year-old man with severe learning difficulties is having an amalgam restoration in his upper right first molar. Upon placement into the cavity, the amalgam appears crumbly and is unusable. What single procedural issue is most likely to have caused this to occur? ★★

A Amalgam contraction

B Moisture contamination

C Out-of-date

D Over-burnished

E Under-triturated

12. A 64-year-old woman is having a new upper complete denture made. She has a hypermobile or 'flabby' anterior ridge, and a window technique is planned for the master impression. What primary property is desired of the impression material used in the flabby area? ★★

A Dimensionally stable

B High elasticity

C High viscosity

D Low elasticity

E Low viscosity

13. A 24-year-old woman requires a replacement crown on her upper right central incisor. as she dislikes the appearance, describing it as 'too dark'. A Vita 3D shade guide™ is used to select the new shade. What element of colour needs to be adjusted, and in which component of the shade guide is this reflected? (Select one answer from the options listed below) ★★

A Chroma, the 'M' value

B Hue, numbers 1 to 5

C Hue, the 'M' value

D Value, the 'L/R' value

E Value, numbers 1 to 5

14. A 72-year-old woman attends a few days after the fit of a replacement complete maxillary denture. She complains of a burning/itchy sensation of her palate. Following examination, it is believed to be a reaction to excess monomer. Which single processing error has most likely occurred? ★★

A Curing temperature of 95°C not attained after an initial slow heating period

B Excess powder in the resin mixture

C Final temperature of 150°C reached too quickly

D Lack of compression during flasking

E Packing process occurred during the 'wet sand' stage

15. A 21-year-old man has undergone endodontic treatment on an upper central incisor with an open apex. He returns after 12 months, with marked discoloration of the crown. Non-setting calcium hydroxide (CH) was used as an intracanal medicament between appointments, and sodium hypochlorite and ethylenediaminetetraacetic acid (EDTA) were used as irrigants. Finally, mineral trioxide aggregate (MTA) was placed as an apical barrier before completing the obturation with gutta percha and subsequently placing a coronal seal of resin-modified glass-ionomer cement (RMGIC). What is the single most likely cause of discoloration in this scenario? ★★

A Interaction of sodium hypochlorite with residual EDTA

B Interaction of CH with residual sodium hypochlorite

C Residual gutta percha within the canal

D Staining of RMGIC

E Use of MTA

16. A 39-year-old woman requires replacement anterior maxillary crowns as part of a full arch rehabilitation. The crowns are to be placed at an increased occlusal vertical dimension (OVD), and following removal of the crowns, there is 1-mm space between the residual core and the desired incisal level. What is the minimum incisal reduction required for the provision of metallo-ceramic crowns in this situation? ★★

A 0.5 mm

B 1 mm

C 1.5 mm

D 2 mm

E 2.5 mm

17. A 31-year-old woman attends with a mesio-incisal fracture of an old composite restoration. The tooth was traumatized playing sport when the patient was 16 years old, and over 80% of the old composite restoration is remaining. Composite resin repair is planned, and the old restoration is air-abraded. After air abrasion, which single agent should be used prior to placement of the bonding agent? ★ ★ ★

A Barium oxide

B Camphorquinone

C Hydroquinone

D Silanizing agent [e.g. gamma-methacryloxypropyl-trimethoxysilane (gamma-MPTS)]

E Tri-ethylene glycol dimethacrylate (TEGMA)

18. The local dental laboratory has recently started providing computer-aided design/computer-aided manufacture (CAD/CAM) cobalt-chrome dentures, produced by selective laser melting (SLM). They recommend clinicians change to them, as they are stronger. What is the primary scientific reason for this? ★ ★ ★

A Greater σ-phase levels of the alloy are produced

B Local heat treating from the laser work hardens the alloy

C Porosities are reduced

D Reduced heating time from the production process improves flexural fatigue

E The quantity of molybdenum can be increased

19. A 52-year-old man recently required a disto-occlusal amalgam restoration adjacent to a gold shell crown. At a subsequent appointment, a silver/brown circular stain is noticed around the contact point on the gold shell crown. Which single process has most likely caused the discoloration? ★ ★ ★

A Electrochemical etching

B Galvanic corrosion

C Intergranular ion exchange

D Mechanical damage during cavity preparation

E Selective leaching

20. A 17-year-old woman with taurodontism requires a direct pulp cap, following an occlusal restoration on their lower right first permanent molar. The supervising consultant recommends using a new calcium silicate cement as pulp-capping material, rather than the conventionally used calcium hydroxide (CH). For which single biological reason is this most appropriate? ★★★★

A Antibacterial

B Forms an ionic bond to the surrounding dentine

C High pH releases proteins and growth factors from the nearby dentine, leading to reparative dentine formation.

D Non-cytotoxic and induces odontoblast proliferation and activity

E Obtundent

21. A 36-year-old man requires multiple composite restorations to restore his worn anterior maxillary teeth. The restorations are to be placed at an increased vertical dimension, using the Dahl approach. Which single type of composite is most appropriate for these restorations? ★★★★

A Compomer

B Flowable composite

C Microfilled composite

D Nanohybrid composite

E Silorane composite

22. A 56-year-old man presents with mild asymptomatic erosion of the palatal aspects of his upper incisors, secondary to acid reflux. What single widely available active ingredient could be recommended in his toothpaste as part of a protective measure? ★★★★

A Arginine 8%

B Casein phosphopeptides–amorphous calcium phosphates (CPP-ACP) 10%

C Sodium fluoride 0.31%

D Sodium lauryl sulfate 0.5%

E Stannous fluoride 0.45%

23. A 66-year-old man is having his edentulous maxilla restored. The residual ridge is a Class III ridge with minor anterior undercut. He attends for an abutment-level, open-tray impression for a full arch implant-supported bridge. Which single impression material is the most appropriate to use? ★ ★ ★ ★

A Addition-cured silicone [polyvinylsiloxane (PVS)]

B Alginate

C Condensation-cured PVS

D Impression plaster

E Polyether

24. A 32-year-old woman with a high smile line requires suturing of the anterior soft tissues after periodontal surgery. Guided bone regeneration has been attempted around the upper left lateral incisor (UL2), using modern microsurgical techniques. Which single type and size of suture would be the most appropriate in this scenario? ★ ★ ★ ★

A Black silk—3.0

B Poliglecaprone—2.0

C Polyester—3.0

D Polyglycolic acid—4.0

E Polypropylene—6.0

25. A 19-year-old woman is having resin infiltration to manage her aesthetic concerns regarding a developmental hypoplastic white spot lesion on her central incisor. By what single mechanism would this technique improve the appearance? ★ ★ ★ ★

A Absorbs blue wavelength light, leading to more light transmitted of a yellow hue

B Increases the refractive index of the lesion by filling the internal porosities

C Increases the transparency of the lesion by occluding the internal porosities

D Lightens the surface colour of adjacent enamel by blending lesion margins

E Provides a matt surface, reducing the reflection of light and masking the appearance

ANSWERS

1. D ★   OHCD 6th ed. → p. 640

An attractive feature of GIC is that it can be placed in bulk and is less technique-sensitive than composite resin. Moisture control should still be maintained, as contamination with blood or saliva can reduce the bond strength.

The use of a conditioning agent on teeth prior to placement of GIC has been demonstrated to improve the bond strength, but the evidence is not conclusive. The main purpose of the conditioner is to remove debris from the surface and facilitate a clean surface for bonding. Strong agents that demineralize the tooth structure surface (such as citric acid or phosphoric acid) should be avoided, as they will reduce the quality of the ionic bond to apatite. Polyacrylic acid 10% is the most commonly recommended conditioner for GICs.

Keywords: GIC, conditioning agent.

→ McCabe J, Walls A. *Applied Dental Materials* (9th ed.). Blackwell Publishing Ltd, Oxford; 2008.

2. E ★   OHCD 6th ed. → p. 644

ZOE cements have a number of properties which facilitate their use as dental material. Primarily, eugenol is thought to leach out from the material and into the surrounding dentine where it is said to have an obtundent or sedative effect upon the dentino-pulpal complex. Its mode of action is primarily attributed to its inhibition of capsaicin receptors. The material is generally supplied as a powder and liquid which has a relatively quick setting time once mixed. The material has historically been used as a lining or base material in deep cavities, as well as a root canal sealer. The material can have antimicrobial properties and has been shown to have good sealability when placed in adequate thickness. However, these would be secondary benefits in this scenario.

Evidence exists to show that dentine bond strengths are negatively affected by ZOE materials. As such, their use should be avoided, or further surface preparation will be required where future adhesive restorations are to be placed. Non-eugenol-containing zinc oxide root canal sealers are available to overcome this issue when restoring the root-treated tooth.

New tricalcium silicate-based restorative materials (e.g. Biodentine™) have a growing wealth of evidence to support their use over ZOE in these clinical situations. However, these materials are more expensive and are yet to be routinely adopted into this clinical scenario.

Keywords: deep amalgam restoration, shooting pain, ZOE.

→ Koch T, Peutzfeldt A, Malinovskii V, Flury S, Häner R, Lussi A. Temporary zinc oxide-eugenol cement: eugenol quantity in dentin and bond strength of resin composite. *European Journal of Oral Sciences*. 2013;**121**:363–9.

3. C ★

Addition-cured silicones are based on polymers of vinylsiloxanes. One half of the material contains polydimethylsiloxane with some methyl groups replaced with hydrogen, and the other half contains polydimethylsiloxane with some methyl groups replaced with a vinyl group. When mixed in the presence of platinum, a cross-linking reaction occurs between the single hydrogen groups and the vinyl groups. Clinically, due to the inherently hydrophobic nature of these polymers, the presence of moisture can result in air blows.

The addition of surfactants (a molecule which reduces the material's surface tension) is one method some manufacturers have used to combat this. Surfactants are bidirectional molecules which have both a hydrophobic and a hydrophilic end. Their addition to PVS materials lowers the surface tension and causes a reduction in the contact angle the material makes with water. This improves the wettability of the material and theoretically decreases the risk of air blows. However, the authors would still recommend that the impression surface is dried thoroughly (particularly in crown and bridge work) to improve the quality of the impression.

Drags may occur when the material is removed before it is set or where undercut is present and high-viscosity material is used.

Folds may occur where the materials do not mix properly or where one material has started to set before the other is placed (when using a two-viscosity technique).

Keywords: PVS, air-dried.

→ Van Noort R. *Introduction to Dental Materials* (4th ed.). Elsevier, Edinburgh; 2013.

4. B ★

Sodium hypochlorite remains the gold standard for chemical disinfection of the root canal system. It is a highly effective antimicrobial agent that dissolves organic matter and helps lubricate the root canal system. The major disadvantage of sodium hypochlorite is that it is unable to remove the smear layer created during mechanical cleaning of the canals. The smear layer (composed primarily of inorganic material and approximately 5 μm in thickness) blocks dentinal tubules and remains a potential reservoir for pathogens. Removal of the smear layer has been shown to improve endodontic outcomes, especially in ReRCT. Alternative irrigants are therefore available to help remove the inorganic matter that remains (e.g. EDTA, citric acid). These irrigants chelate the inorganic components that make up the smear layer and help remove the associated bacteria. Furthermore, the underlying dentinal tubules are exposed, and it is thought that this increases the penetration of the sealer and subsequently improves the adaptation of the root canal filling.

HEBP (1-hydroxyethylidene-1,1-bisphosphonate), or etidronate, is gaining popularity within the endodontic community as a possible alternative chelating agent. However, EDTA remains the most widely used and evidence-based chelating agent at present.

Keywords: inorganic matter, irrigant, root canal.

→ Hülsmann M, Heckendorff M, Lennon A. Chelating agents in root canal treatment: mode of action and indications for their use. *International Endodontic Journal.* 2003;**36**:810–30.

→ Shavravan A, Haghdoost AA, Adl A, Rahimi H, Shadifar F. Effect of smear layer on sealing ability of canal obturation: a systematic review and meta-analysis. *Journal of Endodontics.* 2007;**33**:96–105.

5. A ★

Fibre posts should be bonded into the root canal system. This aids not only retention, but also helps to distribute the forces along the root canal system. In order to do this, resin-based cement is required. Resin-based cements can be light-cured, chemically cured, or dual-cured. The reliable curing depth of conventional composite is around 2 mm, which would not normally be sufficient to cure to the full depth of the post preparation. However, translucent fibre posts can transmit the light along the length of the post and initiate the curing reaction. The problem with this is that the curing reaction will be towards the post. The enormous c-factor could easily lead to the dentine bond being broken. Although there is evidence to suggest that light-cured and dual systems have similar bond strengths along the root regions for this type of post, the authors would argue that dual-cured cement (the chemically cured component) is more likely to reliably achieve full curing throughout the lute and therefore is preferable. Another key element to a successful bond is the use of a dual-cured/chemically cured bonding agent.

It is important to realize that achieving a reliable bond to the root dentine can be challenging, and debonding of fibre posts is a common reason for failure.

Keywords: glass-fibre post, cement.

→ Barfeie A, Thomas MB, Watts A, Rees J. Failure mechanisms of fibre posts: a literature review. *European Journal of Prosthodontics and Restorative Dentistry.* 2015;**3**:115–27.

→ Giachetti L, Scaminaci Russo D, Baldini M, Bertini F, Steier L, Ferrari M. Push-out strength of translucent fibre posts cemented using a dual-curing technique or a light-curing self-adhering material. *International Endodontic Journal.* 2012;**45**:249–56.

6. C ★   OHCD 6th ed. → p. 650

There are various factors influencing patients who have hypersensitive gag reflexes. The gag reflex itself is 'an involuntary contraction of the muscles of the soft palate or pharynx that causes retching'. It is an important protective reflex present in human physiology. It can be described as either somatic (stimulated by touching areas of the mucosa) or psychogenic. The severity of gagging can be graded 1 to 5. Above-moderate gagging (grade 3) routine dental treatment can be challenging. For denture wearers with hypersensitive gag reflexes, coverage of the palate is a frequent complaint that they associate with the problem. However, poor retention and an overly thick palate can contact the dorsum of the tongue and stimulate the gag reflex. Provision of a CoCr denture with good retention and a thin major connector may help from both a physiological and a psychological perspective.

Yield strength is the point at which permanent plastic deformation (proportional limit) occurs within the material. CoCr has a yield strength in the region of 600–700 MPa, giving it good flexural rigidity, and allows denture bases of thin section. Strength in thin section means less palatal coverage and smaller connectors are required.

Keywords: CoCr, property, thinner, major connector.

→ Al-Jabbari Y. Physico-mechanical properties and prosthodontic applications of Co-Cr dental alloys: a review of the literature. *Journal of Advanced Prosthodontics*. 2014;**6**:138–45.

→ Forbes-Hayley C, Blewitt I, Puryer J. Dental management of the 'gagging' patient—an update. *International Journal of Dental and Health Sciences*. 2015;**3**:423–31.

7. E ★ OHCD 6th ed. → p. 638

The increased organic composition of dentine and the presence of dentinal fluid, compared with enamel, mean that a hybrid layer has to be formed in order to allow the hydrophobic resin to bond to the dentinal surface. To allow this to happen, modern bonding systems have three stages: etching, priming, and bonding. Etching demineralizes the enamel or dentine surface to create microporosities or prepare the surface for bonding. It also removes the smear layer. The primer has small hydrophilic monomers, along with solvent molecules, that improve the wettability of tooth structure and allow infiltration of the resin molecules into the exposed collagen fibrils to form a hybrid layer when bonding to the dentine. The bond component is either lightly filled or unfilled resin that combines with the hybrid layer to form a hydrophobic surface for the composite to bond to.

Manufacturers have tried to simplify the bonding process by combining various stages. Self-etching systems have had their priming monomers modified to incorporate carboxylic or phosphate acid groups. When bonding to enamel, in comparison to phosphoric acid, self-etching primers do not produce such high bond strengths, as the acid primers cannot etch as deeply or as uniformly. The results to the dentine are, however, similar to conventional etching methods and furthermore may reduce the technique sensitivity of bonding to the dentine, as there is no risk of overdrying the dentine and collapsing of the exposed collagen fibres. For these reasons, when using a self-etching system for composite restoration, selective etching of enamel is recommended.

Keywords: self-etch adhesive bonding system, modified, etching.

→ Ozer F, Blatz M. Self-etch and etch-and-rinse adhesive systems in clinical dentistry. *Compendium of Continuing Education in Dentistry*. 2013;**34**:12–14.

8. B ★   OHCD 6th ed. → p. 630

Amalgam is commonly classified by the shape of their silver-tin particles, which can be spherical, lathe-cut, or admixed. Lathe-cut amalgam
hardens more slowly and gives a longer working time. The remaining answers refer to properties of spherical amalgam, except answer D which
is another property of lathe-cut amalgams.

Spherical amalgam can achieve a smoother finish because the alloy particles do not impinge upon each other as they do in lathe-cut amalgams.
It is easier to condense because there is less friction between the spherical particles than there is in lathe-cut amalgams. Also, spherical alloys
have less mercury, which results in greater shrinkage, so contacts are
likely to be less tight.

Older amalgams underwent net expansion as the setting reaction progressed. Modern-day amalgams show net contraction, the reasons for
this being:

• Older amalgam had larger alloy particles and a higher mercury content
• Before amalgamators were available, amalgam was mixed by hand trituration, with more vigorous trituration, resulting in more contraction.

Admixed amalgam demonstrates properties between spherical and
lathe-cut amalgams.

Keywords: struggling to pack, before it sets, lathe-cut.

9. C ★

Gold onlays are commonly used in the management of toothwear to
restore posterior teeth because of the limited tooth reduction required.
However, their preparation design frequently lacks retention and resistance form. They therefore rely on adhesive cements to retain them *in
situ*. From the list given, chemically active resin cements are the most
suitable option. All the other options exhibit insufficient strength to
resist the functional forces placed upon a restoration lacking resistance
or retention form. Resin cements are stronger, with high enough bond
strengths to retain onlay-type restorations. It is important to remember
that resin cannot be light-cured through gold restorations and, as such,
dual- or chemically cured resin cement should be used. One of the challenges with bonding to gold is the inherently inert nature of the material
and the lack of an oxide layer produced. Chemically active cements, such
as Panavia®, can bond to noble metals, but methods such as heat treating
or tin plating have been advocated to improve the bond strength.
However, despite these suggestions, evidence exists to show that air-
abrading (sand blasting) the fitting surface alone provides adequate
micromechanical retention to achieve a successful clinical outcome.

Keywords: gold onlays, minimal retention or resistance form,
cementation.

→ Chana H, Kelleher M, Briggs P, Hooper R. Clinical evaluation
of resin-bonded gold alloy veneers. *Journal of Prosthetic Dentistry*.
2000;**83**:294–300.

10. D ★★

The bonding mechanism of the composite is micromechanical. Following demineralization of the surface of the dentine with an etchant, a primer and a bonding agent are used to create a hybrid layer to allow the hydrophobic composite to bond to the 'wet' or hydrophilic dentine surface. This hybrid layer creates resin tags within the exposed dentinal tubules, giving micromechanical retention. The reference listed below gives an excellent summary of the evolution of dentine-bonding agents. The concept of 'wet bonding' was brought about when it was discovered that overdrying of the surface led to a reduction in bond strength. At a microscopic level, when the dentinal surface is etched, the demineralization process leaves a matrix of collagen fibrils exposed, which is supported by residual water. If overdried, this layer collapses (collagen collapse) and the resulting hybrid layer is thin and weak, potentially decreasing the bond strength. Conversely, if the residual water is not expelled, then water globules will form within the resin layer, again resulting in a weaker bond and the risk of future degradation. With modern combined primers and bonding agents, two coats should be applied to thoroughly expel the residual water and optimize the bond. Prevention of collagen collapse is key to the 'wet bonding' principle.

Keywords: composite, wet bonding.

→ Pashley D. The evolution of dentin bonding. *Dentistry Today*. 2003. Available at: http://www.dentistrytoday.com/materials

11. E ★★   OHCD 6th ed. → p. 630

Dental amalgam is an alloy composed primarily of silver, tin, copper, and mercury. Its setting reaction has been refined over many years. The reaction creates a fine balance between various compounds (referred to as gamma phases), with each influencing the property of the amalgam. A crumbly or grainy amalgam has been under-triturated, and the material is often unusable as insufficient wetting of the alloy has occurred. Over-trituration would result in an amalgam mix that is excessively sticky.

Amalgam contraction occurs with all amalgams during the first hour, and this would not noticeably influence the workability of the material.

Moisture contamination remains a problem with zinc-containing amalgams, as this can result in delayed expansion of the amalgam.

Burnishing improves the marginal integrity of amalgams and, as such, reduces the risk of leakage at the margins.

Keywords: amalgam, crumbly, unusable.

12. E ★★

The management of flabby ridges can be difficult. The basic principle comes down to the argument of whether the denture-bearing area should be recorded under compression or relaxation (mucocompressive or mucostatic). With fibrous ridges, it is generally considered that a mucostatic impression of the hypermobile tissue is desirable, as it is more stable during rest (the soft tissue would recoil and dislodge the denture if recorded under compression).

Therefore, a selective pressure technique is used to record the normal tissues under slight compression and the flabby tissue at rest for optimal support and retention. A variety of techniques have been suggested in the literature, each one as an alternative method of achieving a mucostatic impression. They all tend to employ a custom-made tray, with some form of venting or spacing over the flabby tissue. The choice of material is important, as the viscosity is required to be low enough that, when pressure is applied to seat the tray, the resistance of the flabby tissue is greater than the inherent stiffness of the material causing it to flow and not displace the tissue. Traditionally, plaster of Paris was used, but the contemporary replacement is low-viscosity silicone.

Keywords: flabby ridge, window technique.

→ Poonam SR, Agrawal H. A review of prosthodontic management of flabby ridge conditions in maxilla and mandible by noninvasive techniques and with the use of contemporary materials. *Guident*. 2012;**5**:24–32.

13. E ★★

The recognized way of classifying colour was devised by Albert Munsell. He divided colour into three components to precisely define every colour: hue, chroma, and value. Hue is the 'actual' colour and is either red, yellow, green, blue, or purple, or somewhere within that circular scale. This natural order of colour makes up Munsell's colour wheel. Teeth have hues of reds or yellows. This is reflected by the L and R values on the Vita 3D shade guide™; 'L' represents a yellower hue, and 'R' more red (i.e. left and right shifts on the colour wheel). Chroma is the saturation of a colour, i.e. the colour intensity. On the 3D shade guide, this is denoted by the 'M' value. The value is how light or dark an object is (i.e. white to black) and, on the shade guide, is represented by the numbers 1 to 5. When using the shade guide, the value is selected first, then the chroma ('M' value), and finally, if required, the hue is adjusted ('L' and 'R' values). The 3D shade guide provides a comprehensive, systematic chart covering standard tooth colours. In comparison, standard shade guides generally cover a selection of common colours. Modern technological advancements include chairside spectrometers to aid colour selection. Polarized or greyscale images (with shade tabs in them) can help to select the correct hue and value, respectively.

Keywords: dark, element of colour, Vita 3D shade guide™.

→ Vita 3D shade guide user manual. Vita Zahnfabrik. Available at: https://www.vita-zahnfabrik.com/en/VITA-Toothguide-3D-MASTER-26230,27568.html

14. A ★★

Residual monomers in dentures can cause mucosal irritation and theoretical reductions in strength (as the polymerization conversion is reduced). The international standard for residual monomer content is

2.2%. Manufacturers' curing cycles vary in method but typically have a prolonged period of around 1–2 hours at 70°C, followed by a final boil at 100°C for half hour to 1 hour. Despite several traditional studies investigating curing cycle optimization, the reference below demonstrates that there is no scientific basis to account for these two temperatures in the curing cycle. Curing at 95°C overnight would achieve residual monomer levels consistently below the required standard of 2.2%. Achieving similar levels at 70°C would require curing times in excess of 300 hours. The justification for using the protocol outlined above is for practicality, energy efficiency, and concerns of rapid temperature increases boiling the monomer.

Excess powder would lead to granular porosities from unreacted polymer powder. Heating rapidly above acrylics boiling point would lead to gaseous porosities. Packing at the 'wet sand' stage would likely lead to an under-filled mould, and under-compression would result in an overly thick denture base and an unwanted increase in vertical dimension.

Keywords: replacement, denture, burning/itching sensation, excess monomer.

→ Lung C, Darvell B. Minimization of the inevitable residual monomer in denture base acrylic. *Dental Materials*. 2005;**21**:1119–28.

15. E ★★ OHCD 6th ed. → p. 334

MTA has become commonly used for the formation of an apical plug in endodontics, due to its biocompatibility. One of the adverse effects is the resultant discoloration of the tooth. Although the exact mechanism is not yet fully understood, it is suspected to be related to the presence of the radio-opacifier bismuth oxide. A number of potential interactions have been hypothesized. It has been suggested that bismuth oxide can interact with collagen in the dentine to form a dark precipitate. Alternatively, some research suggests that residual sodium hypochlorite can react with bismuth oxide to form a dark precipitate. In efforts to reduce the discoloration of MTA, manufacturers have tried to reduce the content of heavy metals. Iron content has been reduced in white MTA, yet discoloration remains a documented complaint.

Calcium silicate cements with alternative radio-opacifiers, such as zirconium oxide, may reduce discoloration risks in areas of aesthetic concern. One further suggestion has been made that sealing the dentine prior to placement of MTA may reduce discoloration.

Endodontic sealers may cause minor discoloration, but this is not as consistent as with MTA. RMGIC is not known to stain teeth.

Keywords: marked discoloration, MTA.

→ Yun D, Park SJ, Lee SR, Min KS. Tooth discoloration induced by calcium-silicate-based pulp-capping materials. *European Journal of Dentistry*. 2015;**9**:165–70.

16. A ★★   OHCD 6th ed. → p. 252

For a long time, metallo-ceramic crowns were the mainstay of aesthetic indirect restorations due to their greater resilience than traditional porcelain jacket crowns. The advent of dentine bonding and modern high-strength ceramic restorations has led to alternative options becoming available that are generally considered to be more aesthetic due to their optical properties. However, there is still a place for metal-ceramic restorations as they have a proven track record, are durable in high-stress situations, and provide a good compromise between aesthetics and tooth reduction. High-strength ceramics generally require greater circumferential tooth reduction.

The mechanical and aesthetic properties of the materials in metal-ceramic crowns dictate the space. A relatively thin, uniform layer of porcelain supported by metal is the strongest but often does not provide acceptable aesthetics. The absolute minimum requirements for porcelain is 0.7 mm, and metal 0.3–0.5 mm. However, to avoid an opaque-looking restoration, 1.5–2 mm of incisal reduction is advocated. Therefore, in this scenario, as 1 mm of incisal clearance already exists, a minimum of 0.5-mm further reduction is needed.

Keywords: 1 mm of space, desired incisal level, metallo-ceramic crowns.

→ Ricketts D, Barlett D. *Advanced Operative Dentistry: A Practical Approach* (1st ed.). Churchill Livingstone, London; 2013.

17. D ★★★   OHCD 6th ed. → p. 632

Composite is primarily composed of a resin matrix and an inorganic filler. The filler improves the material characteristics by reducing shrinkage, increasing compressive strength, and improving wear rate. Fillers are commonly composed of glass particles (e.g. aluminoborosilicate), and the size of the particles is used to classify the type of composite (e.g. microfilled, nanofilled, nano-hybrid, etc.). The composition of the filler particles significantly influences the physical properties of the resultant composite.

Unfortunately, resins and fillers do not bond chemically, and as such, an intermediary silane coupling agent is required. Silanes have both an inorganic and an organic end to their molecule, allowing the chemical linkage of the resin and filler. Contact of the composite with air inhibits the polymerization process, leaving an unreacted surface that can be used for future bonding. However, in old composites, this is inevitably worn (or polished) away, leaving a surface layer predominantly composed of exposed inorganic filler. The original silane coating again will have been worn away from exposure to the oral environment, and therefore, to optimize the bond when repairing composites, a fresh silane layer should be applied. Some newer universal bonding agents may already contain silane.

Barium oxide is added for its radio-opacifying properties. Camphorquinone is the source of free radicals for the polymerization reaction of light-cured composites. Hydroquinone prevents premature polymerization. TEGMA is a low-weight resin monomer added to improve handling characteristics and reduce viscosity.

Keywords: composite, repair, prior to bonding.

→ Staxrud F, Dahl J. Silanising agents promote resin-composite repair. *International Dental Journal*. 2015;**65**:311–15.

18. C ★★★

Traditionally, dental alloys have been produced by casting methods utilizing the lost wax technique; this method is labour-intensive and time-consuming. CAD/CAM has become readily available in dentistry for prosthesis production. CAD/CAM methods can either be subtractive (i.e. milling of pre-manufactured blocks) or additive (SLM, stereolithography, etc.). SLM works by high-powered lasers selectively fusing areas of a metal powder, layer upon layer, to the designed 3D structure. This process has the advantage over milling of being able to produce hollow 3D structures. In comparison to traditional casting methods, porosities are greatly reduced, which significantly improves the alloy's physical properties. The accuracy is also comparable, if not better, than casting.

The σ-phase of Co-Cr makes the material more brittle. This is related to the composition of the alloy, and not the production process. The addition of molybdenum increases the γ-phase (which demonstrates improved strength), but this is not related to the manufacturing process. The addition of tungsten helps to reduce the σ-phase.

Keywords: CAD/CAM, SLM, stronger.

→ Koutsoukis T, Zinelis S, Eliades G, Al-Wazzan K, Rifaiy MA, Al Jabbari YS. Selective laser melting technique of Co-Cr dental alloys: a review of structure and properties and comparative analysis with other available techniques. *Journal of Prosthodontics*. 2015;**24**:303–12.

19. B ★★★

Various types of corrosion can affect dental materials, and the surrounding environment plays a role in this. When dissimilar metals are placed within an electrolytic solution, there is potential to create an electrochemical cell (e.g. a chemical battery), otherwise known as a galvanic cell. It has been reported that when amalgam is placed adjacent to gold in saliva, a galvanic cell can be induced, leading to galvanic corrosion. This leads to surface staining with a silver brown colour in a ring around the contact point. However, it is suspected that it is the presence of free mercury that results in galvanic corrosion. This reaction is short-lived, with little mercury remaining after about 1 hour and almost no residual current after 1 day.

The effects of this corrosion are clinically insignificant with regard to the alloy properties, but it has been reported that this galvanic current can occasionally cause short-lived mild pain. Replacement of the restoration is not normally required.

Keywords: amalgam, gold, silver/brown circular stain, contact point.

→ Fusayama T, Katayori T, Nomoto S. Corrosion of gold and amalgam placed in contact with each other. *Journal of Dental Research*. 1963;**42**:1183–97.

→ Upadhyay D, Panchal AD, Dubey RS, Srivastava VK. Corrosion of alloys used in dentistry: a review. *Materials Science and Engineering*. 2006;**432**:1–11.

20. D ★★★★ OHCD 6th ed. → p. 334

In vital pulp therapy, CH was traditionally the gold standard until newer materials, such as MTA [a type of bioactive endodontic cement (BEC)], became available. When applied directly to pulp tissues, CH forms a superficial layer of necrosis, which contains calcium deposits. These act as foci for calcification, and subjacent pulp cells differentiate into odontoblasts to produce reparative dentine and a hard tissue barrier. Furthermore, the high pH is thought to solubilize proteins and growth factors trapped in the adjacent dentine, which stimulates pulp cell differentiation. BECs have been shown to release a greater number of growth factors than CH.

BECs differ in that they have been demonstrated to induce less inflammation at the interface and cause greater proliferation of odontoblasts. Some research suggests that the formation of CH within BECs is responsible for this finding (again solubilizing cytokines from the surrounding dentine). Additionally, BECs biocompatibility have been linked with the material's ability to form hydroxyapatite. Biologically, BECs are more biocompatible, and results suggest that histologically dentine formation is more regular, less porous, and in increased amounts.

Additionally, the ability to bond to dentine is important in the success of pulp capping. Mechanically, BECs have been shown to have an ionic bond to the dentine, which may limit bacterial penetration. Both materials display antibacterial properties, and neither material has been shown to be obtundent.

Keywords: direct pulp cap, new calcium silicate, calcium hydroxide, biological reason.

→ Modena KC, Casas-Apayco LC, Atta MT, *et al*. Cytotoxicity and biocompatibility of direct and indirect pulp capping materials. *Journal of Applied Oral Sciences*. 2009;**17**:544–54.

21. D ★★★★ OHCD 6th ed. → p. 632

Composites placed at an increased occlusal vertical dimension (OVD) for toothwear are becoming common practice. The chosen material needs to have good mechanical properties to resist the increased occlusal loads placed on these 'proud' restorations, along with good aesthetic properties. Traditional microhybrid composites combine large and small filler particulars to increase the filler content. Higher filler contents generally improve the mechanical properties and reduce polymerization shrinkage. Old microfill composites utilized smaller filler particles, which reduced the size of surface irregularities and improved surface smoothness and appearance. However, this negatively impacted on mechanical properties, as the glass content was reduced.

The introduction of nanoparticles to modern composites has been claimed to maintain the mechanical properties of the microhybrid, but also to harness the aesthetic properties of microfill composites. Therefore, in a case like in the scenario, a nanohybrid composite would be the most appropriate choice of materials. A conventional microhybrid material would be a suitable alternative, as it has a proven track record.

Keywords: composite, worn, teeth, increased OVD.

→ Moraes RR, Gonçalves L de S, Lancellotti AC, Consani S, Correr-Sobrinho L, Sinhoreti MA. Nanohybrid resin composite: nanofiller loaded materials or traditional microhybrid resins. *Operative Dentistry*. 2009;**34**:551–7.

22. E ★★★★

Various active ingredients have been investigated to assess their potential to protect against erosion, with limited conclusive results. Some compounds, such as CPP-CAP, calcium nanophosphate, titanium fluoride, and stannous fluoride, have shown potential in reducing the impact of erosion. Over time, these compounds build a protective glaze/coatings on the tooth surface. Alternatively, some clinicians would prescribe higher-strength sodium fluoride (1.1% in patients over 16 years of age), but this would help to remineralize the lost ions, rather than prevent dissolution. Although the actual quality of the evidence is weak and there are numerous methodological challenges which reduce the external validity of results, stannous fluoride toothpastes are readily available on the high street and may provide greater benefit to patients over sodium fluoride alone. Furthermore, as the product cost is low (compared to CPP-ACP or a prescription) and this type of fluoride formulation is not detrimental, then the authors would suggest its use to supplement a preventative programme until further evidence is available. Clinicians should also remember that standard dietary advice and any necessary medical management are necessary and more important than the active ingredient of toothpaste.

Arginine is generally used as a desensitizing agent, and sodium lauryl sulfate is a foaming agent in toothpastes.

Keywords: erosion, widely available, toothpaste, protective.

→ Carvalho FG, Brasil VL, Silva Filho TJ, Carlo HL, Santos RL, Lima BA. Protective effect of calcium nanophosphate and CPP-ACP agents on enamel erosion. *Brazilian Oral Research*. 2013;**27**:463–70.

→ Hove LH, Holme B, Young A, Tveit AB. The protective effect of TiF4, SnF2 and NaF against erosion-like lesions *in situ*. *Caries Research*. 2008;**42**:68–72.

→ Wang X, Megert B, Hellwig E, Neuhaus KW, Lussi A. Preventing erosion with novel agents. *Journal of Dentistry*. 2011;**39**:163–70.

23. E ★★★★ OHCD 6th ed. → p. 646

Fixed and removable prostheses rely upon the accuracy of working impressions. In implant dentistry, this accuracy has greater relevance, particularly where suprastructures are used to join implants. Any discrepancies prevent passivity of fit and may cause complications (e.g. fracture of veneering material or marginal bone loss).

Contemporary elastomeric materials have high accuracy and good dimensional stability. Polyethers are generally favoured over addition PVS in the scenario, as they have greater rigidity and therefore are thought to better retain the impression copings in the correct position during casting. It is important though that polyethers are poured within 1 hour, as moisture absorption can cause distortion. PVS materials are suitable alternatives, as studies have shown similar accuracy to polyethers. However, results are less reproducible.

Some clinicians may still use impression plaster for the above situation, but it is only applicable to edentulous cases with no undercut. Furthermore, there is significant cumulative distortion, following the pouring of the master model.

Hydrocolloids are not accurate or rigid enough for this application.

The era of digital dentistry is beginning to revolutionize prosthodontics, and with future advances, intraoral scanning may supersede conventional impression techniques.

Keywords: minor undercut, open-tray impression, implants.

→ Donavon T, Chee W. Impression materials: a comparative review of impression materials most commonly used in restorative dentistry. *Dental Clinics of North America.* 2004;**48**:445–70.

→ Hoods-Moonsammy V, Owen P, Howes D. A comparison of the accuracy of polyether, polyvinyl siloxane, and plaster impressions for long-span implant-supported prostheses. *International Journal of Prosthodontics.* 2014;**27**:433–8.

24. E ★★★★ OHCD 6th ed. → p. 362

A vast array of suture materials are available in modern medicine, and often numerous materials will be appropriate for a given situation. In relation to modern periodontal microsurgery (particularly in the aesthetic zone), a number of basic principles apply to material choice. In general, monofilament sutures are preferential to multifilament fibres, as they do not 'wick' bacteria into the wound, which aggravates the inflammatory response. Secondly, in delicate tissues (e.g. the dental papilla), finer and less traumatic sutures are recommended, as this promotes quicker wound healing and causes less chance of disruption to the blood supply.

Synthetic monofilament fibres are usually considered the material of choice, as they are least traumatic and only induce mild tissue reactions. Despite this, some clinicians favour the use of polyglycolic acid, as good knot tension can be achieved.

Black silk is a braided multifilament material which produces one of the higher tissue reactions, and although it has good handling properties, it is infrequently used. Polyester is again a multifilament fibre and not frequently used in dentistry. Vicryl® (polyglycolic acid) is a multifilament, synthetic, resorbable material. In smaller sizes, it may be appropriate for the task at hand; however, #4.0 is generally considered too large. It is frequently used in dento-alveolar surgery.

Poliglecaprone (e.g. Monocryl®) would be a more suitable resorbable material, as it is a monofilament fibre and has high initial strength during the first few days of wound healing. It is, however, more expensive. The most appropriate choice would therefore be 6.0 polypropylene (Prolene®), a small monofilament, non-resorbable suture which induces minor tissue reactions. Being non-resorbable, there is less risk of dislodgement and wound dehiscence during the critical early healing stages, compared with resorbable sutures.

Keywords: periodontal surgery, microsurgical, suture.

→ Kurtsmann G. Suturing for success. *Dentistry Today*. Available at: http://www.dentistrytoday.com/periodontics/359-suturing-for-surgical-success

→ Velvart P, Peters C. Soft tissue management in endodontic surgery. *Journal of Endodontics*. 2005;**31**:4–16.

25. B ★★★★

The management of developmental white spot lesions is frequently an aesthetic concern and can be challenging to manage. The four traditional management strategies are remineralization, masking with bleaching, microabrasion, or restoration. Most clinicians would wish to avoid formal restoration, if possible, particularly in younger patients. However, the most conservative measures are inconsistent in their results, and furthermore, microabrasion can remove up to 360 µm of enamel and leave a rough surface.

Resin infiltration is a contemporary technique that uses low-viscosity resin to fill subsurface porosities. It was initially developed for preventing progression of early carious lesions. In white spot lesions, the resin fills the subsurface porosities, increasing the refractive index to a value similar to that of the surrounding enamel (1.52). Prior to infiltration, the porosities are filled with air or water, which has a much lower index (air has a refractive index of 1) and makes the lesion more obvious to the eye. Although results are not 100% successful, they are promising and can provide acceptable results without the need for further treatment.

Keywords: resin infiltration, aesthetic concerns.

→ Kim S, Kim EY, Jeong TS, Kim JW. The evaluation of resin infiltration for masking labial enamel white spot lesions. *International Journal of Paediatric Dentistry*. 2011;**21**:241–8.

Head and neck syndromes

Nicholas Longridge

'How many teeth should I have?'

A comparatively small chapter, syndromes of the head and neck are generally rare. It is unlikely that the majority of clinicians will diagnose or treat patients affected by many of the syndromes discussed. However, it is highly likely that clinical findings or presenting features may find their way into undergraduate academic examinations.

Most syndromes are presented in the literature as a specific list of associated clinical findings, and many are still referred to eponymously. Some of the syndromes with oral manifestations can also be associated with more sinister conditions and, as such, a broad knowledge of the common syndromes with orofacial manifestations is important. It is highly advised to read the chapter on syndromes of the head and neck in the *Oxford Handbook of Clinical Dentistry*.

Key topics include:

- Syndromes associated with hypodontia
- Syndromes affecting orofacial development
- Syndromes linked with gastrointestinal conditions
- Syndromes subsequent to infections.

QUESTIONS

1. A 9-year-old boy has multiple retained deciduous teeth, a prominent brow, and a wide nasal bridge. Multiple supernumeraries are evident on the orthopantomogram (OPT), and the mother informs you that her son has recently seen a specialist regarding the lack of collarbones. Which single condition is this child most likely to have? ★

A Apert's syndrome

B Cleidocranial dysostosis

C Melkerson–Rosenthal syndrome

D Pfeiffer syndrome

E Pierre–Robin sequence

2. A 7-year-old girl attends with her mother for a routine examination (see Figure 13.1). The patient's mother has read that her child may have congenitally missing teeth and that they have an increased prevalence for periodontitis. You also note the girl has low-set ears, upward sloping palpebral fissures, brachycephaly, and a tendency for tongue protrusion. What is the single most likely diagnosis? ★

A 45,XO

B Trisomy 13

C Trisomy 18

D Trisomy 21

E XXY

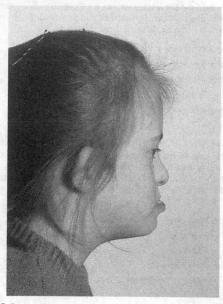

Figure 13.1

Reproduced from Welbury R, et al, *Paediatric Dentistry* fourth edition, Figure 17.2, page 286, Copyright (2012) by permission of Oxford University Press.

3. A 27-year-old woman has marked mandibular prognathism and multiple basal cell carcinomas. She has previously been diagnosed with Gorlin–Goltz syndrome (naevoid basal cell carcinoma syndrome). An orthopantomogram (OPT) is taken to investigate cystic change in the mandible. Which single type of lesion are you most likely to identify? ★★

A Ameloblastomas

B Dentigerous cysts

C Odontogenic keratocysts

D Radicular cysts

E Solitary bone cyst

4. A 17-year-old adolescent girl has multiple hard, bony lumps on her maxilla. She says that her mother had similar lumps and had a colectomy. Which is the single most likely diagnosis? ★★

A Gardner's syndrome

B Heerfordt syndrome

C Melkerson–Rosenthal syndrome

D Paterson–Brown-Kelly syndrome

E Peutz–Jeghers syndrome

5. A 6-year-old girl has pronounced facial asymmetry and large unilateral café-au-lait spots on her skin. She has attended her dentist for regular examinations since the early loss of her primary central incisors, which exfoliated with her entire roots intact. She has recently recovered from a fractured right femur. What is the single most likely diagnosis? ★★★

A Crouzon syndrome

B Down's syndrome

C Eagle's syndrome

D Gardner's syndrome

E McCune–Albright syndrome

6. An 8-year-old boy attends for a new patient consultation. He is under the care of the local Paediatric Maxillofacial Unit for a cleft palate. His appearance can be seen in Figure 13.2. Which is the single most likely diagnosis? ★★★

A Cherubism

B Ectodermal dysplasia

C Marfan's syndrome

D Pierre–Robin sequence

E Treacher–Collins syndrome

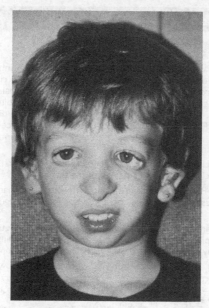

Figure 13.2
Reproduced from Traboulsi E.I., *Genetic diseases of the eye*, 2nd ed, Figure 12.13, Chapter 12, Copyright (2012), by permission of Oxford University Press USA.

ANSWERS

1. B ★   OHCD 6th ed. → p. 754

Cleidocranial dysostosis (cleidocranial dysplasia) is an inherited genetic condition that typically presents with hypoplastic clavicles, delayed closure of fontanelles, and dento-alveolar abnormalities. Dental abnormalities can include a high-arched palate, multiple supernumeraries, retained deciduous teeth, and crown/root dilacerations. Frontal and parietal bossing is common, with mid-face hypoplasia also noted. The condition is autosomal dominant and mainly affects membranous bones.

Apert's and Pfeiffer syndromes are genetic conditions which result in the premature closure of specific sutures of the skull vault.

Melkerson–Rosenthal syndrome is an autosomal dominant condition that can present with swollen or cracked lips, fissured tongue, and facial paralysis.

Pierre–Robin sequence is another first branchial arch genetic condition, which can present with similar features to Treacher–Collins. The mandibular body is shown to be considerably shorter in this condition.

Keywords: lack of collarbones, prominent brow, multiple supernumeraries.

2. D ★   OHCD 6th ed. → p. 755

Trisomy 21 is more commonly referred to as Down's syndrome. As the most common of all malformations, the features described above are most likely to be encountered with this syndrome. Prevalence is approximately 1 in 700 births, with a 50% increase in incidence when the mother exceeds 40 years of age. It occurs as a result of an extra copy of all or part of chromosome 21.

Developmental delay, auditory problems, and congenital cardiac defects are common occurrences. Greater than 50% live to 50 years of age. Hypodontia is a common feature and may complicate dental management. An increased susceptibility to periodontal disease, infection, and haematological disorders, e.g. leukaemia, is also reported, whilst caries incidence is reduced. Taurodontism, delayed eruption of teeth, or teeth with short roots are additional oral features that may be evident.

The other answers listed are alternatively known as the following:

- 45,XO—Turner's syndrome
- Trisomy 13—Patau or D-syndrome
- Trisomy 18—Edward's syndrome
- XXY—Klinefelter's syndrome.

Keywords: congenitally missing teeth, periodontitis, brachycephaly, upward sloping palpebral fissures, tongue protrusion.

3. C ★★

Gorlin–Goltz syndrome (naevoid basal cell carcinoma syndrome) is a rare autosomal dominant condition brought about by a mutation in the PTCH gene. Patients have multiple skin lesions known as basal cell carcinomas that are locally invasive neoplasms. Jaw lesions are common and occur in the majority of patients diagnosed with the syndrome. These lesions are odontogenic keratocysts, which develop from remnants of the dental lamina. They are locally aggressive cysts/neoplasm (the true classification is heavily debated within the profession!) that are often excised surgically.

Ameloblastomas are generally multiloculated tumours of the posterior mandible. Unilocular ameloblastoma accounts for a small percentage of ameloblastomas.

Dentigerous cysts are considered developmental cysts that arise from remnants of the dental follicle (reduced enamel epithelium). They are associated with the amelodentinal junction (ADJ/EDJ) of unerupted teeth, often third molars, and can vary significantly in size and expansion. Radiographically, a follicular space exceeding 5 mm should be investigated as a potential dentigerous cyst.

Radicular cysts are associated with the apices of non-vital teeth. They can vary in size quite significantly but are often well circumscribed, with cortication at the margins.

Solitary bone cysts in the mandible are often unilocular in nature and present with scalloping around the root apices of multiple teeth. They may develop as a result of previous trauma and are often void of epithelium upon surgical exploration.

Keywords: Gorlin–Goltz, cystic change.

→ El-Naggar AK, Chan JKC, Grandis JR, Takata T, Slootweg PJ. *WHO Classification of Head and Neck Tumours* (4th ed.). International Agency for Research on Cancer Press, Lyon; 2017.

4. A ★★   OHCD 6th ed. → p. 755

Gardner's syndrome (familial adenomatous polyposis) is a rare autosomal dominant condition. Multiple osteomas, fibrous tumours, sebaceous cysts, and polyposis of the colon are features of Gardner's syndrome. Multiple osteomas would require further investigation, as the intestinal polyps in Gardner's syndrome can undergo malignant change and require surgical removal. Intraoral osteomas can impede or delay eruption and can complicate denture provision. It is highly unlikely that Gardner's syndrome would be diagnosed following a dental visit, but investigation of gastrointestinal symptoms and referral to a Gastroenterology Department may be required if suspicions were aroused.

Heerfordt syndrome is associated with sarcoidosis and can present with uveitis, parotitis, fever, and possible facial palsy.

Paterson–Brown-Kelly syndrome is associated with oesophageal webbing, glossitis, cheilitis, and difficulty swallowing.

Peutz–Jeghers syndrome would present with multiple hyperpigmented macules, often affecting the hands and perioral tissues. The syndrome is associated with benign intestinal polyposis and has low malignant potential.

Melkerson–Rosenthal syndrome is discussed within other questions in this chapter.

Keywords: multiple bony lumps, maxilla, colectomy.

5. E ★★★   OHCD 6th ed. → p. 754

McCune–Albright syndrome is diagnosed with two of the following three clinical traits:

- Polyostotic fibrous dysplasia
- Café-au-lait spots
- Autonomous endocrine abnormality.

The condition is caused by a genetic mutation and is rare, occurring in <1 in 100,000. Fibrous dysplasia involves replacement of trabecular bone with immature bone and fibrous tissue and can often result in significant bone deformities or fractures. The craniofacial bones are thought to be involved in approximately 50% of cases. The radiographic appearance of bone in patients with fibrous dysplasia is often described as 'ground-glass' in appearance. Management of fibrous dysplasia can be complex and protracted.

Skin pigmentation is often unilateral and can cover large areas of the body.

Endocrine abnormalities are traditionally referred to as being precocious puberty but can include goitres, hyperthyroidism, and Cushing's syndrome, to name a few. Hypophosphataemia has also been reported with this syndrome.

Crouzon syndrome is a first branchial arch syndrome, which primarily presents with craniosynostosis, exophthalmus, and hypertelorism.

Eagle's syndrome results from a misshapen styloid process. It can present with pain in the jaw and neck region that can occur with movement of the neck or swallowing. Associated calcification of the stylohyoid ligament can lead to syncope from temporary occlusion of the carotid vessels when looking sideways.

Keywords: café-au-lait spots, facial asymmetry.

6. E ★★★   OHCD 6th ed. → p. 760

Treacher–Collins syndrome (mandibulofacial dysostosis) is an autosomal dominant condition that affects the first branchial arch, and thus craniofacial development. Genetic mutation affects the *TCOF-1* gene, which encodes the Treacle protein. Structures derived from the first arch are therefore affected. Hypoplastic zygomas and a retrognathic mandible, with downsloping palpebral fissures, are characteristic features. Generally, normal cognitive development occurs. However, speech and hearing abnormalities can delay development. Cleft palate is identified in approximately one-third of cases. The mandibular ramus is particularly affected, and a high gonial angle results.

Cherubism is often referred to as familial fibrous dysplasia and is associated with painless swelling of the jaws. Delayed eruption of the teeth is common, and improvement can occur over time or with surgery post-puberty when the condition becomes self-limiting.

Ectodermal dysplasia is a common condition which can have dramatic effects on dentition, including hypodontia, small conical teeth, and maxillary hypoplasia. Very fine or abnormal hair and the inability to sweat are additional identifiable features.

Marfan's syndrome is a connective tissue disorder that results in the production of defective fibrillin-1. Several clinical features can be present, but patients are often tall and thin, with arachnodactyly (spider-like fingers).

Pierre–Robin sequence is discussed within other questions in this chapter.

Keywords: malar hypoplasia, deformed pinnas, coloboma.

Radiology and radiography

Raheel Aftab

'X-ray vision, your greatest superpower.'

When you consider that, with direct vision alone, you can only see the coronal few millimetres of teeth and none of the surrounding alveolus, it becomes clear that, without additional visual aids, we can only assess and treat a relatively small proportion of our patient's oral health needs.

In 1895, only months after the very first medical radiograph, Dr Otto Walkhoff recorded the very first dental radiograph. This exposure was of his own dentition and lasted a lengthy 25 minutes.

Since then, radiography has become a staple tool of the profession and refinement of the technology has allowed us to reduce exposure times down to milliseconds, with radiation doses smaller than those experienced by people taking short-haul flights. Further advances in dose reduction and reformatting protocols have allowed for computed tomography to become increasingly popular for diagnostics and treatment planning in endodontic, oral surgery, and orthodontic cases.

The benefits of dental radiography make them an indispensable resource, but since all types of radiation pose some degree of risk to human health, the clinician must consider how useful the information from the proposed exposure will be. There are no shortages of tragic stories of employees working with radiation who suffered ill health years after stopping work.

Today dental radiography can be performed routinely and safely as a result of the valuable lesson learnt from the debilitating consequences suffered by past medical professionals, nuclear workers, and even the 'radium girls' who painted luminous material onto watch faces.

Key topics include:

- Limitations of radiographs
- Image selection criteria
- Radiation physics, protection, and legislation
- Radiographic interpretation
- Types of dental radiographic imagery.

QUESTIONS

1. A radiographer is discussing the importance of aluminum filtration in standard X-ray tubes. As part of the lecture, the dental students are informed that X-rays and gamma rays are classified as ionizing radiation and occupy a specific section on the electromagnetic spectrum. Following the seminar, one of the students asks what properties of X-rays enable them to avoid being attenuated by the aluminium filter. ★

A Long wavelength and high photon energy

B Long wavelength and low photon energy

C Medium wavelength and high photon energy

D Short wavelength and high photon energy

E Short wavelength and low photon energy

2. A 45-year-old woman has undergone post-operative radiotherapy following resection and selective neck dissection of a T2N1M0 squamous cell carcinoma of the right retromolar pad. At her 6-month review, she is showing signs of xerostomia. Which single physical interaction between radiation and tissue would predominantly explain the clinical signs? ★

A Attenuation

B Compton effect

C Ionization

D Photoelectric effect

E Unmodified scatter

3. A dental student has accidentally taken a right bitewing on an average-build 52-year-old man at 50 kV. The radiographer discusses the risk of low-energy photons and advises that a kilovoltage of 60–70 is generally advised. However, following the incident, the student is now confused why an even higher kilovoltage (80–90 kV) is not used to investigate for interproximal caries. What is the main diagnostic disadvantage of using a kilovoltage of >70? ★

A Darkens the image

B Decreases the contrast

C Improves the resolution

D Increases the ionization

E Lightens the image

4. A 53-year-old woman has vertical bitewings requested to assess her bone levels, following a basic periodontal examination (BPE), as shown in Table 14.1:

Table 14.1		
3	2	3
3	2	3

The radiographer performing the exposure accidentally performed a panoramic radiograph instead, because that is what is usually performed in the department for periodontal bone-level assessment. The patient would now like to discuss any potential sequelae of this error. The risk of which single effect has been increased? ★

A Carcinogenic

B Deterministic

C Heritable

D Metastatic

E Stochastic

5. A radiation protection advisor has recently visited a number of local practices and has recommended that changes are made to their X-ray machines. He advises converting from a round to a rectangular collimator. Making this change to radiography equipment is related to which single International Commission on Radiological Protection's (IRCPs) key principles? ★

A Authorization

B Justification

C Limitation

D Optimization

E Restriction

6. A 32-year-old woman attends for consultation in the local Restorative Dentistry Department where she is assessed by a specialty registrar (StR). She is subsequently sent to the Radiology Department for the radiographs to be carried out by a radiographer. Under the Ionising Radiation Medical Exposure) Regulations (IR(ME)R 2018), the StR is acting as which of the following agents? (Select one answer from the options listed below.) ★ ★

A Operator

B Operator and practitioner

C Practitioner

D Referrer

E Referrer and practitioner

7. A 44-year-old woman has had bitewing radiographs to investigate for interproximal caries. The film was positioned using the 'stick-on-tab' bitewing holding technique. Following development, it is noticed all the mesial and distal contact points of all teeth appear blurry and overlapped. If the image is to be retaken, which single factor should be corrected to improve the image? ★★

A Film positioning

B Horizontal angulation of the collimator

C Length of exposure

D Patient movement

E Vertical angulation of the beam-aiming device

8. A 14-year-old girl has a periapical radiograph taken of her lower right first permanent molar (LR6) with a digital photostimulable phosphor (PSP) plate. When the image is processed, there is a ghost image overlying the LR6. Which single action is most appropriate to correct this problem? ★★

A Dispose of the PSP, and retake the image with a new plate

B Ensure that the PSP data are fully erased, and repeat

C Repeat the radiograph, and ensure the patient does not move during the exposure

D Turn the PSP around to ensure the front surface is facing the X-ray tube, and retake

E Use the software to correct the fault

9. A foundation dentist is updating their practice radiation folder. They notice that no radiation protection advisor (RPA) is recorded, and their foundation trainer wishes to know which single piece of documentation makes this mandatory. ★★★

A Health and Safety at Work etc. Act (HSW) 1974

B Ionising Radiation Regulations (IRR) 2017

C Ionising Radiation (Medical Exposure) Regulations (IR(ME)R) 2018

D Radiation and Health Protection (RHP) 1998

E Royal College of Radiologists Guidelines (RCRG) 2008

10. An 11-year-old boy is assessed in a Paediatric Trauma Clinic, following a fall off his scooter. The referring general dental practitioner has provided a periapical radiograph suggestive of a horizontal mid-third root fracture of the upper right central incisor (UR1), but it is not conclusive. The tooth is grade 1, mobile, and non-tender and gave a negative response to sensibility testing. What is the single most appropriate next step to confirm the diagnosis? ★ ★ ★

A Request a cone beam computed tomography (CBCT)

B Request a dentopantomogram (DPT)

C Request a supplemental periapical radiograph

D Request an upper midline occlusal radiograph

E Request to use an electronic apex locator to detect a fracture

11. An 18-year-old man attends the local Emergency Department (ED) after a blow to the right cheek playing rugby. Clinical signs suggest a zygomatic complex fracture, and there is no diplopia, loss of visual acuity, or restriction of eye movements. Which single plain film radiographic images are most likely to provide the greatest diagnostic information? ★ ★ ★ ★

A Dentopantomogram (DPT) and posteroanterior (PA) mandible

B DPT and reverse Townes

C DPT and submentovertex

D Lateral skull and PA skull

E Occipitomental (OM) and OM 30

12. A 56-year-old man reports recurrent swelling under the right angle of the jaw every time he eats a meal. The swelling presents with pain and eventually reduces in size after several hours. Bimanual palpation reveals a firm bony lump immediately adjacent to the submandibular gland. A salivary gland calculus or sialolith is made as the provisional diagnosis. Which single plain film radiograph would be the most appropriate first-line image for visualizing the potential salivary stone? ★ ★ ★ ★

A Dentopantomogram

B Lateral oblique

C Lower oblique occlusal

D Lower occlusal 45°

E Lower occlusal 90°—'true occlusal'

ANSWERS

1. D ★

Each packet of X-ray energy is termed a photon. X-ray photons have short wavelengths and high photon energy. These photons are produced when high-powered electrons are fired at a tungsten target. Resultant deflection of these electrons or ejection of target electrons results in photons of energy being emitted. Low-energy photons are removed within the X-ray tube by an aluminum filter, to reduce irradiation from photons with poor penetrating power.

Collision of these photons with different structures within the body can have a variety of effects, which ultimately results in differential penetrance through tissues. This provides a radiographic image.

Radiowaves occupy a position at the opposite end of the electromagnetic spectrum, characterized by long wavelengths and low photon energy.

Keywords: X-rays, gamma rays, electromagnetic spectrum.

→ Whaites E, Drage N. *Essentials of Dental Radiography and Radiology* (5th ed.). Churchill Livingstone, London; 2013.

2. D ★

Collision of an X-ray photon with electrons within the tissues results in the ejection of photoelectrons. The X-ray photon gives up all energy upon collision and is therefore absorbed by the tissue. Photoelectrons can continue to collide with other electrons within the tissue, producing further photoelectrons. Ionization brought about by these electrons is thought to be linked to the damaging effect of X-rays. This is known as the photoelectric effect.

Attenuation refers to the process of absorption and scattering, as the beam passes through organic tissues. This process reduces the intensity of the X-ray.

The Compton effect, or scatter, refers to the interaction of a moderate-to high-energy X-ray photon with an outer shell electron. The effects are similar across all tissues. X-ray photons can be scattered in any direction but are dependent on the energy of the incoming photon. Compton scatter is very difficult to minimize and can decrease the contrast of, or fog, the resultant image.

Ionization refers to the process of producing a charged atom or ion.

Unmodified scatter refers to the change in direction of a low-energy photon, without ionization. This process may result in loss of energy but has little effect upon the resultant radiographic image.

Keywords: radiotherapy, xerostomia, physical.

→ Whaites E, Drage N. *Essentials of Dental Radiography and Radiology* (5th ed.). Churchill Livingstone, London; 2013.

3. B ★

Kilovoltage reflects the penetrating power of an X-ray—in other terms, the higher the kilovoltage, the higher the energy of the beam. Contrast refers to the optical density differences visualized on a radiograph—think fifty shades of grey—it is the contrast that enables us to analyse the different tissues irradiated on a radiograph. Density is the degree of darkening of a film.

Increasing the kilovoltage will decrease the contrast of the resultant image. Conversely, decreasing the kilovoltage will increase the contrast. This is because low-energy photons are more likely to be absorbed or scattered by the tissues being irradiated. As a result, fewer photons reach the film and the ratio between radio-opaque and radiolucent areas of the film will be more significant.

High kilovoltage will also affect the density of the film and, as such, a balance between kilovoltage, milliamperage, and time of exposure must be sought. Most modern periapical and bitewing radiographs use between 60 and 70 kV. Kilovoltage is kept the same for most standard intraoral views, but adjusted for panoramic radiographs where the time cannot be changed.

In simple terms, altering the milliamperage changes the quantity of X-rays produced. The relationship between milliamperage and exposure time is inversely proportional, i.e. increasing the milliamperage and decreasing the exposure time by the same amounts will result in the same image. Milliamperage is generally set (6–8 mA) on most modern X-ray machines. Therefore, alterations in exposure time will be a major factor in the resultant optical density of intraoral images.

Keywords: higher kilovoltage.

4. E ★

Stochastic effects occur by chance. The probability of these effects occurring increases with exposure to more irradiation. However, they could occur at any point and there is no known threshold which is assumed to be safe. The relationship between dose and risk is linear in nature, with no association between severity and dose. Cancer induction (somatic effects and carcinogenic effects) and heritable diseases (genetic effects) are two subcategories of stochastic effects.

Deterministic effects are dose-dependent and will occur following a specified dose of radiation. These can include erythema, hair loss, xerostomia, and cataracts, which are common deterministic effects after radiotherapy to the head and neck region.

Metastatic effects refer to pathology that has spread from its primary site to an additional site within the body. See Figure 14.1 which shows the sequence of events when radiation is absorbed by a biological medium.

Keywords: bitewings, panoramic, sequelae.

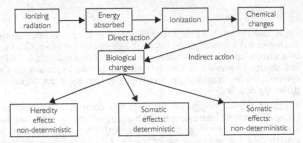

Figure 14.1
Reproduced from Mason R, and Bourne S, *A Guide to Dental Radiography* Fourth Edition, Figure 1.5, page 7, Copyright (1998) by permission of Oxford University Press.

5. D ★

Justification, optimization, and dose limitation are three key principles of radiation protection, as outlined by the IRCP.

- 'The Principle of Justification: any decision that alters the radiation exposure situation should do more good than harm.
- The Principle of Optimization of Protection: the likelihood of incurring exposure, the number of people exposed, and the magnitude of their individual doses should all be kept as low as reasonably achievable, taking into account economic and societal factors.
- The Principle of Application of Dose Limits: the total dose to any individual from regulated sources in planned exposure situations other than medical exposure of patients should not exceed the appropriate limits specified by the Commission.'

In this scenario, changing from a round to a rectangular collimator would reduce the field of exposure, thus lowering the received dose.

Keywords: round, rectangular collimator, IRCP's key principles.

→ International Commission on Radiological Protection. *The 2007 Recommendations of the International Commission on Radiological Protection.* 2007. Available at: http://www.icrp.org

6. D ★★

The IR(ME)R 2018 are designed to provide protection for patients who require radiographic imaging. The regulations discuss the role of clinicians in justifying and taking radiographs, as well as diagnostic reference levels. The regulations also provide information on how to report medical exposures that have exceeded the required dose.

The role of individuals is broken down into the referrer, practitioner, and operator. The referrer is the clinician who is entitled to refer for an image and must supply sufficient information to justify the exposure. The practitioner is the health professional who takes responsibility for the medical exposure and ensures that it complies with the principles of IR(ME)R 2018. The operator is an adequately individual who takes the radiograph.

In many radiological departments, the operator would be a radiographer.

The referrer, as in this scenario, would be any dentist or medical professional who refers a patient for a radiographic exposure.

According to IR(ME)R 2018, 'The primary responsibility of the practitioner is to justify medical exposures'. The practitioner in a hospital setting is often designated by the employer. However, the power to justify the exposure is often delegated to the operator, assuming the request complies with pre-existing local guidelines. General dental practitioners could therefore occupy all three roles.

Keywords: sent to radiology department, IR(ME)R 2018, agent.

7. B ★★

Overlapping of the contact points occurs when there is inappropriate horizontal angulation of the X-ray tube. The tube should be positioned at 90° to the film, which needs to be carefully positioned to ensure the beam passes directly through the interproximal regions. Use of a beam-aiming device will assist with positioning of the X-ray tube at 90° to the film. However, incorrect placement of the film could still result in a poor radiograph.

Extremely curved or aberrant tooth positioning may result in more than one bitewing being required.

Incorrect vertical angulation of the collimator could result in foreshortening or lengthening of the teeth. Movement by the patient would result in global blurring of the whole image. See Figure 14.2 which shows a faulty bitewing radiograph with an inaccurate horizontal angulation. Figure 14.3 shows the same region with the fault corrected.

Keywords: blurry/overlapped, mesial and distal contact points.

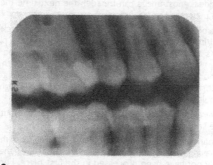

Figure 14.2

Reproduced from Mason R, and Bourne S, *A Guide to Dental Radiography* Fourth Edition, Figure 4.4a, page 60, Copyright (1998) by permission of Oxford University Press.

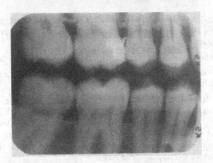

Figure 14.3
Reproduced from Mason R, and Bourne S, *A Guide to Dental Radiography* Fourth Edition, Figure 4.4b, page 60 Copyright (1998) by permission of Oxford University Press.

8. B ★★

The majority of dental practices use digital radiography because processing is fast and more economical and there is less chance of processing errors. Additionally, the dose of radiation received per image is typically less than for the conventional counterpart. Two main types of digital systems exist: PSP plates and charge-coupled devices (CCDs). The benefits of PSP plates are that the films are of a similar size to conventional films and are often better tolerated by the patient. CCDs are linked to the computer by a lead and are bulkier. However, the image can be viewed immediately without additional processing steps or a separate processing machine.

For PSP plates, residual energy remains on the plate following scanning. Exposure to a bright light source removes the residual energy and allows the film to be reused. If this process has failed or has not been done, then a residual ghost image can be seen the next time the plate is exposed and processed.

Manufacturer-dependent, a small metal disc on the back of the film is involved in the automated mechanism that draws the plate into the scanner. As a result, if the film is positioned back to front, a white disc will appear on the image, which can obscure the view of the final radiograph. If no such disc is present, the image will be back to front. This could be corrected using the computer software, but it might cause confusion if multiple contralateral images are being taken.

The software can be used to change the contrast without altering the kilovoltage settings but cannot remove double images.

In this scenario, the ghost image could have resulted from the processing machine having not fully erased the previous image, or the plate might accidentally not have been processed in the first place. For this reason, option B is the most appropriate answer, although the plate might be faulty and might need replacing if no fault can be found with the processor. PSP plates are expensive and reusable, so they should *not* be thrown away.

Keywords: periapical PSP, ghost image.

9. B ★★★

The Ionising Radiation Regulations 2017 (IRR17) is a piece of legislation intended to protect members of staff working with radiation and the general public. It is essential to comply with these guidelines. Dose limits, risk assessment, staff training, and quality assurance are key components of these guidelines, along with the appointment of an RPA. An RPA is a legal requirement whose role is to ensure compliance and provide advice on complying with the IRR 2017. These may be an external person but could also be a staff role within the company or practice.

IRR 2017 superseded the IRR 1999, whilst the Ionising Radiation (Medical Exposure) Regulations 2018 are designed to protect the *patient* from ionizing radiation.

Keywords: radiation protection advisor, documentation.

10. D ★★★

Root fractures are a well-recognized occurrence following dental trauma. They are commonly described by their location within the root of the tooth, with apical third root fractures displaying better outcomes than coronal third root fractures.

Most fractures occur obliquely due to the vector of forces applied to the tooth during the traumatic incident. Since radiographs are two-dimensional, unless there is displacement between the fractured segments or the X-ray beam is travelling in the same direction as the fracture line, the fracture will not be clearly seen.

For these reasons, two radiographs are recommended to ensure that a fracture is not missed. Ideally, a vertical parallax view is advised, since most oblique fractures will travel in a vertical direction. An upper midline occlusal radiograph provides a wide field of view, which is useful following trauma, but many practices will not have the facilities to perform this, so a periapical radiograph taken at an acute angle could be an alternative. See Figure 14.4a which shows X-rays not passing through a fracture, so the fracture line is indistinct on the radiograph. Figure 14.4b shows X-rays passing through a fracture line, so it is more obvious on the radiograph.

A panoramic radiograph (DPT/OPG) is not advised due to the risk of the C-spine obscuring the midline. The dose of radiation from a CBCT could not be justified at this stage, although it would provide a conclusive diagnosis.

Keywords: periapical radiograph, root fracture, central incisor, confirm diagnosis.

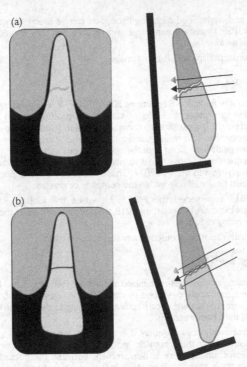

Figure 14.4

11. E ★★★★

Like most trauma scenarios, two plain film radiographs are indicated to ensure fractures are not missed. In this case, facial views are likely to be requested, which usually comprise OM 0° and OM 30° views. This is sometimes supplemented with a submentovertex or 'jug-handle view', which gives good visualization of the zygomatic arch. However, isolated zygomatic arch fractures are less common than complex fractures.

In this scenario, an OM 0° will provide the best image of the facial bones. It provides good visualization of the orbital floor, naso-ethmoidal complex, paranasal sinuses, and zygomatic complex. See Figure 14.5a which shows the position of the head for the OM projection. Figure 14.5b shows an OM view to demonstrate fractures of the right zygomatico-maxillary complex.

Like the OM 0°, the OM 30° helps identify Le Fort fractures and fractures of the coronoid processes. See Figure 14.6a which shows the position of

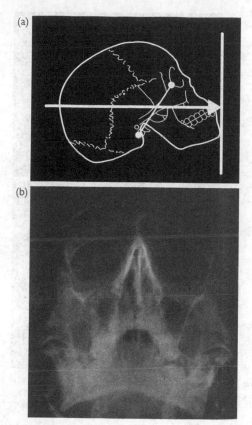

Figure 14.5a, b

Reproduced from Mason R, and Bourne S, *A Guide to Dental Radiography* Fourth Edition, Figure 10.5a, page 166, Copyright (1998) by permission of Oxford University Press.

the head for the 30° OM projection. Figure 14.6b shows a 30° OM view to demonstrate the fracture patterns in the floor of the orbit and on the inferior surface of the zygomatic arch.

Lateral skull is good for identifying the cranial base and paranasal air sinuses. A PA skull shows the calvarium and helps to identify conditions such as multiple myeloma and Paget's disease of the bone.

A DPT is a standard dental imaging system for dento-alveolar issues and mandibular fractures or condylar issues. This often combined with either a PA mandible or reverse Townes when assessing for mandibular fractures.

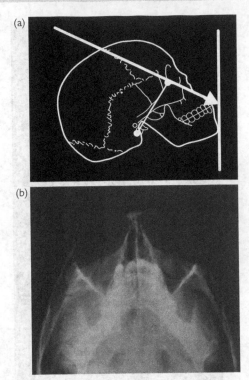

Figure 14.6a, b
Reproduced from Mason R, and Bourne S, *A Guide to Dental Radiography* Fourth Edition, Figure 10.6a, page 167, Copyright (1998) by permission of Oxford University Press.

Computed tomography is often used for complex mid-facial fractures, but it is unlikely to be a first-line image requested in Accident and Emergency (unless there are other neurological indications).

Keywords: zygomatic complex fracture, plain film, images.

12. C ★★★★

The history of the presenting complaint, combined with the clinical examination findings, is highly indicative of salivary gland or duct pathology. Unilateral recurrent mealtime swelling would be pathognomonic for salivary gland pathology. A lower oblique occlusal is a lower occlusal view taken with the head rotated away from the X-ray tube. This enables good visualization of the submandibular gland and the posterior submandibular duct, as the primary beam passes from the angle of the jaw through the gland onto the film positioned between the maxillary and mandibular teeth. Radio-opaque calculi are often visible on these films (see Figure 14.7 which shows a lower occlusal for the posterior part of the submandibular duct, showing a calculi). However, not all blockages are radio-opaque. Historically, these images have also been used to identify impacted wisdom teeth; however, this has largely been superseded by panoramic radiographs and cone beam computed tomography (CBCT).

A lateral oblique is more frequently used to assess caries in patients unable to tolerate intraoral films or dentopantomograms (DPTs).

A lower occlusal 90°—or lower true occlusal—would be the first-line plain film radiograph to investigate a blockage within the anterior floor of the mouth, closer to the opening of the submandibular duct. This image would not visualize the area in question in this scenario, as it is too far posterior.

A lower occlusal 45° involves setting the X-ray tube at 45° to the film through the anatomical menton to enable visualization of the anterior mandible.

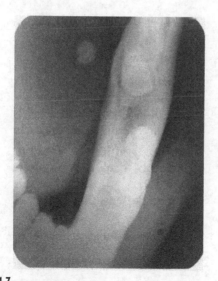

Figure 14.7

Reproduced from Mason R, and Bourne S, *A Guide to Dental Radiography* Fourth Edition, Figure 13.1d, page 204, Copyright (1998) by permission of Oxford University Press.

A DPT is often taken to investigate large facial swellings and abscesses, as well as for assessment of the developing dentition in orthodontics. It would not be first line in the identification of calculi/swellings in the floor of the mouth; however, it is possible to identify calcifications within the gland using this image.

Sialography involves injecting a radio-opaque dye into the submandibular duct prior to imaging. This would often be undertaken to assist in diagnosis and treatment planning, following suggestion of salivary gland pathology. Ultrasound or magnetic resonance imaging (MRI) would be another approach to investigate swellings of the neck.

Keywords: submandibular gland, calculus or sialolith, plain film, first line.

Statistics, epidemiology, and dental public health

Peter Clarke

'There's lies, more lies and then there's statistics.'

The content of this subject is frequently overlooked, as it is often 'not seen as pertinent' to practitioners' day-to-day work. However, the impact of dental public health (DPH) as a discipline can be far reaching. DPH is concerned with improving the oral health of the population, rather than the individual. It has been described as the science and art of preventing oral disease, promoting oral health, and improving quality of life through the organized efforts of society.

DPH teams have numerous responsibilities, including oral health surveillance, developing and monitoring quality dental services, oral health improvement, policy and strategy development and implementation, and strategic leadership and collaborative working for health. As such, the impact of DPH can frequently been seen at a local level, e.g. through health promotion campaigns or provision of new/redistribution of services (in conjunction with commissioners) to meet local needs.

DPH is predominantly a postgraduate subject, and although the undergraduate curriculum does not cover the whole topic, some core knowledge is valuable. In particular, understanding research methodology and basic statistics is a useful skill to help interpret the dental literature appropriately. This is ever more necessary in the modern era of evidence-based dentistry.

The questions in this chapter will predominantly cover the fundamentals of statistics relevant to medical research, along with the basics of study design. Additional questions will touch on the concepts of health promotion and epidemiology, with further reading suggested to supplement the content.

Key topics include:

- Study design
- Data analysis
- Critical appraisal
- Epidemiology
- Health promotion
- Strategic working and collaboration
- Assessing evidence on oral health and dental interventions, programmes, and services
- Developing and monitoring quality dental services.

QUESTIONS

1. A local public health team is collecting data on caries from a group of schoolchildren. A sample of the data collected is shown in Table 15.1. Calculate the mean, mode, and median for the data collected below. (Select one answer from the options listed below.) ★

A Mean—6, mode—6, median—6

B Mean—7, mode—6, median—6

C Mean—7, mode—7, median—6

D Mean—7, mode—7, median—9

E Mean—8, mode—6, median—8

Table 15.1	
Name	**Diseased, missing, filled teeth (DMFT)**
Amit	3
Andy	9
Chloe	6
Francesca	10
Heather	6
Josephine	6
Kat	5
Kate	5
Mani	8
Matty	6
Peter	9
Vish	11

2. A local Maxillofacial Unit are working on a clinical trial to develop a screening blood test which will help identify patients at risk of oral squamous cell carcinoma. The chief investigator informs the group that current tests available have a very low sensitivity and a high specificity. What single term is 'sensitivity' also commonly known as? ★ ★

A False negatives

B False positives

C True negatives

D True positives

E Type I error

3. A senior lecturer in oral and maxillofacial surgery is discussing the use of different types of data (variables) that can be recorded. Her most recent epidemiological research collected the TMN stage of all oral squamous cell carcinomas diagnosed in the Head and Neck Department. Which single type of data does this staging system represent? ★★

A Continuous

B Discrete

C Nominal

D Ordinal

E Qualitative

4. A study aiming to identify whether alcohol consumption and smoking during pregnancy increase the risk of the development of cleft lip and palate is being conducted. After selecting 50 newborn babies with cleft lip and palate from a local database, a questionnaire is provided to their parents to investigate the above health-related behaviours. A further 50 individuals born without cleft lip and palate are matched for age, sex, and social demographics and provided with the same questionnaire. Medical records are also examined. What single type of study design is being utilized in this scenario? ★★

A Case-control

B Cross-sectional

C Prospective cohort

D Randomized controlled trial

E Retrospective cohort

5. A junior dental student is presenting the outcomes from their elective research project. They refer to the Ottawa Charter on multiple occasions, and a colleague asks to which principle of public health the Ottawa Charter refers. (Select one answer from the options listed below.) ★★

A Amalgam safety

B Caries prevention

C Health promotion

D Infection control

E Sustainable development

6. A cross-sectional study investigating the prevalence of tooth brushing abrasion is being conducted locally. The team develops a new index, as it felt previous measurement tools were not fit for purpose. During the clinical training and calibration exercise, examiner feedback stated that descriptors were too vague. What single characteristic of the index needs to be readdressed? ★★

A Acceptability

B Objectivity

C Reliability

D Simplicity

E Validity

7. A dental public health consultant is running an oral health promotion project focusing on periodontal disease reduction. They decide to join with another public health team focusing on health promotion for diabetes to help promote a unified message. What single approach is being taken to manage the risk factors? ★★★

A Common risk factor approach

B Disease-centred approach

C Medical model approach

D Settings approach to health promotion

E Single-message approach

8. A longitudinal study aiming to identify the link between smoking and periodontal disease is being carried out. During data collection, a large number of participants did not return for follow-up. Statistical analysis showed no significant link between the two variables, but previous research does. What single statistical problem may account for this finding? ★★★

A Negative likelihood ratio

B Positive likelihood ratio

C True positive rate

D Type I error

E Type II error

9. A local research group is conducting an observational study, as a randomized controlled trial was deemed unethical. The group uses the Bradford Hill criteria to help with its conclusions. What is the single core aspect of observational studies that these criteria were developed to evaluate? ★★★

A Bias

B Causation

C Incidence

D Randomization

E Selection

10. An observational study investigating the effect of different toothbrushing regimes is being conducted within the local dental school. The study involves two consultants observing a sample of dental students brushing their teeth. During construction of the protocol, a concern is raised that students may perform differently because they are being observed (i.e. more likely to brush for longer). What single term is used to describe this effect? ★★★

A Berksom effect

B Butterfly effect

C Central tendency effect

D Hawthorne effect

E Measurement effect

11. Statistical analysis of data collected during a research project investigating the age and onset of aggressive periodontitis is being performed. Exploratory data analysis using a histogram identifies a positive skew in the distribution of the variable 'age' (i.e. more in younger patients). When presenting the data, which paired summary measures are the most appropriate to report the location and spread of age? (Select one answer from the options listed below.) ★★★

A Mean and interquartile range

B Mean and standard deviation

C Median and interquartile range

D Median and standard deviation

E Mode and proportion

12. A study to compare the effect of two surgical interventions on the reduction of mobility in periodontally involved teeth is being conducted. Outcome data were recorded using Miller's classification of tooth mobility. Which single statistical test is the most appropriate to compare tooth mobility between the two intervention groups? ★★★★

A Analysis of variance (ANOVA)

B Fisher's exact test

C Kruskal–Wallis test

D Mann–Whitney U test.

E Spearman's rank coefficient

13. Public Health England are working with the local clinical commissioning groups to reorganize the out-of-hours dental services. Before continuing, the commissioners require some further information on the current dental services. What primary investigation should initially be conducted prior to the commissioning of any new dental service? ★★★★

A Cost-effectiveness analysis (CEA)

B Cost utility analysis (CUA)

C Joint strategic needs assessment (JSNA)

D Oral health needs assessment (OHNA)

E Root cause analysis (RCA)

14. During hospital induction, a member of the clinical governance team discusses the importance of continually assessing standards to improve patient care. The Caldicott Principles are highlighted multiple times. Following the talk, a junior colleague asks to which single 'pillar' of clinical governance these principles relate. ★★★★

A Audit

B Information governance

C Research

D Risk management

E Staff training

ANSWERS

1. B ★

The mean is the sum of the value of numbers divided by the quantity of numbers (in this case, 84/12 = 7). Commonly, the mean is referred to as 'the average'. However, the mean, mode, and median range are all averages.

The mode is the most frequent value, which, in this case, is 6, which appears four times in the data set.

The median is the middle value in the data set when placed in sequential order. In this sequence, the sixth and seventh number is 6, so the median is 6. If the data set has an even number of data points, then the median value is calculated as being halfway between the two middle data points.

Keywords: data, sample, mean, mode, median.

2. D ★★

Sensitivity refers to the ability of a test to correctly identify the proportion of subjects with disease. A test which is considered to have 'high sensitivity' is good at identifying patients with disease. A 100% sensitivity would identify all patients with disease. If this test (with 100% sensitivity) were negative, it is safe to assume that the patient is disease-free.

Specificity reflects the 'true negative rate', i.e. the patients correctly identified as not having active disease. Tests with a high specificity help identify patients free from disease, who would record a negative result to the test. A positive result in a test with 100% specificity would be a strong indicator of disease.

False positives (otherwise known as type I error) and false negatives are used to help calculate the specificity and sensitivity of tests. In reality, tests combine sensitivity and specificity to reduce the risk of misdiagnosis. Tests which display 100% specificity and 100% sensitivity would identify all healthy patients and all patients with disease. However, whilst this is mathematically possible, it is practically highly unlikely. Frequently, a choice has to be made as to whether to accept a test where the sensitivity or specificity are less than ideal. For example, if a screening test was being developed for diagnosing cancer, it would be better to have a higher sensitivity and accept a lower specificity, so that cases are not missed. The choice of what level of sensitivity and specificity to accept is often dictated by the purpose of the test (i.e. screening or diagnosis) and the severity of the disease.

Keywords: sensitivity.

3. D ★★

Ordinal data are data which are ranked in order of importance or sequence. This is in contrast to nominal data, which are unordered categorical data. The numerical ranking provided is arbitrary and bears no relation to the actual measurement or distance between the data points presented. The value assigned to each rank is intended to reflect a sequence. TNM staging is one example of this (e.g. T1, 2, 3, 4), which reflects the size and extent of invasion of the tumour. Council tax banding (A, B, C, D, E) and the Glasgow coma scale (3–15) are other examples of ordinal data.

Data can generally be classified as 'qualitative' or 'quantitative'. Qualitative data are traditionally non-numerical data, e.g. eye colour, and are presented as categorical data. Quantitative data are numerical data which can assume different forms. Continuous (synonym: scalar) data, such as periodontal pocket depths or attachment loss, are data recorded on a continuous scale.

Discrete quantitative data, such as diseased, missed, filled teeth (DMFT), are numerical data with discrete data points.

Keywords: types of variables, TMN.

4. A ★★

A case-control study design begins by identifying patients (cases) with the condition under investigation (e.g. cleft lip and palate). Patients without the condition (controls) are subsequently sought to enable comparisons between the groups regarding the occurrence of possible risk factors. This study design retrospectively analyses the various risk factors/exposures (e.g. smoking and alcohol intake) to identify a possible causal relationship. They are more commonly used when uncommon and rare conditions or diseases are the outcome of interest.

Case-control studies are often quicker and less costly to conduct, but are less robust in identifying true causal relationships, as multiple risk factors may be involved and recall bias can be a significant confounding factor. Randomized controlled trials (RCTs) provide a higher level of evidence concerning causation, but like cohort studies, they are more time-consuming and considerably more expensive.

Odds ratios are often calculated from case-control studies to estimate the association between two factors. An odds ratio equal to '1' would imply the risk for the disease is similar between exposed and non-exposed participants. An odds ratio above '1' would imply an increased risk of those with the disease to be exposed to the risk factor. These studies and statistics are frequently encountered in the dental literature, and identifying the limitations of the study and interpreting the results are important.

This is in contrast to a cohort study, which may be retrospective but is typically prospective, in which those exposed to a certain risk factor are identified and prospectively monitored for disease development over time. RCTs involve random assignment of subjects into either a control or an experimental arm, which are then prospectively followed for a specified time period.

Keywords: risk, with, without, matched, questionnaire, medical records.

→ Daly B, Batchelor P, Treasure E, Watt R. *Essential Dental Public Health* (2nd ed.). Oxford University Press, Oxford; 2013.

5. C ★★

The Ottawa Charter is an international document published in 1986 by the World Health Organization. Prevention of diseases and health promotion should be the fundamental components of all public health organizations. The five key principles of health promotion include:

1. Creating supportive environments
2. Building healthy public policy
3. Strengthening community action
4. Developing personal skills
5. Reorienting health services.

These principles were developed following international consultation in Ottawa and are subsequently referred to as the Ottawa Charter. Since 1986, these principles have been utilized to improve oral health, and a number of different approaches and models of change have been proposed.

Keywords: Ottawa Charter, principle, public health.

→ World Health Organization. *The Ottawa Charter for Health Promotion*. 1986. Available at: http://www.who.int/healthpromotion/conferences/previous/ottawa/en/

6. B ★★

Different aspects should be considered when conducting an epidemiological study, including costs, sample size, and ethical considerations. In some circumstances, it is not feasible or appropriate to conduct a full examination with specific tests on all participants. Therefore, researchers often use a measurement tool, or a health index, to assess health condition. To be effective, an index should ideally have the following properties:

- *Simple*—the index should be easy to learn and apply. A large number of clinicians can therefore be taught to use the tool quickly and obtain consistent results.
- *Objective*—descriptors should leave little room for individual interpretation; otherwise, results are likely to be unreliable.
- *Valid*—the index should measure what it intends to; otherwise, measurement bias can be introduced.
- *Reliable/reproducible*—each time the index is used, the result should be similar (consistent), assuming the disease state has not changed. Reliability refers to any deviation inherent to the index, whereas reproducibility relates to discrepancies with intra-/inter-examiner use.
- *Quantifiable*—the index should provide categorical or numerical data, allowing statistical analysis.

- *Sensitive*—the index should allow the detection of small variations of the condition between individuals and small changes over time (discriminatory capacity).
- *Acceptable*—the index should be acceptable to patients.

Few dental indices have all these properties. In the example in the scenario, the examiner's feedback suggested the category descriptors were too vague. Therefore, they need to be made less subjective and more objective.

Keywords: index, descriptors, too vague.

7. A ★★★

The traditional approach to health promotion was for individual organizations to promote health messages for their individual disease (disease-centred approach); this is now outdated and no longer recommended. Given the prevalence and relevance of several chronic diseases (such as cardiovascular disease, diabetes, caries, periodontal disease, and obesity), which all have common risk factors, a new public health proposal has been conceived—the common risk factor approach. This affords several benefits. Firstly, it reduces wastage by avoiding duplication of similar health messages for different diseases. Secondly, it reduces conflicting health messages from different organizations only focusing on 'their' disease. Thirdly, it improves the reach of these shared health promotion messages to the most deprived and socially excluded, due to improved cost-effectiveness of the programmes. Together, these benefits maximize the impact of preventive activities, increasing the effectiveness and efficacy.

The settings approach to health promotion refers to the implementation of health promotion campaigns in specific environments or places, e.g. oral health promotion in schools. This approach may be used as a subset to the common risk factor approach or disease-centred approach.

Keywords: health promotion, unified message.

→ Chestnutt I. *Dental Public Health At a Glance*. Wiley Blackwell, Chichester; 2016.

→ Sheiham A, Watt R. The common risk factor approach: a rational basis for promoting oral health. *Community Dentistry and Oral Epidemiology*. 2000;**28**:399–406.

8. E ★★★

In research, the null statistical hypothesis assumes there is no differences between the two variables being investigated. A hypothesis cannot be proven, only rejected, as a sample is being taken, and therefore, data for the entire population are not available. Rejecting the null hypothesis means that the difference between the two groups should not be discarded or denied. As the statistical analysis is undertaken on a sample of the total population, then the results may not actually reflect what happens in the population. When the null hypothesis is falsely rejected, it is termed a type I error or alpha (α) error, which is sometimes referred to as a 'false positive'. In this situation, the researchers would be incorrectly claiming that a difference is present. In contrast, a type II error or a beta (β) error (false negative) would occur if the null hypothesis was incorrectly accepted.

The power of the study (sensitivity of the test) and significance level (p value) will dictate the probability of type I and II errors. It is generally accepted that a power of 80% and a significance level of 0.05 are used, but this may vary, depending on the investigation and the relative importance of type I and II errors in the circumstance. These can be used to determine the sample size required for the study by conducting a sample size calculation. During the sample size calculation, a dropout rate is usually accounted for. However, if the dropout rate is greater than expected, the sample size will be insufficiently large to detect the expected differences and the study is underpowered. This will increase the risk of a type II error, and the sample may be too small to reliably detect a difference between the two groups when it exists.

Keywords: participants, did not return, no significant link.

9. B ★★★

The Bradford Hill criteria aim to assist with identifying causation between an exposure (risk factor) and a disease or health condition. Many factors can occur together, which could erroneously be considered a causative factor if not investigated correctly. Nine aspects were initially proposed:

1. Strength of the association
2. Consistency with other investigators
3. Specificity
4. Temporality (time sequence)
5. Biological gradient (dose-dependent relationship)
6. Plausibility (biological credibility)
7. Coherence
8. Experimental evidence
9. Analogy.

Modern epidemiological and statistical methods have changed considerably since these considerations were proposed in 1965, but whilst the interpretation of each aspect may develop, the criteria are still considered relevant today.

Keywords: observational, Bradford Hill criteria.

→ Fedak K, Bernal A, Capshaw ZA, Gross S. Applying the Bradford Hill criteria in the 21st century: how data integration has changed causal inference in molecular epidemiology. *Emerging Themes in Epidemiology*. 2015;**12**:14.

→ Hill AB. The environment and disease: association or causation? *Proceedings of the Royal Society of Medicine*. 1965;**58**:295–300.

10. D ★★★

Observational studies can be considered descriptive (i.e. case reports) or analytical (i.e. case-control). These study designs are susceptible to different types of bias. Observational bias represents errors in the study design or data collection that have not occurred by chance. There are a number of types of observational bias, one of which is response bias. Response bias occurs when the participants respond how they believe they should respond.

The Hawthorne effect is a type of response bias in which participants change their behaviour in response to their awareness of being observed.

Berksom (effect) bias refers to a selection bias that results when a study design only assesses patients admitted to a certain facility. These subjects are likely to be from a very specific group of patients and, as such, they are unlikely to represent the population accurately.

Central tendency (effect) bias is the tendency for a participant to provide a score towards the middle of a scale, rather than the limits. For example, if providing patients with a visual analogue scale to rate satisfaction, they are more likely to place a mark in the middle of the scale.

Keywords: observing, perform differently.

11. C ★★★

After data collection, it is important for researchers to review their data and gain a greater understanding of the type of data they have collected. This process is referred to as exploratory data analysis. A histogram enables the researcher to examine continuous data (such as age) visually. A typical bell-shaped curve is considered a normal distribution, but data can also be skewed to the left (positive) and to the right (negative), suggesting a non-normal distribution.

Summary measures or statistics enable researchers to present large amounts of data in a format that is easy to understand and visualize, e.g. mean and standard deviation. These measures help researchers and readers to understand the location (centre) and spread of the data. The mean, median, and mode are commonly used to present the average or central values of the data set, whilst the standard deviation and interquartile range present the spread of the data. Data that are more spread out would have a wider standard deviation, and this may help identify how accurately the data represent the population. Much greater information is provided when both summary measures are presented together, i.e. the mean and standard deviation.

Continuous data with skewed distribution are more accurately reported using the median and interquartile ranges, whilst the mean and standard deviation are recommended for normally distributed continuous data. Categorical data are often presented using percentages.

Keywords: exploratory data analysis, positive skew, summary measures.

12. D ★★★★

There are various statistical tests available for hypothesis testing. Overall, the choice of the most appropriate statistical test will depend on the:

- Normality of the distribution (parametric vs non-parametric)
- Type of data (continuous, ordinal, nominal)

292   CHAPTER 15 Statistics, epidemiology, and DPH

- Number of comparison groups
- Dependence of the data (e.g. independent variables, paired data, etc.).

For ordinal or categorical data (such as Miller's classification—a common classification for tooth mobility based on severity), the distribution is generally non-parametric (i.e. not normally distributed), and therefore, a non-parametric test is the correct choice. When assessing two independent groups, the Mann–Whitney U test is appropriate. Should there have been more interventions and then more groups to compare, then the Kruskal–Wallis test would be the most appropriate.

Where data are binary, then the chi-squared test tends to be employed. To compare two groups of binary data with a small sample size (where the expected value is <5), the Fisher's exact test is more accurate than the chi-squared test.

ANOVA is used for normally distributed continuous data where there are >2 independent groups to compare.

Spearman's coefficient is used to assess the correlation between a dependent variable and one or more independent variables (i.e. a known risk factor and the outcome of interest). It is a non-parametric test. When data are normally distributed, Pearson's correlation coefficient can be used (parametric test).

Keywords: two interventions, Miller's classification (ordinal data).

→ Gosall N, Gosall G. *The Doctor's Guide to Critical Appraisal* (4th ed.). PasTest, Knutsford; 2015.

13. D ★★★★

Before treating an individual patient, a clinical examination and diagnostic phase is undertaken. Similarly, in public health, when commissioning new dental services, an examination of current services is needed; for dental services, this will be an OHNA. This process will look at elements such as the population demographics (e.g. ageing population), the current dental service provision (availability, cost, location), disease occurrence (prevalence, trends), service users (demands and priority groups), and current evidence base. This information is then used in the planning process. In the example given in the scenario, an OHNA would advise the commissioners on the options available and how to contract out-of-hours emergency dental care. Ideally, health service planning should be considered as a cycle. Needs assessment should precede policymaking and also should be performed after evaluation of the new implementation, to restart the cycle.

The JSNA looks at the wider picture, beyond dental health. With the 2012 Health and Social Care Act reforms in the UK, it became a statutory requirement for local health and well-being boards to conduct them. The JSNA looks at the health of the population, including negative health behaviours (e.g. smoking), identifies health inequalities, and attempts to define what the health and social care needs of the population are now and in the future. The aim is to aid planning and commissioning of services to meet the needs of the local population.

Options A and B are more related to health economics, rather than commissioning of services. RCA is a problem-solving technique used following adverse incidents, to help identify potential human and systemic factors that may have contributed to the event.

Keywords: commissioning, reorganize, new service.

→ Chestnutt I. *Dental Public Health At a Glance*. Wiley Blackwell, Chichester; 2016.

→ Department of Health and Social Care. *Joint strategic needs assessment and joint health and wellbeing strategies explained*. 2011. Available at: https://www.gov.uk/government/publications/joint-strategic-needs-assessment-and-joint-health-and-wellbeing-strategies-explained

14. B ★★★★

The Caldicott Principles were established following the Caldicott Report into the 'use of patient identifiable data' in 1997. These guidelines relate to information governance, i.e. the way in which we use, handle, and share patient information.

The key principles are:

1. Justify the purpose(s)
2. Do not use patient-identifiable information, unless it is absolutely necessary
3. Use minimal necessary patient-identifiable information
4. Access to patient-identifiable information should be on a strict need-to-know basis
5. Everyone with access to patient-identifiable information should be aware of their responsibilities
6. Understand and comply with the law.

Since 1998, NHS organizations have appointed a Caldicott guardian who is responsible for ensuring an organization uses the personal information of its service users in a legal, ethical, confidential, and appropriate manner. The underpinning legal framework for information sharing within the UK is currently the Data Protection Act 2018. Legislation is always liable to change, and the authors would advise all clinicians to keep up-to-date with any changes within their country.

Keywords: Caldicott.

→ UK Caldicott Guardian Council. *A Manual for Caldicott Guardians*. 2017. Available at: https://www.gov.uk/government/groups/uk-caldicott-guardian-council

Index

Tables and figures are indicated by *t* and *f* following the page number.